Clinical Manual of Geriatric Psychiatry

Edited by

Mugdha E. Thakur, M.D.

Dan G. Blazer, M.D., Ph.D.

David C. Steffens, M.D., M.H.S.

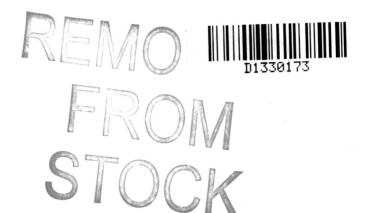

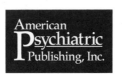

American Psychiatric Publishing, Inc.

Washington, DC
London, England

If you would like to buy between 25 and 99 copies of this or any other American Psychiatric Publishing title, you are eligible for a 20% discount; please contact Customer Service at appi@psych.org or 800-368-5777. If you wish to buy 100 or more copies of the same title, please e-mail us at bulksales@psych.org for a price quote.

Copyright © 2014 American Psychiatric Association
ALL RIGHTS RESERVED
Manufactured in the United States of America on acid-free paper
17   16   15   14   13   5   4   3   2   1
First Edition
Typeset in Adobe Garamond Pro and Helvetica LT Std.

American Psychiatric Publishing
A Division of American Psychiatric Association
1000 Wilson Boulevard
Arlington, VA 22209-3901
www.appi.org

Library of Congress Cataloging-in-Publication Data
Clinical manual of geriatric psychiatry / edited by Mugdha E. Thakur, Dan G. Blazer, David C. Steffens. — First edition.
    p. ; cm.
Includes bibliographical references and index.
ISBN 978-1-58562-441-6 (pbk. : alk. paper)
    I. Thakur, Mugdha E., editor of compilation. II. Blazer, Dan G., II (Dan German), editor of compilation. III. Steffens, David C., editor of compilation. IV. American Psychiatric Publishing, issuing body.
    [DNLM: 1. Aged. 2. Mental Disorders—diagnosis. 3. Mental Disorders—therapy. 4. Age Factors. 5. Aging—psychology. WT 150]
    RC451.4.A5
    618.97'689—dc23
                                                                2013023270
British Library Cataloguing in Publication Data
A CIP record is available from the British Library.

Contents

4   **Dementia and Milder Cognitive Syndromes. . . . 99**

Constantine G. Lyketsos, M.D., M.H.S.

5   **Mood Disorders. 125**

*David C. Steffens, M.D., M.H.S., Dan G. Blazer, M.D., Ph.D.,
and John L. Beyer, M.D.*

6   **Schizophrenia and Paranoid Disorders 159**

*Ipsit V. Vahia, M.D., Nicole M. Lanouette, M.D., and
Dilip V. Jeste, M.D.*

List of Tables and Figures

Contributors

Carmen Andreescu, M.D.
Department of Psychiatry, University of Pittsburgh, Western Psychiatric Institute and Clinic, Pittsburgh, Pennsylvania

John L. Beyer, M.D.
Assistant Professor and Director, Duke Mood and Anxiety Disorder Clinic, Department of Psychiatry and Behavioral Sciences, Duke University School of Medicine, Durham, North Carolina

Dan G. Blazer, M.D., Ph.D.
J.P. Gibbons Professor of Psychiatry and Behavioral Sciences, Department of Psychiatry and Behavioral Sciences; Professor of Community and Family Medicine; and Vice Chair of Academic Development, Duke University School of Medicine, Durham, North Carolina

Jack D. Edinger, Ph.D.
Professor, Department of Medicine, National Jewish Health, Denver, Colorado

Dawn E. Epstein, B.S.
Department of Psychology and Neuroscience, Duke University, Durham, North Carolina

Li-Wen Huang, M.D.
Department of Internal Medicine, Duke University Medical Center, Durham, North Carolina

Sharon K. Inouye, M.D., M.P.H.
Professor of Medicine, Department of Medicine, Beth Israel Deaconess Medical Center, Harvard Medical School, Boston, Massachusetts; Milton and Shirley F. Levy Family Chair; Director, Aging Brain Center, Institute for Aging Research, Hebrew SeniorLife, Boston, Massachusetts

Dilip V. Jeste, M.D.
Estelle and Edgar Levi Chair in Aging, Distinguished Professor of Psychiatry and Neurosciences, University of California, San Diego, La Jolla, California

Andrew D. Krystal, M.D., M.S.
Professor of Psychiatry, Department of Psychiatry and Behavioral Sciences, Duke University School of Medicine, Durham, North Carolina

Nicole M. Lanouette, M.D.
Assistant Clinical Professor of Psychiatry, University of California, San Diego, La Jolla, California

Eric J. Lenze, M.D.
Department of Psychiatry, Washington University School of Medicine, St. Louis, Missouri

Constantine G. Lyketsos, M.D., M.H.S.
The Elizabeth Plank Althouse Professor and Chairman, Department of Psychiatry, Johns Hopkins Bayview Medical Center; Vice Chairman, Department of Psychiatry and Behavioral Sciences, The Johns Hopkins Hospital, Baltimore, Maryland; Co-Director, Division of Geriatric Psychiatry and Neuropsychiatry

Thomas R. Lynch, Ph.D.
School of Psychology, University of Southampton, Southampton, United Kingdom

Shahrzad Mavandadi, Ph.D.
Adjunct Assistant Professor, University of Pennsylvania and Philadelphia VA Medical Center VISN 4 Mental Illness Research, Education, and Clinical Center, Philadelphia, Pennsylvania

Benoit H. Mulsant, M.D.
Centre for Addiction and Mental Health and Professor, Department of Psychiatry, Faculty of Medicine, University of Toronto, Toronto, Ontario, Canada

David W. Oslin, M.D.
Professor, University of Pennsylvania and Philadelphia VA Medical Center VISN 4 Mental Illness Research, Education, and Clinical Center, Philadelphia, Pennsylvania

Bruce G. Pollock, M.D., Ph.D.
Centre for Addiction and Mental Health and Professor, Department of Psychiatry, Faculty of Medicine, University of Toronto, Toronto, Ontario, Canada

Moria J. Smoski, Ph.D.
Department of Psychiatry and Behavioral Sciences, Duke University School of Medicine, Durham, North Carolina

David C. Steffens, M.D., M.H.S.
Professor and Chairman, Department of Psychiatry, University of Connecticut Health Center, Farmington, Connecticut

Joel E. Streim, M.D.
Professor of Psychiatry, Geriatric Psychiatry Section, University of Pennsylvania; VISN 4 Mental Illness Research Education & Clinical Center, Philadelphia Veterans Affairs Medical Center, Philadelphia, Pennsylvania

Mugdha E. Thakur, M.D.
Associate Professor, Department of Psychiatry and Behavioral Sciences, Duke University School of Medicine, Durham, North Carolina

Ipsit V. Vahia, M.D.
Assistant Professor of Psychiatry, Stein Institute for Research on Aging, University of California, San Diego, La Jolla, California

Julie Loebach Wetherell, Ph.D.
VA San Diego Healthcare System and University of California, San Diego, La Jolla, California

William K. Wohlgemuth, Ph.D.
Miami VA Healthcare System, Miami, Florida

Disclosure of Competing Interests

The following contributors to this book have indicated a financial interest in or other affiliation with a commercial supporter, a manufacturer of a commercial product, a provider of a commercial service, a nongovernmental organization, and/or a government agency, as listed below:

John L. Beyer, M.D.—*Research support:* AmGen, Forest, Janssen, Takeda.

Andrew D. Krystal, M.D., M.S.—*Grants/research support:* Abbott, Astellas, Brainsway, National Institutes of Health, Neosynch, Pfizer, Phillips-Respironics, Sunovion/Sepracor, Teva/Cephalon, Transcept; *Consultant:* Abbott, Astellas, AstraZeneca, Bristol-Myers-Squibb, Eisai, Eli Lilly, GlaxoSmith-Kline, Jazz, Johnson & Johnson, Kingsdown Inc., Merck, Neurocrine, Novartis, Ortho-McNeil-Janssen, Respironics, Roche, Sanofi-Aventis, Somnus, Sunovion/Sepracor, Somaxon, Takeda, Teva/Cephalon, Transcept.

Eric J. Lenze, M.D.—*Grant support:* Johnson & Johnson, Lundbeck, Roche.

Constantine G. Lyketsos, M.D., M.H.S.—*Grant support (research or CME):* Associated Jewish Federation of Baltimore, Astra-Zeneca, Bristol-Myers, Eisai, Elan, Forest, Functional Neuromodulation Inc., Glaxo-Smith-Kline, Lilly, National Football League, National Institute of Mental Health, National Institute on Aging, Novartis, Ortho-McNeil, Pfizer, Weinberg Foundation; *Consultant/advisor:* Adlyfe, Astra-Zeneca, Avanir, Bristol-Myers-Squibb, Eisai, Elan, Forest, Genentech, Glaxo-Smith-Kline, Lilly, Lundbeck, Merz, NFL Benefits Office, NFL Players Association, Novartis, Pfizer, Supernus, Takeda, Wyeth, Zinfandel; *Honorarium or travel support:* Forest, Glaxo-Smith-Kline, Health Monitor, Pfizer.

Benoit H. Mulsant, M.D.—Dr. Mulsant currently receives research support from the Canadian Institutes of Health Research, the U.S. National Institutes of Health (NIH), Bristol-Myers-Squibb (medications for a NIH-funded clinical trial), and Pfizer/Wyeth (medications for a NIH-funded clinical trial). He directly owns stocks of General Electric (less than $5,000). Within the past 3 years, he has also received some travel support from Roche. He has no intellectual property, patent ownership, copyright, or trademarks. He is a member of the Board of Trustees of the Centre for Addiction and Mental Health (CAMH) (Toronto, Ontario, Canada) and a member of the Board of Directors of the CAMH Foundation (Toronto, Ontario, Canada).

Bruce G. Pollock, M.D., Ph.D.—Dr. Pollock receives research support from the U.S. National Institutes of Health and the Canadian Institutes of Health Research. Within the past 5 years, he has been a member of the advisory board of Lundbeck Canada (final meeting was May 2009) and Forest Laboratories (final meeting was March 2008). Dr. Pollock has served one time as a consultant for Wyeth (October 2008) and Takeda (July 2007). He was also a faculty member of the Lundbeck International Neuroscience Foundation (final meeting was April 2010).

The following contributors to this book indicated that they have no competing interests or affiliations to declare:

Dan G. Blazer, M.D., Ph.D.
Jack D. Edinger, Ph.D.
Li-Wen Huang, M.D.
Sharon K. Inouye, M.D., M.P.H.
Dilip V. Jeste, M.D.
Nicole M. Lanouette, M.D.
Thomas R. Lynch, Ph.D.
Shahrzad Mavandadi, Ph.D.
David W. Oslin, M.D.
David C. Steffens, M.D., M.H.S.
Joel E. Streim, M.D.
Mugdha E. Thakur, M.D.
Ipsit V. Vahia, M.D.
Julie Loebach Wetherell, Ph.D.

Preface

C*linical Manual of Geriatric Psychiatry* comes from a rich tradition; it is the newest book from the editors of the authoritative *The American Psychiatric Publishing Textbook of Geriatric Psychiatry.* The manual was produced specifically to address the needs of busy clinicians from various specialties who are involved in the care of older adults. There are many geriatricians, internists, family practice specialists, physician extenders, social workers, and nurses who are at the forefront of delivering psychiatric care to our elderly population and educating their families. Our hope is that this handy book will become a field guide of sorts for these busy professionals and help guide their care of vulnerable patients. We hope this volume will be on their desks or in their pockets, rather than sitting on bookshelves.

The contributors to this volume are experts in their fields who have helped update and focus this manual on what is clinically most relevant. A variety of disorders are covered, as are general principles of interviewing older adults, psychopharmacology in older adults, and practice in nursing homes.

One important consideration is the transition from DSM-IV to DSM-5 that happened as this manual was in its last stages of editing. We made a decision not to overhaul the entire manual based on the changes between DSM editions and to continue to largely rely on DSM-IV. We based our decision on the fact that diseases have not actually changed since the last DSM edition. What *has* changed is some of the terminology and descriptors. Clinically one would still approach patients the same way as before. With this is mind, we have provided a succinct DSM-5 update for each of the disorders where applicable. The treatments of all disorders are based on the latest evidence available at the time of publication.

Finally, readers are referred to a variety of references for additional reading if they find something in the manual to be particularly interesting and worthy of further exploration. We hope you enjoy this guide.

Mugdha E. Thakur, M.D.
Dan G. Blazer, M.D., Ph.D.
David C. Steffens, M.D., M.H.S.

1

The Psychiatric Interview of Older Adults

Dan G. Blazer, M.D., Ph.D.

The foundation of the diagnostic workup of an older adult experiencing a psychiatric disorder is the diagnostic interview. In this chapter, I review the core of the psychiatric interview, including history taking, assessment of the family, and the mental status examination; describe structured interview schedules and rating scales that are of value in the assessment of older adults; and outline techniques for communicating effectively with older adults.

History

The elements of a diagnostic workup of an elderly patient are presented in Table 1–1. To obtain historical information, the clinician should first interview the patient, if that is feasible, and then ask the patient's permission to interview family members. If the patient has difficulty providing an accurate

Table 1–1. Diagnostic workup of the elderly patient

History

    Current illness

    Past history

    Family history

    Context

    Medication history

    Medical history

Family assessment

Mental status examination

or understandable history, the clinician should concentrate especially on eliciting the symptoms or problems that the patient perceives as being most disabling, then fill the historical gap with data from the family.

Current Illness

DSM-5 (American Psychiatric Association 2013) provides the clinician with a useful catalogue of symptoms and behaviors of psychiatric interest that are relevant to the diagnosis of the current illness. The clinician must include in the initial interview a review of the more important psychiatric symptoms in a relatively structured format as shown in Table 1–2.

The review of symptoms is most valuable when considered in the context of symptom presentation, including onset, duration, severity and fluctuation, precipitating factors, prior efforts at addressing the symptoms and their success, diurnal or seasonal variation, whether symptoms cluster together, and whether they are ego-syntonic or ego-dystonic. Defining a 1-month or 6-month window enables the patient to review symptoms and events temporally—an approach not usually taken by distressed elders, who tend to concentrate on immediate sufferings.

Critical to the assessment of the current illness is an assessment of function and change in function. The two parameters that are most important are *social functioning* and *activities of daily living* (ADLs). Questions should be asked about the social interaction of the older adult, such as the frequency of his or her

Table 1–2.   Review of symptoms during the initial interview

Common symptoms

    Excessive weakness or lethargy

    Depressed mood or "the blues"

    Memory problems or difficulty concentrating

    Feelings of helplessness, hopelessness, and uselessness

    Isolation

    Suspicion of others

    Anxiety and agitation

    Sleep problems

    Appetite problems and weight loss

Critical symptoms that should be reviewed

    Presence or absence of suicidal thoughts

    Profound anhedonia

    Impulsive behavior ("I can't control myself")

    Confusion

    Delusions and hallucinations

visits outside the home, telephone calls, and visits from family and friends. The clinician must ask about the patient's ability to get around (e.g., walk inside and outside the house), to perform certain physical activities independently (e.g., bathe, dress, shave, brush teeth, and select clothes), and to do instrumental activities (e.g., cook, maintain a bank account, shop, and drive). It is also important to assess how often the elder actually engages in these activities.

The clinician must take care to avoid accepting the patient's explanation for a given problem or set of problems. Statements such as "Most people slow down when they get to be my age" can lull the clinician into complacency about what may be a treatable psychiatric disorder. Also, the advent of new and disturbing symptoms in an older adult between office visits can exhaust the clinician's patience, thereby derailing pursuit of the problem. Distress over changes in functioning, such as sexual functioning, may overwhelm the older adult patient and, especially if the clinician is perceived as unconcerned, may precipitate self-medication or even a suicide attempt.

Past History

Next, the clinician must review the history of symptoms and episodes. The frequency, duration, and timing of prior episodes must be clarified. The perspective of the family is especially valuable in the attempt to link current and past episodes.

Other psychiatric and medical problems should be reviewed as well, especially medical illnesses that have led to hospitalization and the use of medication, including significant illnesses in young adulthood. Previous periods of overt disability in usual activities may flag prior psychiatric difficulties that may have been forgotten. An older person sometimes becomes angry or irritated when the clinician continues to probe. Reassurance regarding the importance of obtaining this information will generally suffice, except when the clinician is working with a patient who cannot tolerate the discomfort and distress, even for brief periods. Older persons who have chronic and moderately severe anxiety or a histrionic personality style, as well as distressed patients with Alzheimer's disease, tolerate their symptoms poorly.

Family History

A history should be obtained about institutionalization, significant memory problems in family members, hospitalization for a nervous breakdown or depressive disorder, suicide, alcohol use disorder, electroconvulsive therapy, long-term residence in a mental health facility (and possibly a diagnosis of schizophrenia), and use of mental health services by family members (Blazer 1984). The older person with symptoms consistent with senile dementia or primary degenerative dementia is likely to have a family history of dementia.

Of relevance to the pharmacological treatment of certain disorders—especially depression—in older adults is the tendency of individuals in a family to respond therapeutically to the same pharmacological agent. Therefore, relevant treatment history of family members should be elicited.

Context

Psychiatric disorders occur in a biomedical and psychosocial context. Although the clinician will try to determine what medical problems the patient has experienced, it is possible to overlook a variation in the relative contribution of these medical disorders to psychopathology or to overlook the psychosocial contribution to the onset and continuance of the problem. Environmental precipitants remain important in the web of causation leading to the onset of an episode of emotional distress and are critical to the assessment of the older adult.

Medication History

Evaluating the medication history of the older adult is essential. The older person should be asked to bring to the appointment all pill bottles, a list of both prescription and nonprescription medications taken, and the dosage schedule. A comparison between the written schedule and the pill containers will frequently expose some discrepancy.

Older persons are less likely than younger persons to abuse alcohol, but a careful history of alcohol intake is essential to the diagnostic workup. Substance use disorder beyond alcohol and prescription drugs is rare in older adults but not entirely absent.

Medical History

Given the high likelihood of comorbid medical problems associated with psychiatric disorders in late life, a comprehensive medical history is essential. Most older persons see a primary care physician regularly (although decreasing payments from Medicare render this assumption less accurate each year). The geriatric psychiatrist should obtain medical records, if possible. Major illnesses should be recorded. A brief telephone call to the primary care physician can be extremely useful.

Family Assessment

Clinicians working with older adults must be equipped to evaluate the family—both its functionality and its potential as a resource for the older adult. Geriatric psychiatry, almost by definition, is family psychiatry.

A primary goal of the clinician, as advocate for the older adult with psychiatric disturbance, is to facilitate family support for the elder during a time of disability. At least four parameters of support are important for the clinician to evaluate as the treatment plan evolves: 1) the availability of family members to the older person over time, 2) the tangible services provided by the family to the older person, 3) the perception of family support by the older patient (and therefore the willingness of the patient to cooperate and accept support), and 4) tolerance by the family of specific behaviors that derive from the psychiatric disorder.

Assessing the range and extent of service delivery by the family to the older person with functional impairment provides a convenient barometer of the economic, social, and emotional burdens placed on the family and also serves as a segue to discuss respite care with the primary caregiver if indicated.

Family tolerance of specific behaviors may not correlate with overall support. Sanford (1975) found that the following behaviors were tolerated by families of older persons with impairments (in decreasing percentages): incontinence of urine (81%), personality conflicts (54%), falls (52%), physically aggressive behavior (44%), inability to walk unaided (33%), daytime wandering (33%), and sleep disturbance (16%).

Mental Status Examination

The mental status examination of the older psychiatric patient is central to the diagnostic workup. Many aspects of this examination can be assessed during the history-taking interview.

Appearance may be affected by the older patient's psychiatric symptoms (e.g., the depressed patient may neglect grooming), cognitive status (e.g., the patient with dementia may not be able to match clothes or even put on clothes appropriately), and environment (e.g., a nursing home patient may not be groomed as well as a patient living at home with a spouse).

Affect and mood usually can be assessed by observing the patient during the interview. *Affect* is the feeling tone that accompanies the patient's cognitive output (Linn 1980). Affect may fluctuate during the interview; however, the older person is more likely to have a constriction of affect. *Mood,* the state that underlies overt affect and is sustained over time, is usually apparent by the end of the interview. For example, the affect of a depressed older adult may not reach the degree of dysphoria seen in younger persons (as evidenced by crying spells or protestations of uncontrollable despair), yet the depressed mood is usually sustained and discernible from beginning to end.

Psychomotor activity may be agitated or retarded. Psychomotor retardation or underactivity is characteristic of major depression and severe schizophreniform symptoms, as well as of some variants of primary degenerative dementia. Psychiatrically impaired older persons, except some who have advanced dementia, are more likely to show hyperactivity or agitation. Those who are depressed will appear uneasy, move their hands frequently, and have difficulty remaining seated through the interview. Patients with mild to moderate dementia, especially those with vascular dementia, will be easily distracted, rise from a seated position, and/or walk around the room or even out of the room. Pacing is often observed when the older adult is admitted to a hospital ward. Agitation usually can be distinguished from anxiety—the agitated individual does not complain of a sense of impending doom or dread. In patients with psychomotor dysfunction, movement generally relieves the immediate discomfort, although it does not correct the underlying disturbance. Occasionally, the older adult with motor retardation may actually be experiencing a disturbance in consciousness and may even reach an almost stuporous state. The patient may not be easily aroused, but when aroused, he or she will respond by grimacing or withdrawal.

Perception is the awareness of objects in relation to each other and follows stimulation of peripheral sense organs (Linn 1980). Disturbances of perception include hallucinations—that is, false sensory perceptions not associated with real or external stimuli. Hallucinations often take the form of false auditory perceptions, false perceptions of movement or body sensation (e.g., palpitations), and false perceptions of smell, taste, and touch. The older patient who is severely depressed may have frank auditory hallucinations that condemn or encourage self-destructive behavior.

Disturbances in thought content are the most common disturbances of cognition noted in older patients with psychosis. The depressed patient often develops beliefs that are inconsistent with objective information obtained from family members about the patient's abilities and social resources. Older patients appear less likely to experience delusional remorse, guilt, or persecution.

Even if delusions are not obvious, *preoccupation with a particular thought or idea* is common among depressed elderly persons. Such preoccupation is closely associated with obsessional thinking or irresistible intrusion of thoughts into the conscious mind. Although the older adult rarely acts on these thoughts compulsively, the guilt-provoking or self-accusing thoughts may occasionally become so difficult to bear that the person considers, attempts, or succeeds in committing suicide.

Disturbances of thought process accompany disturbances of content. There may be problems with the structure of associations, the speed of associations, and the content of thought. The older adult who is compulsive or has schizophrenia may pathologically repeat the same word or idea in response to a variety of probes, as may the patient who has primary degenerative dementia. Some older adults with dementia have circumstantiality—that is, the introduction of many apparently irrelevant details to cover a lack of clarity and memory problems. On other occasions, elderly patients may appear incoherent, with no logical connection of their thoughts, or they may produce irrelevant answers. The intrusion of thoughts from previous conversations into a current conversation is a prime example of the disturbance in association found in patients with primary degenerative dementia (e.g., Alzheimer's disease). This symptom is not typical of other dementias, such as the dementia of Huntington's disease. However, in the absence of dementia, even paranoid older adults do not generally show a significant disturbance in the structure of associations.

Suicidal thoughts are critical to assess in the elderly patient with psychiatric impairment. Although thoughts of death are common in late life, spontaneous revelations of suicidal thoughts are rare. A stepwise probe is the best means of assessing the presence of suicidal ideation (Blazer 1982). First, the clinician should ask the patient if he or she has ever thought that life was not worth living. If so, has the patient considered acting on that thought? If so, how would the patient attempt to inflict such harm? If the patient has definite plans, the clinician should probe to determine whether the implements for a suicide attempt are available. Suicidal ideation in an older adult is always of concern, but intervention is necessary when suicide has been considered seriously and the implements are available.

Assessment of memory and cognitive status is most accurately performed through psychological testing. However, the psychiatric interview of the older adult must include a reasonable assessment. *Testing of memory* is based on three essential processes: 1) registration (the ability to record an experience in the central nervous system), 2) retention (the persistence and permanence of a registered experience), and 3) recall (the ability to summon consciously the registered experience and report it) (Linn 1980). Registration apart from recall is difficult to evaluate directly. Registration usually is not impaired except in patients with one of the more severely dementing illnesses.

Retention, on the other hand, can be blocked by both psychic distress and brain dysfunction. Lack of retention is especially relevant to the unimportant data often asked for in a mental status examination. For example, requesting the older adult to remember three objects for 5 minutes will frequently identify a deficit if the older adult has little motivation to attempt the task.

Disturbances of recall can be tested directly in several ways. The most common tests assess orientation to time, place, person, and situation. Immediate recall can be tested by asking the older person to repeat a word, phrase, or series of numbers.

During the mental status examination, intelligence can be assessed only superficially. The classic test for calculation is to ask a patient to subtract 7 from 100 and to repeat this operation on the succession of remainders. Usually, five calculations are sufficient to determine the older adult's ability to complete this task. If the older adult fails the task, a less exacting test is to request the patient to subtract 3 from 20 and to repeat this operation on the succession of remainders until 0 is reached. This is also a test of attention because the patient needs to stay focused on the task. These examinations must not be rushed, for older persons may not perform as well when they perceive time pressure. A capacity for abstract thinking is often tested by asking the patient to interpret a well-known proverb, such as "A rolling stone gathers no moss." A more accurate test of abstraction, however, is classifying objects in a common category. For example, the patient is asked to state the similarity between an apple and a pear. Whereas the ability to name objects from a category, such as fruits, is retained despite moderate and sometimes marked declines in cognition, the opposite process of classifying two different objects in a common category is not retained as well.

Rating Scales and Standardized Interviews

Rating scales and standardized or structured interviews have increased in popularity as the need has increased for systematic, reproducible diagnoses for third-party carriers (part of the impetus for the dramatic change in nomenclature evidenced in DSM-IV [American Psychiatric Association 1994] and, most recently, DSM-5) and for a standard means of assessing change in clinical status. A thorough review of all instruments that are used is not possible in this chapter. Therefore, selected instruments are presented and evaluated in this section.

Cognitive Dysfunction and Dementia Schedules

Several standardized assessment methods for delirium have emerged. Perhaps the best and the most easily used is the Confusion Assessment Method (Inouye 1990). The scale assesses nine characteristics of delirium, including acute onset (evidence of such onset), fluctuating course (behavior change during the day), inattention (trouble in focusing), disorganized thinking (presence of rambling or irrelevant conversations and illogical flow of ideas), and altered level of consciousness (rated from alert to comatose). Diagnosis of delirium according to DSM-IV criteria can be derived from the scale.

Two interviewer-administered cognitive screens for dementia have been popular in both clinical and community studies. The first is the Short Portable Mental Status Questionnaire (SPMSQ; Pfeiffer 1975), a derivative of the Mental Status Questionnaire developed by Kahn et al. (1960). The SPMSQ consists of 10 questions designed to assess orientation, memory, fund of knowledge, and calculation. For most community-dwelling older adults, ≤2 errors indicates intact functioning; 3–4 errors, mild impairment; 5–7 errors, moderate impairment; and ≥8 errors, severe impairment. The ease of administration of this instrument and its reliability as supported by accumulated epidemiological data make it useful for both clinical and community screens.

The Mini-Mental State Examination (Folstein et al. 1975) is a 30-item screening instrument that assesses orientation, registration, attention and calculation, recall, and language. It requires 5–10 minutes to administer and includes more items of clinical significance than does the SPMSQ. Seven to 12 errors suggests mild to moderate cognitive impairment, and 13 or more errors indicate severe impairment. This instrument is perhaps the most frequently used standardized screening instrument in clinical practice.

Depression Rating Scales

Several self-rating depression scales have been used to screen for depression in patients at all stages of the life cycle; most of these scales have been studied in older populations. The most widely used of the current instruments in community studies is the Center for Epidemiologic Studies Depression Scale (CES-D; Radloff 1977). The scale consists of ratings of 20 behaviors and feelings, and the patient indicates how frequently each was experienced over the past week (from no days to most days). In a factor-analytic study of the CES-D in a community population, four factors were identified: somatic symptoms, positive affect, negative affect, and interpersonal relationships (Ross and Mirowsky 1984). The somatic items (e.g., loss of interest, poor appetite) have been shown to be more likely to be associated with a course of depressive episodes similar to that described for major depression with melancholia, and the positive-affect items are more likely to be associated with higher life satisfaction scores.

The Geriatric Depression Scale (GDS) was developed because the scales discussed earlier present problems for older persons who have difficulty in selecting one of four forced-response items (Yesavage et al. 1983). The 30-item GDS permits patients to rate items as either present or absent; it includes questions about symptoms such as cognitive complaints, self-image, and losses. Items selected were thought to have relevance to late-life depression.

Of the scales used by interviewers to rate patients, the Hamilton Rating Scale for Depression (Ham-D; Hamilton 1960) is by far the most commonly used. The advantage of having ratings based on clinical judgment has made the Ham-D a popular instrument for rating outcome in clinical trials. For example, a reduction in the score to one-half the initial score or to a score below a certain value would indicate partial or complete recovery from an episode of depression.

A scale that has received considerable attention clinically, having been standardized in clinical but not community populations, is the Montgomery-Åsberg Rating Scale for Depression (Montgomery and Åsberg 1979). This scale follows the pattern of the Ham-D and concentrates on 10 symptoms of depression; the clinician rates each symptom on a scale of 0–6 (for a range of scores between 0 and 60). The symptoms include apparent sadness, reported sadness, inattention, reduced sleep, reduced appetite, concentration difficulties, lassitude, inability to feel, pessimistic thoughts, and suicidal thoughts. Theoretically, this scale is an improvement over the Ham-D in that it appears to better differentiate between responders and nonresponders to intervention for depression.

General Assessment Scales

Several general assessment scales (occasionally combined with functioning in other areas) have been found useful in both community and clinical populations. Many of these scales are available in DSM-5 online materials and are listed in DSM-5 (American Psychiatric Association 2013). One of the more frequently used scales is the Global Assessment of Functioning Scale (American

Psychiatric Association 2000). On this scale, the rater makes a single rating, from 0 to 100, that best describes—on the basis of his or her clinical judgment—the lowest level of the subject's functioning in the week before the rating. The scale has not been standardized for older adults, but its common use in psychiatric studies suggests the need for standardization. The scale was incorporated as Axis V in DSM-IV-TR to measure overall functioning. Newer scales have been planned for DSM-5 (American Psychiatric Association 2013).

The Older Americans Resources and Services (OARS) Multidimensional Functional Assessment Questionnaire (Multidimensional Functional Assessment 1978), administered by a lay interviewer, produces functional impairment ratings in five dimensions: mental health, physical health, social functioning, economic functioning, and ADLs. In one community survey that used OARS (Blazer 1978a), 13% of the persons in the community were found to have mental health impairment.

Effective Communication With the Older Adult

The clinician who works with the older adult should be cognizant of factors relating to both the patient and the clinician that may produce barriers to effective communication (Blazer 1978b). Many older persons experience a relatively high level of anxiety yet do not complain of this symptom. Stress deriving from a new situation, such as visiting a clinician's office or being interviewed in a hospital, may intensify such anxiety and subsequently impair effective communication. Perceptual problems, such as hearing and visual impairments, may exacerbate disorientation and complicate the communication of problems to the clinician. Elders are more likely to withhold information than to hazard answers that may be incorrect—in other words, older persons tend to be more cautious. They frequently take longer to respond to inquiries and resist the clinician who attempts to rush through the history-taking interview.

The elderly patient may perceive the physician unrealistically, on the basis of previous life experiences (i.e., transference may occur). Also, the clinician may perceive the older adult patient incorrectly because of fears of aging and death or because of previous negative experiences with his or her own parents. For a clinician to work effectively with older adults, his or her personal feelings should be discussed during training—and afterward.

Certain techniques have generally proved to be valuable in communicating with the elderly patient. First, the older person should be approached with respect. The clinician should knock before entering a patient's room and should greet the patient by surname (e.g., Mr. Jones, Mrs. Smith) rather than by a given name.

After taking a position near the older person—near enough to reach out and touch the patient—the clinician should speak clearly and slowly and use simple sentences in case the person's hearing is impaired. The interview should be paced so that the older person has enough time to respond to questions. Nonverbal communication is frequently a key to effective communication with elderly persons because they may be reticent about revealing affect verbally. The patient's facial expressions, gestures, postures, and long silences may provide clues to the clinician about issues that are unspoken.

One key to successful communication with an older adult is a willingness to continue working as a professional with that person. Older adults place a great deal of stress on loyalty and continuity.

References

American Psychiatric Association: Diagnostic and Statistical Manual of Mental Disorders, 4th Edition. Washington, DC, American Psychiatric Association, 1994

American Psychiatric Association: Diagnostic and Statistical Manual of Mental Disorders, 4th Edition, Text Revision. Washington, DC, American Psychiatric Association, 2000

American Psychiatric Association: Diagnostic and Statistical Manual of Mental Disorders, 5th Edition. Washington, DC, American Psychiatric Association, 2013

Blazer DG: The OARS Durham surveys: description and application, in Multidimensional Functional Assessment: The OARS Methodology—A Manual, 2nd Edition. Durham, NC, Duke University Center for the Study of Aging and Human Development, 1978a, pp 75–88

Blazer DG: Techniques for communicating with your elderly patient. Geriatrics 33:79–80, 83–84, 1978b

Blazer DG: Depression in Late Life. St Louis, MO, CV Mosby, 1982

Blazer DG: Evaluating the family of the elderly patient, in A Family Approach to Health Care in the Elderly. Edited by Blazer D, Siegler IC. Menlo Park, CA, Addison-Wesley, 1984, pp 13–32

Folstein MF, Folstein SE, McHugh PR: "Mini-mental state": a practical method for grading the cognitive state of patients for the clinician. J Psychiatr Res 12:189–198, 1975

Hamilton M: A rating scale for depression. J Neurol Neurosurg Psychiatry 23:56–62, 1960

Inouye SK: Clarifying confusion: the Confusion Assessment Method—a new method for detection of delirium. Ann Intern Med 113:941–950, 1990

Kahn RL, Goldfarb AI, Pollack M, et al: Brief objective measures for the determination of mental status in the aged. Am J Psychiatry 117:326–328, 1960

Linn L: Clinical manifestations of psychiatric disorders, in Comprehensive Textbook of Psychiatry, 3rd Edition, Vol 1. Edited by Kaplan HI, Freedman AM, Sadock BJ. Baltimore, MD, Williams & Wilkins, 1980, pp 990–1034

Montgomery SA, Åsberg M: A new depression scale designed to be sensitive to change. Br J Psychiatry 134:382–389, 1979

Multidimensional Functional Assessment: The OARS Methodology—A Manual, 2nd Edition. Durham, NC, Duke University Center for the Study of Aging and Human Development, 1978

Pfeiffer E: A Short Portable Mental Status Questionnaire for the assessment of organic brain deficit in elderly patients. J Am Geriatr Soc 23:433–441, 1975

Radloff LS: The CES-D Scale: a self-report depression scale for research in the general population. Appl Psychol Meas 1:385–401, 1977

Ross CE, Mirowsky J: Components of depressed mood in married men and women: the CES-D. Am J Epidemiol 119:997–1004, 1984

Sanford JRA: Tolerance of debility in elderly dependents by supporters at home: its significance for hospital practice. Br Med J 3:471–473, 1975

Yesavage JA, Brink TL, Rose TL, et al: Development and validation of a geriatric depression screening scale: a preliminary report. J Psychiatr Res 17:37–49, 1983

Suggested Readings

Blazer DG: Techniques for communicating with your elderly patient. Geriatrics 33:79–80, 83–84, 1978

Folstein MF, Folstein SE, McHugh PR: "Mini-mental state": a practical method for grading the cognitive state of patients for the clinician. J Psychiatr Res 12:189–198, 1975

Inouye SK: Clarifying confusion: the Confusion Assessment Method—a new method for detection of delirium. Ann Intern Med 113:941–950, 1990

Othmer E, Othmer SC, Othmer JP: Psychiatric interview, history and mental status examination, in Kaplan and Sadock's Comprehensive Textbook of Psychiatry, 8th Edition, Vol 1. Edited by Sadock BJ, Sadock VA. Philadelphia, PA, Lippincott Williams & Wilkins, 2005, pp 794–826

2

Psychopharmacology

Benoit H. Mulsant, M.D.
Bruce G. Pollock, M.D., Ph.D.

Pharmacological intervention in late life requires special care. Elderly patients are more susceptible to drug-induced adverse events. Particularly troublesome among older persons are peripheral and central anticholinergic effects such as constipation, urinary retention, delirium, and cognitive dysfunction; antihistaminergic effects such as sedation; and antiadrenergic effects such as postural hypotension. Sedation and orthostatic hypotension not only interfere with basic activities but also pose a significant safety risk to elderly patients because they can lead to falls and fractures. Increased susceptibility to adverse effects in elders may be a result of the pharmacokinetic and pharmacodynamic changes associated with aging, such as diminished glomerular filtration, changes in the density and activity of target receptors, reduced liver size and hepatic blood flow, and decreased cardiac output (Pollock et al. 2009; Uchida et al. 2009) (Table 2–1).

Table 2–1. Physiological changes in elderly persons associated with altered pharmacokinetics

Organ system	Change	Pharmacokinetic consequence
Circulatory system	Decreased concentration of plasma albumin and increased α_1-acid glycoprotein	Increased or decreased free concentration of drugs in plasma
Gastrointestinal tract	Decreased intestinal and splanchnic blood flow	Decreased rate of drug absorption
Kidney	Decreased glomerular filtration rate	Decreased renal clearance of active metabolites
Liver	Decreased liver size; decreased hepatic blood flow; variable effects on cytochrome P450 isozyme activity	Decreased hepatic clearance
Muscle	Decreased lean body mass and increased adipose tissue	Altered volume of distribution of lipid-soluble drugs, leading to increased elimination half-life

Source. Adapted from Pollock 1998.

Illnesses that affect many elderly persons (e.g., diabetes) further diminish the processing and removal of medications from the body. In addition, polypharmacy and the associated risk of drug interactions add another level of complexity to pharmacological treatment in older patients. Poor adherence to treatment regimens—which can be a result of impaired cognitive function, confusing drug regimens, or lack of motivation or insight associated with the psychiatric disorder being treated—is a significant obstacle to effective and safe pharmacological treatment. Finally, it should be appreciated that psychotropic medications are not as extensively studied in elders as in younger individuals or those without comorbid medical illness with respect to pharmacokinetic and dosing information (Pollock et al. 2009). For example, fewer than one-third of the package inserts for the drugs most commonly prescribed in elderly patients have specific dosing recommendations (Steinmetz et al. 2005). New methodologies such as population pharmacokinetics can help to address this lack of information about dosage and drug-drug interactions (Bigos et al. 2006; Jin et al. 2010). Nonetheless, even with currently available knowledge, medications cause considerable morbidity in elders. In a study by Laroche et al. (2007), 66% of the admissions to an acute geriatric medical unit were preceded by the prescription of at least one inappropriate medication; even among patients taking appropriate medications, the prevalence of adverse drug reactions was 16%.

Despite these challenges, psychiatric disorders can be treated successfully in late life with psychotropic drugs. In this chapter, we summarize relevant data on the efficacy, tolerability, and safety of the major psychotropic drugs.

Antidepressant Medications

Selective Serotonin Reuptake Inhibitors

Six selective serotonin reuptake inhibitors (SSRIs) are available in the United States (see Table 2–2). They are approved by the U.S. Food and Drug Administration (FDA) for the treatment of major depressive disorder (all except fluvoxamine) and several anxiety disorders (generalized anxiety disorder: escitalopram, paroxetine; obsessive-compulsive disorder: fluoxetine, fluvoxamine, paroxetine, sertraline; panic disorder: fluoxetine, paroxetine, sertraline; posttraumatic stress disorder: paroxetine, sertraline; and social anxiety disorder: paroxetine, sertraline) in adults. In older adults, SSRIs remain first-line antidepressants (Sonnenberg et al. 2008) because of this broad spectrum of action, high efficacy (Mukai and Tampi 2009; Pinquart et al. 2006), ease of use, good tolerability, and relative safety. More than 40 randomized controlled trials of SSRIs involving more than 6,000 geriatric patients with depression have been published (Table 2–2). However, as with most drugs, few clinical trials of SSRIs have been conducted in "real-life" geriatric situations (e.g., in long-term-care facilities) or in very old patients. Overall, published trials support the efficacy and tolerability of SSRIs in older patients with major depression. These patients are at high risk for relapse and recurrence, and maintenance therapy with escitalopram or paroxetine has been shown to be effective in their prevention (Gorwood et al. 2007; Reynolds et al. 2006). Many open studies and some small controlled trials in special populations also have concluded that SSRIs are reasonably efficacious, safe, and well tolerated

Table 2–2. Summary of published randomized controlled trials of selective serotonin reuptake inhibitors for acute treatment of geriatric depression

	No. of published trials (cumulative no. of older participants)	Dosages studied (mg/day)	Comments
Citalopram	7[a] (1,343)	10–40	Citalopram was more efficacious than placebo in one of two trials and as efficacious as amitriptyline and venlafaxine. It was better tolerated than nortriptyline but associated with a lower remission rate. Several trials included patients with stroke and dementia.
Escitalopram	2[b] (781)	10–20	In one failed trial, escitalopram and fluoxetine were well tolerated but not superior to placebo. In another trial, escitalopram did not differ from placebo.
Fluoxetine	13[c] (2,092)	10–80	Fluoxetine was more efficacious than placebo in two of five trials and as efficacious as amitriptyline, doxepin, escitalopram, paroxetine, sertraline, trimipramine, and venlafaxine. In patients with dysthymic disorder, fluoxetine was marginally superior to placebo. In patients with dementia of the Alzheimer's type, fluoxetine did not differ from placebo.
Fluvoxamine	4[d] (278)	50–200	Fluvoxamine was more efficacious than placebo and as efficacious as dothiepin, imipramine, mianserin, and sertraline.
Paroxetine	9[e] (1,474)	10–60	Paroxetine was more efficacious than placebo and as efficacious as amitriptyline, bupropion, clomipramine, doxepin, fluoxetine, and imipramine. Paroxetine was less efficacious than venlafaxine in older patients (n=30) who had previously failed to respond to two other antidepressants. Mirtazapine was marginally superior to paroxetine. In very old long-term-care patients with minor depression, paroxetine was not more efficacious but was more cognitively toxic than placebo. One trial included patients with dementia.

Table 2–2. Summary of published randomized controlled trials of selective serotonin reuptake inhibitors for acute treatment of geriatric depression (*continued*)

	No. of published trials (cumulative no. of older participants)	Dosages studied (mg/day)	Comments
Sertraline	11[f] (1,948)	50–200	Sertraline was more efficacious than placebo and as efficacious as amitriptyline, fluoxetine, fluvoxamine, imipramine, nortriptyline, and venlafaxine. Sertraline was better tolerated than imipramine and venlafaxine. Greater cognitive improvement occurred with sertraline than with nortriptyline or fluoxetine. Some trials included long-term-care patients. In one small single-site trial, sertraline was more efficacious than placebo for the treatment of depression associated with Alzheimer's dementia. However, this finding was not replicated in a larger multicenter trial.

[a]Allard et al. 2004; Andersen et al. 1994; Kyle et al. 1998; Navarro et al. 2001; Nyth and Gottfries 1990; Nyth et al. 1992; Roose et al. 2004b; Rosenberg et al. 2007.

[b]Bose et al. 2008; Kasper et al. 2005.

[c]Altamura et al. 1989; Devanand et al. 2005; Doraiswamy et al. 2001; Evans et al. 1997; Feighner and Cohn 1985; Finkel et al. 1999; Kasper et al. 2005; Petracca et al. 2001; Schatzberg and Roose 2006; Schone and Ludwig 1993; Taragano et al. 1997; Tollefson et al. 1995; Wehmeier et al. 2005.

[d]Phanjoo et al. 1991; Rahman et al. 1991; Rossini et al. 2005; Wakelin 1986.

[e]Burrows et al. 2002; Dunner et al. 1992; Geretsegger et al. 1995; Guillibert et al. 1989; Katona et al. 1998; Mazeh et al. 2007; Mulsant et al. 2001b; Rapaport et al. 2003; Schatzberg et al. 2002; Schone and Ludwig 1993.

[f]Bondareff et al. 2000; Cohn et al. 1990; Doraiswamy et al. 2003; Finkel et al. 1999; Forlenza et al. 2001; Lyketsos et al. 2003; Newhouse et al. 2000; Oslin et al. 2000, 2003; Rosenberg et al. 2010; Rossini et al. 2005; Schneider et al. 2003; Sheikh et al. 2004a; Weintraub et al. 2010.

in older patients with mild cognitive impairment (Devanand et al. 2003; Reynolds et al. 2011), minor depression (Lavretsky et al. 2010; Rocca et al. 2005), schizophrenia (Kasckow et al. 2001), cardiovascular disease (Glassman et al. 2002; Serebruany et al. 2003), cerebrovascular disease (Y. Chen et al. 2007; Murray et al. 2005; Rampello et al. 2004; Rasmussen et al. 2003; Robinson et al. 2000, 2008), Parkinson's disease (Barone et al. 2006; Devos et al. 2008), or other medical conditions (Arranz and Ros 1997; Evans et al. 1997; Goodnick and Hernandez 2000; Karp et al. 2005; Lotrich et al. 2007; Trappler and Cohen 1998) and in family dementia caregivers with minor or major depression (Lavretsky et al. 2010).

Two published placebo-controlled trials of citalopram (Lenze et al. 2005) and escitalopram (Lenze et al. 2009) support the efficacy of SSRIs in older patients with generalized anxiety disorder. The use of SSRIs to treat other anxiety disorders is based on small open trials (Flint 2005; Lenze et al. 2002; Sheikh et al. 2004b; Wylie et al. 2000) or extrapolation from studies in younger adults.

Some published studies—including two randomized controlled trials—suggest that SSRIs may be efficacious in the treatment of behavioral disturbances associated with dementia, including not only agitation and disinhibition but also delusions and hallucinations (Nyth and Gottfries 1990; Nyth et al. 1992; Pollock et al. 1997, 2002, 2007). Some older open studies and small single-site controlled trials also supported the use of SSRIs for the treatment of depression associated with Alzheimer's dementia (Katona et al. 1998; Lyketsos et al. 2003; Nyth and Gottfries 1990; Nyth et al. 1992; Olafsson et al. 1992; Petracca et al. 2001; Taragano et al. 1997). However, a larger multicenter trial failed to confirm these results; in this study, sertraline was not more efficacious and was less well tolerated than placebo for the treatment of depression in Alzheimer's disease (Rosenberg et al. 2010; Weintraub et al. 2010). Another recent multicenter study also showed no differences among sertraline, mirtazapine, and placebo in treating depression in patients with Alzheimer's disease. Tolerability of either drug was worse than with placebo (Banerjee et al. 2011).

Some administrative or quasi-experimental geriatric data suggest that escitalopram may be more efficacious or better tolerated than other SSRIs (Wu et al. 2008a, 2008b). However, available data from head-to-head randomized comparisons indicate that all SSRIs currently available have similar efficacy and tolerability in the treatment of depression (see Table 2–2). Nevertheless, experts favor the use of citalopram, escitalopram, or sertraline over fluvoxamine, fluoxetine, or paroxetine (Alexopoulos et al. 2001; Mulsant et al. 2001a; Rajji et al. 2008) because of their favorable pharmacokinetic profiles (Table 2–3) and their lower potential for clinically significant drug interactions (Table 2–4). Some data also suggest that they may be better tolerated (Cipriani et al. 2009) and more beneficial in terms of cognitive improvement (Burrows et al. 2002; Doraiswamy et al. 2003; Furlan et al. 2001; Jorge et al. 2010; Newhouse et al. 2000; Savaskan et al. 2008). However, some recent data suggest that citalopram—like other SSRIs—may have deleterious cognitive effects in some very old patients (Culang et al. 2009) and that those with executive dysfunction may not benefit from citalopram and other SSRIs (Sneed et al. 2010).

Also, in August 2011, the FDA issued a warning, updated in March 2012, against the use of dosages of citalopram above 40 mg/day in any person and above 20 mg/day in individuals older than 60 years because of a risk of prolonged QTc and torsade de pointes (see footnote b in Table 2–3).

In older patients, SSRI starting dosages are typically half the minimal efficacious dosage (see Table 2–3), and the dosage is usually doubled after 1 week. All of the SSRIs can be administered in a single daily dose except fluvoxamine, which should be given in two divided doses. Even though frail older patients typically tolerate these drugs relatively well (Oslin et al. 2000), some patients experience some gastrointestinal distress (e.g., nausea) during the first few days of treatment. Significant hyponatremia resulting from the syndrome of inappropriate secretion of antidiuretic hormone (SIADH) is a rare but potentially dangerous adverse effect that is observed almost exclusively in elderly patients (Fabian et al. 2004).

SSRIs may directly affect platelet activation (Pollock et al. 2000), and they are associated with a small increase in the risk of gastrointestinal or postsurgical bleeding (Dalton et al. 2006; Looper 2007). They act synergistically with other medications that increase the risk of gastrointestinal bleeding, such as nonsteroidal anti-inflammatory drugs (NSAIDs) and low-dose aspirin. Thus, SSRIs should be used cautiously in older patients taking these medications, and the prophylactic use of acid-suppressing agents should be considered in some high-risk patients (de Abajo and Garcia-Rodriguez 2008; Yuan et al. 2006).

Table 2–3. Pharmacokinetic properties of selective serotonin reuptake inhibitors and serotonin-norepinephrine reuptake inhibitors

	Half-life (days), including active metabolites	Proportionality of dosage to plasma concentration	Risk of uncomfortable withdrawal symptoms	Efficacious dosage range in elderly (mg/day)[a]
Citalopram	1–3	Linear across therapeutic range	Low	20[b]
Desvenlafaxine	0.5	Linear up to 600 mg/day	High	50
Duloxetine	0.5	Linear across therapeutic range	Moderate	60–120
Escitalopram	1–2	Linear across therapeutic range	Low	10–20
Fluoxetine	7–10	Nonlinear at higher dosages	Very low	20–40
Fluvoxamine	0.5–1	Nonlinear at higher dosages	Moderate	50–300
Paroxetine	1	Nonlinear at higher dosages	Moderate	20–40
Sertraline	1–3	Linear across therapeutic range	Low	50–200
Venlafaxine XR	0.2	Linear across therapeutic range	High	75–300

Note.   XR = extended-release.

[a]Starting dosage is typically half of the lowest efficacious dosage; all the selective serotonin reuptake inhibitors can be administered in single daily doses except for fluvoxamine, which should be given in two divided doses.

[b]In March 2012, the U.S. Food and Drug Administration updated a drug safety communication originally issued in August 2011, stating the following: "The maximum recommended dose of citalopram is 20 mg per day for patients with hepatic impairment, patients who are older than 60 years of age, patients who are CYP 2C19 poor metabolizers, or patients who are taking concomitant cimetidine (Tagamet®) or another CYP2C19 inhibitor, because these factors lead to increased blood levels of citalopram, increasing the risk of QT interval prolongation and Torsade de Pointes" (U.S. Food and Drug Administration 2012).

Table 2–4. Newer antidepressants' inhibition of cytochrome P450 (CYP) and potential for causing clinically significant drug-drug interactions

	CYP1A2	CYP2C9/2C19	CYP2D6	CYP3A4	Potential for causing clinically significant drug-drug interaction
Bupropion	0	0	++	0	Low
Citalopram	+	0	+	0	Low
Desvenlafaxine	0	0	+	0	Minimal
Duloxetine	0	0	++	+	Low
Escitalopram	+	0	+	0	Minimal
Fluoxetine	+	++	+++	++	High
Fluvoxamine	+++	+++	+	++	High
Mirtazapine	0	0	0	+	Low
Nefazodone	0	+	0	+++	High
Paroxetine	+	+	+++	+	Moderate
Sertraline	+	+	+	+	Low
Venlafaxine	0	0	0	0	Low

Note.   0 = minimal or no inhibition; + = mild inhibition; ++ = moderate inhibition; +++ = strong inhibition.

SSRIs also can be associated with bradycardia and should be started with caution in patients with low heart rates (e.g., patients taking β-blockers). They rarely cause extrapyramidal symptoms (Mamo et al. 2000), and they are well tolerated by most patients with Parkinson's disease (P. Chen et al. 2007). The risk of falls and hip fractures does not differ among different classes of antidepressants (Liu et al. 1998), and there is concern that chronic use of SSRIs may contribute to the risk of fractures through their direct effects on bone metabolism (Diem et al. 2007; Richards et al. 2007).

A large pharmacoepidemiological study in elders found that SSRIs, compared with non-SSRI antidepressants, are associated with a greater risk for suicide during the first month of therapy (Juurlink et al. 2006). However, the absolute risk is low, which suggests that there may be a vulnerable subgroup at risk for an idiosyncratic response. A very large meta-analysis and controlled data available to the FDA indicated a substantial reduction in the risk for suicidal ideation in older patients taking SSRIs compared with those taking placebo (Barbui et al. 2009; Friedman and Leon 2007; Nelson et al. 2007).

Serotonin-Norepinephrine Reuptake Inhibitors

As of June 2013, there are three serotonin-norepinephrine reuptake inhibitors (SNRIs) approved by the FDA for the treatment of major depressive disorder in adults: desvenlafaxine, duloxetine, and venlafaxine. Duloxetine and venlafaxine have also been approved for the treatment of generalized anxiety disorder; duloxetine for diabetic peripheral neuropathic pain and fibromyalgia; and venlafaxine for panic disorder and social anxiety disorder. Because of their usually favorable side-effect profile in younger patients and their dual mechanism of action (Chalon et al. 2003; Harvey et al. 2000), SNRIs have become the preferred alternatives to SSRIs. Some meta-analyses have suggested that venlafaxine is associated with a higher rate of remission than are SSRIs in younger depressed patients (Shelton et al. 2005; Smith et al. 2002; Stahl et al. 2002; Thase et al. 2001, 2005a). However, several other meta-analyses and head-to-head trials have contradicted these results or challenged their clinical significance in both younger (Cipriani et al. 2009; Hansen et al. 2005; Kornstein et al. 2010a; Lam et al. 2010; Papakostas et al. 2007; Vis et al. 2005) and older (Mukai and Tampi 2009; Nelson et al. 2008; Rajji et al. 2008) patients. Also, the risk-benefit ratio of SNRIs may be different in younger and older patients and may change the relative desirability of these medications in the treatment of older patients.

The efficacy, tolerability, and relative safety of SNRIs in the treatment of late-life depression are supported by 10 published controlled trials involving about 1,300 older patients (9 trials with venlafaxine and 1 with duloxetine; Table 2–5). Two additional analyses of geriatric data pooled from randomized placebo-controlled trials conducted in mixed-age adults support the efficacy of desvenlafaxine and duloxetine for late-life depression (Kornstein et al. 2010a; Nelson et al. 2005). In randomized comparisons of desvenlafaxine with escitalopram and placebo in perimenopausal and postmenopausal women ages 40–70 years with major depressive disorder, desvenlafaxine and escitalopram had similar efficacy and tolerability (Kornstein et al. 2010b; Soares et al. 2010). Additional data from open-label studies and case series support the efficacy of SNRIs in older patients, including those with atypical depression (Roose et al. 2004a), treatment-resistant depression (Mazeh et al. 2007), dysthymic disorder (Devanand et al. 2004), poststroke depression (Dahmen et al. 1999), generalized anxiety disorder (Katz et al. 2002), chronic pain syndromes (Grothe et al. 2004), stress urinary incontinence (Mariappan et al. 2005), or pain symptoms associated with geriatric depression (Karp et al. 2010; Raskin et al. 2007; Wohlreich et al. 2009).

SNRIs do not inhibit significantly any of the major cytochrome P450 (CYP) isoenzymes and thus are unlikely to cause clinically significant drug-drug interactions (Oganesian et al. 2009) (see Table 2–4). However, venlafaxine and duloxetine are metabolized by CYP2D6, and their concentrations can increase markedly in genetically poor metabolizers or in patients who are taking drugs that inhibit this isoenzyme (Whyte et al. 2006). The concentration of duloxetine also can be increased by drugs that inhibit CYP1A2. Dose adjustments of SNRIs are not recommended on the basis of age (see Table 2–3), but SNRIs should be used with caution in older patients with renal or liver disease (Dolder et al. 2010).

SNRIs inhibit the reuptake of serotonin. Thus, they share the side-effect profile of SSRIs, including not only nausea, diarrhea, headaches, and excessive sweating but also sexual dysfunction (Montejo et al. 2001), SIADH and hyponatremia (Kirby et al. 2002), upper gastrointestinal tract bleeding (de Abajo and Garcia-Rodriguez 2008), serotonin syndrome (McCue and Joseph 2001; Perry 2000), and discontinuation symptoms (Montgomery et al. 2009). SNRIs

Table 2–5.   Summary of published randomized controlled trials of serotonin-norepinephrine reuptake inhibitors (desvenlafaxine, duloxetine, venlafaxine), bupropion, and mirtazapine for acute treatment of geriatric depression

	No. of published trials (cumulative no. of older participants)	Dosages studied (mg/day)	Comments
Bupropion	2[a] (163)	100–450	Bupropion was as efficacious as imipramine and paroxetine.
Desvenlafaxine	0	NA	No published geriatric randomized trials as of December 2010.
Duloxetine	1[b] (311)	20–60	Duloxetine was more efficacious than and as well tolerated as placebo. Duloxetine also showed efficacy on pain and cognitive measures.
Mirtazapine	2[c] (370)	15–45	Mirtazapine was as efficacious as low-dose (total daily dose=30–90 mg) amitriptyline and marginally superior to paroxetine.

Table 2–5. Summary of published randomized controlled trials of serotonin-norepinephrine reuptake inhibitors (desvenlafaxine, duloxetine, venlafaxine), bupropion, and mirtazapine for acute treatment of geriatric depression *(continued)*

	No. of published trials (cumulative no. of older participants)	Dosages studied (mg/day)	Comments
Venlafaxine	9[d] (1,032)	50–300	Venlafaxine did not differ from placebo in one trial. Venlafaxine was as efficacious as citalopram, clomipramine, dothiepin, fluoxetine, nortriptyline, and sertraline and was more efficacious than paroxetine (in 30 older patients who had previously failed to respond to two other antidepressants) and trazodone. It was less well tolerated than placebo, fluoxetine, and sertraline; tolerated as well as citalopram and dothiepin; and better tolerated than clomipramine, nortriptyline, and trazodone.

Note. NA=not applicable.
[a]Branconnier et al. 1983; Doraiswamy et al. 2001; Weihs et al. 2000.
[b]Raskin et al. 2007; Wohlreich et al. 2009.
[c]Hoyberg et al. 1996; Schatzberg et al. 2002.
[d]Allard et al. 2004; Gasto et al. 2003; Kok et al. 2007; Mahapatra and Hackett 1997; Mazeh et al. 2007; Oslin et al. 2003; Schatzberg and Roose 2006; Smeraldi et al. 1998; Trick et al. 2004.

are also associated with adverse effects that can be linked to their action on the adrenergic system, including dry mouth, constipation, urinary retention, increased ocular pressure, cardiovascular problems, and transient agitation (Aragona and Inghilleri 1998; Benazzi 1997; Dolder et al. 2010). These adverse effects appear to be dose dependent (Clayton et al. 2009; Liebowitz and Tourian 2010; Thase 1998), and they are usually self-limiting. However, cardiovascular effects of SNRIs are of special concern in the elderly. SNRIs can cause not only some increase in blood pressure (Clayton et al. 2009; Thase 1998; Thase et al. 2005c; Zimmer et al. 1997) but also clinically significant orthostatic hypotension, syncope, electrocardiographic changes, arrhythmia, acute ischemia, and death in overdose (Clayton et al. 2009; Davidson et al. 2005; Johnson et al. 2006; Lessard et al. 1999; Reznik et al. 1999). At this time, it is not known whether the cardiovascular risks of the three SNRIs differ. However, venlafaxine has been used for the longest time, and the bulk of the relevant available data implicate venlafaxine. In the United Kingdom, the National Institute for Clinical Excellence has recommended that venlafaxine not be prescribed to patients with preexisting heart disease, that an electrocardiogram be obtained at baseline, and that blood pressure and cardiac functions be monitored in those patients taking higher doses (National Collaborating Centre for Mental Health 2004). Overall, duloxetine and venlafaxine may be less well tolerated than escitalopram and sertraline (Cipriani et al. 2009), and a randomized trial conducted under double-blind conditions in older nursing home residents found that venlafaxine was less well tolerated and less safe than sertraline, without evidence for an increase in efficacy (Oslin et al. 2003).

In conclusion, it seems prudent not to use SNRIs as first-line agents in older patients but to reserve SNRIs for those whose symptoms do not respond to SSRIs (Alexopoulos et al. 2001; Cooper et al. 2011; Karp et al. 2008; Mulsant et al. 2001a; Whyte et al. 2004) or those who present with depression and chronic pain (Karp et al. 2010; Raskin et al. 2007; Wohlreich et al. 2009). This recommendation is congruent with the results from the Sequenced Treatment Alternatives to Relieve Depression (STAR*D) study (Rush et al. 2006). In this large study, mixed-age patients who had failed to respond to a first-line SSRI had similar outcomes when the next treatment step was to augment the SSRI with sustained-release bupropion or buspirone, switch to another SSRI, or switch to an agent from another class (i.e., bupropion or venlafaxine extended-release [XR]). The following steps included using a combination of venlafaxine XR and mirtazapine, with outcomes similar to those associated with switching to the monoamine oxidase inhibitor (MAOI) tranylcypromine (Rush et al. 2006).

Other Newer Antidepressants

Only limited controlled data support the efficacy and safety of bupropion or mirtazapine in older patients (see Table 2–5). Nevertheless, because of their usually favorable side-effect profiles and their different mechanisms of action, these two drugs are often used in older patients whose symptoms do not respond to or who cannot tolerate SSRIs (Alexopoulos et al. 2001).

Bupropion

Published data supporting the safety and efficacy of bupropion in geriatric depression are limited to two small controlled trials (see Table 2–5) and one small open study (Steffens et al. 2001). Expert consensus favors the use of bupropion—alone or as an augmentation agent—in older depressed patients whose symptoms have not responded to SSRIs or who cannot tolerate them (Alexopoulos et al. 2001). In particular, bupropion can be helpful for patients who complain of nausea, diarrhea, unbearable fatigue, or sexual dysfunction during SSRI treatment (Nieuwstraten and Dolovich 2001; Thase et al. 2005b). Although augmentation with bupropion has been reported to be helpful in patients who were partial responders to SSRIs or venlafaxine (Bodkin et al. 1997; Spier 1998), the safety of this combination in older patients has not been established (Joo et al. 2002). Controlled data on the use of bupropion in patients with heart disease (Kiev et al. 1994; Roose et al. 1991), in smokers (Tashkin et al. 2001), and in patients with neuropathic pain (Semenchuk et al. 2001) confirm clinical experience that bupropion is relatively well tolerated by medically ill patients. Bupropion is contraindicated in patients who have or are at risk for seizure disorders (e.g., poststroke patients). However, the sustained-release preparation of bupropion appears to be associated with a very low incidence of seizure, comparable to that of other antidepressants (Dunner et al. 1998). Bupropion also has been associated with the onset of psychosis in case reports (Howard and Warnock 1999), and the prudent action is to avoid this medication in psychotic patients or in agitated patients at risk for the development of psychotic symptoms. The propensity of bupropion to induce psychosis in at-risk patients has been attributed to its action on dopaminergic neurotransmission (Howard and Warnock 1999). The same mechanism has been hypothesized to underlie the association of bupropion with gait disturbance and falls in some patients (Joo et al. 2002; Szuba and Leuchter 1992). Bupropion is a moderate inhibitor of CYP2D6 (Kotlyar et al. 2005). It appears to be metabolized by CYP2B6 (Hesse et al. 2004), and adverse effects of bupropion such as seizures or gait disturbance may be more likely in patients who take drugs that inhibit CYP2B6, such as fluoxetine or paroxetine (Joo et al. 2002).

Mirtazapine

The antidepressant activity of mirtazapine has been attributed to its blockade of α_2 autoreceptors, resulting in a direct enhancement of noradrenergic neurotransmission and an increase in the synaptic levels of serotonin (5-hydroxytryptamine [5-HT]), indirectly enhancing neurotransmission mediated by serotonin type 1A (5-HT$_{1A}$) receptors. In addition, like the antinausea drugs granisetron and ondansetron, mirtazapine inhibits 5-HT$_2$ and 5-HT$_3$ receptors. Thus, mirtazapine could be particularly helpful for patients who do not tolerate SSRIs because of sexual dysfunction (Gelenberg et al. 2000; Montejo et al. 2001), tremor (Pact and Giduz 1999), or severe nausea (Pedersen and Klysner 1997). In one case series, mirtazapine was used successfully to treat depression in 19 mixed-age oncology patients who were receiving chemotherapy (Thompson 2000). It also has been combined with SSRIs (Pedersen and Klysner 1997); however, these combinations should be used cautiously because they have been associated with a serotonin syndrome in an older patient (Benazzi 1998). The STAR*D study found that a combination of mirtazapine and venlafaxine XR had modest efficacy in patients with treatment-resistant depression, comparable to the efficacy of the MAOI tranylcypromine (Rush et al. 2006); however, only a few STAR*D participants were elderly, and the safety of this combination has not been established in older patients.

No published placebo-controlled trials and only two comparator-controlled trials of mirtazapine in geriatric depression have been done (see Table 2–5). Consistent with this paucity of controlled data, experts favor the use of mirtazapine as a third-line drug in older depressed patients who cannot tolerate or whose symptoms have not responded to SSRIs or venlafaxine (Alexopoulos et al. 2001). Mirtazapine also has been used to treat depression in frail nursing home patients (Roose et al. 2003) and in older patients with dementia (Raji and Brady 2001), but there are concerns about its effect on cognition. It has been shown to impair driving performance in two placebo- and active comparator–controlled trials in healthy volunteers (Ridout et al. 2003; Wingen et al. 2005) and to cause delirium in older patients with organic brain syndromes (Bailer et al. 2000). This deleterious effect on cognition is possibly a result of mirtazapine's antihistaminergic and sedative effects. Other adverse effects of mirtazapine include weight gain with lipid increase (Nicholas et al. 2003), hyponatremia (Cheah et al. 2008), and, very rarely, neutropenia or even agranulocytosis (Hutchison 2001).

Nefazodone

Given the absence of any controlled trials of nefazodone in geriatric depression, mediocre outcomes in an open study (Saiz-Ruiz et al. 2002), potentially problematic drug-drug interactions caused by its strong inhibition of CYP3A4 (see Table 2–4), and reports that the incidence of hepatic toxicity or even liver failure is 10- to 30-fold higher with nefazodone than with other antidepressants (Carvajal García-Pando et al. 2002), nefazodone should not be used in older patients.

Tricyclic Antidepressants and Monoamine Oxidase Inhibitors

As is the case in younger patients (Rush et al. 2006), tricyclic antidepressants (TCAs) and MAOIs have become third- and fourth-line drugs in the treatment of late-life depression because of their adverse effects and the special precautions that their use entails (Mottram et al. 2006; Mulsant et al. 2001a; Rajji et al. 2008; Wilson and Mottram 2004). The tertiary-amine TCAs— amitriptyline, clomipramine, doxepin, and imipramine—can cause significant orthostatic hypotension and anticholinergic effects, including cognitive impairment, and they should be avoided in elderly persons (Beers 1997). The secondary amines desipramine and nortriptyline are preferred in older patients. They have a lower propensity to cause orthostasis and falls, in addition to having linear pharmacokinetics and more modest anticholinergic effects (Chew et al. 2008). Their relatively narrow therapeutic index (i.e., the plasma level range separating efficacy and toxicity) necessitates monitoring of plasma levels and electrocardiograms in older patients. A single dose is given at bedtime; 5–7 days after initiation of desipramine at 50 mg or nortriptyline at 25 mg, plasma levels should be measured and dosages adjusted linearly, with targeted plasma levels of 200–400 ng/mL for desipramine and 50–150 ng/mL for nortriptyline. These narrow ranges ensure efficacy while decreasing risks of cardiac toxicity and other side effects. Like the tertiary-amine TCAs, desipramine and nortriptyline are type 1 antiarrhythmics: they have quinidine-like effects on cardiac conduction and should not be used in patients who have or are at risk for cardiac conduction defects (Roose et al. 1991). Most anticholinergic side effects of desipramine and nortriptyline (e.g., dry mouth, constipation) resolve with time or usually can be mitigated with symptomatic treatment (Rosen et al. 1993). However, TCAs have been associated with cognitive worsening (Reifler et al. 1989) or with less cognitive improvement than occurs with sertraline (Bondareff et al. 2000; Doraiswamy et al. 2003) or other SSRIs.

Even though MAOIs have been found to be efficacious in older depressed patients (Georgotas et al. 1986), and they may have a special role in patients with atypical or treatment-resistant depression, these medications are now rarely used in older patients (Shulman et al. 2009). This is in large part because they can cause significant hypotension or life-threatening hypertensive or serotonergic crises as a result of dietary or drug interactions. When MAOIs are used in older patients whose symptoms have typically failed to respond to SSRIs, SNRIs, and TCAs, phenelzine is preferred to tranylcypromine because it has been more extensively studied in older patients (Georgotas et al. 1986). A typical starting dosage would be 15 mg/day, with a target dosage of 45–90 mg/day in three divided doses. Patients need to follow dietary restrictions (Shulman and Walker 2001) and to inform any health care providers (including pharmacists) that they are taking an MAOI. Another option is the selegiline transdermal patch. It was developed to deliver selegiline at blood concentrations sufficient to inhibit monoamine oxidase A and B (MAO-A and MAO-B) in the brain without inhibiting MAO-A in the gastrointestinal tract, thereby reducing the risk of hypertensive crisis (Nandagopal and DelBello 2009). No geriatric data are available, but dietary restrictions are not needed at the 6-mg/24-hour dosage. However, they are recommended with higher dosages (Robinson and Amsterdam 2008), and potentially lethal drug interactions remain a concern.

Psychostimulants

Even though psychostimulants are used in the treatment of late-life mood disorders by some clinicians, this practice has minimal empirical support. A few small double-blind trials suggested that methylphenidate is generally well tolerated and modestly efficacious for medically burdened depressed elders (Satel and Nelson 1989; Wallace et al. 1995). Methylphenidate also has been used for the treatment of apathy and anergia associated with late-life depression or dementia (Herrmann et al. 2008). SSRIs inhibit dopamine release and may contribute to apathy and fatigue. A small study suggested that methylphenidate can be used to augment SSRIs in older depressed patients (Lavretsky et al. 2006). The wakefulness-promoting agent modafinil, which appears to induce a calm alertness through nondopaminergic mechanisms, also may have utility when targeting apathy and fatigue in patients taking SSRIs (Dunlop et al. 2007; Fava et al. 2007), but geriatric data are currently nonexistent. Caution is advised regarding the possible exacerbation by methylphenidate and other psychostimulants of anxiety, psychosis, anorexia, or hypertension and potential interactions with warfarin. Experience with other dopaminergic medications, such as pergolide, piribedil, pramipexole, and ropinirole, in the elderly has been limited, but there have been several encouraging controlled trials in patients with Parkinson's disease and depression (Aiken 2007; Barone et al. 2006, 2010; Rektorová et al. 2003) and in elderly patients with cognitive impairment (Nagaraja and Jayashree 2001).

Antipsychotic Medications

In older adults, as in other age groups, atypical antipsychotics are being prescribed as first-line drugs for the treatment of psychotic symptoms of any etiology. Studies support the efficacy of these agents in the treatment of late-life schizophrenia and late-onset psychoses (Scott et al. 2011), but their role in the treatment of behavioral and psychological symptoms of dementia is being questioned (Ballard and Corbett 2010; Salzman et al. 2008; Siddiqi et al. 2007). A highly publicized report and an FDA warning have indicated a nearly twofold increase in the rate of deaths in older patients with behavioral and psychological symptoms of dementia treated with atypical antipsychotics when compared with placebo (Kuehn 2005; Schneider et al. 2005). These reports have led to a reexamination of the safety of both conventional and atypical antipsychotics in older patients. A series of studies emphasize their association with mortality (Ballard et al. 2009; Ray et al. 2009; Wang et al. 2005), stroke (Gill et al. 2005; Herrmann et al. 2004), severe hyperglycemia in patients with diabetes (Lipscombe et al. 2009), femur fractures (Liperoti et al. 2007), and venous thromboembolism (Kleijer et al. 2010). The relative safety of atypical compared with conventional antipsychotics remains unclear: atypical antipsychotics may cause fewer falls (Hien le et al. 2005; Landi et al. 2005) and fewer extrapyramidal symptoms (Lee et al. 2004; Rochon et al. 2005; van Iersel et al. 2005), but they may cause more cerebrovascular events (Percudani et al. 2005), venous thromboembolism (Liperoti et al. 2005), and pancreatitis (Koller et al. 2003). Given the current uncertainty regarding the safety of antipsychotics—and, for most indications, the absence of consistent evidence supporting the efficacy or safety of drugs from alternative classes (Ballard and Corbett 2010; Sink et al. 2005)—clinicians need to consider the risk-benefit ratio for each individual patient (Gauthier et al. 2010; Rabins and Lyketsos 2005).

Risperidone

Of the atypical antipsychotics currently available in the United States, risperidone has the most published geriatric data for a variety of conditions (Schneider et al. 2005, 2006a; Sink et al. 2005). The efficacy and safety of risperidone in the treatment of behavioral and psychological symptoms of dementia have been reported in several randomized placebo-controlled trials (e.g., Brodaty et al. 2003; De Deyn et al. 1999, 2005b; Katz et al. 1999; Schneider et al. 2006a, 2006b; Sink et al. 2005); in randomized comparisons with haloperidol (Chan et al. 2001; De Deyn et al. 1999; Suh et al. 2004), promazine and olanzapine (Gareri et al. 2004), and olanzapine (Fontaine et al. 2003; Mulsant et al. 2004); and in many uncontrolled studies and large case series.

The efficacy and tolerability of risperidone in the treatment of late-life schizophrenia are supported by one randomized comparison with olanzapine (Harvey et al. 2003; Jeste et al. 2003) and one randomized open-label study of crossover from conventional antipsychotics to risperidone or olanzapine (Ritchie et al. 2003, 2006). The parallel study showed similar efficacy between olanzapine and risperidone but more weight gain and less cognitive improvement with olanzapine. In the crossover study, patients who were switched to olanzapine were more likely to complete the switching process and to show an improvement in psychological quality of life. The results from these two controlled trials are supported by a large body of uncontrolled data in older patients with schizophrenia and other psychotic disorders (e.g., Davidson et al. 2000; Madhusoodanan et al. 1999). In addition, an analysis of the patients with schizophrenia age 65 and older ($N=57$) who participated in randomized studies of the long-acting injectable ("depot") risperidone (Risperdal Consta) found that it was well tolerated and produced significant symptomatic improvements (Lasser et al. 2004).

One randomized comparison with haloperidol (Han and Kim 2004) and some uncontrolled data (e.g., Mittal et al. 2004; Parellada et al. 2004) support the efficacy and tolerability of risperidone in the treatment of delirium. However, there have been several case reports of delirium induced by risperidone. One small randomized comparison with clozapine ($N=10$) (Ellis et al. 2000) and several open trials of low-dose risperidone in the treatment of Parkinson's disease and drug-induced psychosis or Lewy body dementia have had inconsistent results, with clear worsening of parkinsonian symptoms in some studies (e.g., Culo et al. 2010; Ellis et al. 2000; Leopold 2000). Thus, risperidone should be used with great caution in the treatment of these disorders (Parkinson Study Group 1999).

As with other atypical antipsychotics, the efficacy and tolerability of risperidone in younger patients with bipolar disorder (and possibly other mood disorders) (Andreescu et al. 2006) are well established. However, no efficacy data in older patients with bipolar disorder would favor the selection of a specific atypical antipsychotic for these patients. As a result, experts continue to favor the use of mood stabilizers as first-line agents except in the presence of severe mania or mania with psychosis, in which case they favor combining risperidone, olanzapine, or quetiapine with a mood stabilizer (Sajatovic et al. 2005b; Young et al. 2004).

Commonly reported side effects of risperidone include orthostatic hypotension (on initiation of treatment) and extrapyramidal symptoms that are dose dependent (Katz et al. 1999). At a given dosage, concentrations of risperidone (and possibly its active metabolite paliperidone or 9-hydroxyrisperidone) seem to increase with age (Aichhorn et al. 2005). Therefore, typical dosages should be between 0.5 and 2 mg/day for older patients with dementia and lower than 4 mg/day for older patients without dementia. Of all the atypical antipsychotics, risperidone appears to be the most likely to be associated with hyperprolactinemia (Kinon et al. 2003). Risperidone causes only moderate electroencephalographic abnormalities (Centorrino et al. 2002), and it is rarely associated with cognitive impairment, probably because of its low affinity for muscarinic receptors (Chew et al. 2006; Harvey et al. 2003; Mulsant et al. 2004). Like other antipsychotics, risperidone can cause weight gain, diabetes, or dyslipidemia. It is more likely to do so than are aripiprazole and ziprasidone but less likely than are clozapine, olanzapine, and quetiapine (American Diabetes Association et al. 2004; Feldman et al. 2004; Zheng et al. 2009).

Paliperidone

Paliperidone is the active 9-hydroxy metabolite of risperidone, and therefore its pharmacological action, efficacy, and side effects should be very similar to those of risperidone. It is being marketed as a once-daily XR formulation that takes 24 hours to reach a maximum concentration. Paliperidone clearance is not affected by hepatic impairment or CYP2D6 metabolism, but it is affected by renal function. FDA approval was based on three 6-week trials that included a total of only 125 subjects age 65 years and older (e.g., Davidson et al. 2007; Kane et al. 2007). Limited available data indicate that paliperidone may be effective in the treatment of schizophrenia in elderly patients (Madhusoodanan and Zaveri 2010). However, paliperidone has not yet been studied in patients with dementia, and doses remain speculative for this population.

Olanzapine

Next to risperidone, olanzapine has the most published geriatric data. Its efficacy and tolerability in the treatment of behavioral and psychological symptoms of dementia have been reported in several randomized placebo-controlled trials (e.g., Clark et al. 2001; De Deyn et al. 2004; Schneider et al. 2006b; Street et al. 2000) and in randomized comparisons with haloperidol (Verhey et al. 2006), promazine and risperidone (Gareri et al. 2004), and risperidone (Fontaine et al. 2003; Mulsant et al. 2004). However, a meta-analysis of published and nonpublished placebo-controlled trials of olanzapine in the treatment of behavioral and psychological symptoms of dementia concluded that "olanzapine was not associated with efficacy overall" (Schneider et al. 2006a, p. 205). Also, the study by Street et al. (2000) found an inverted dose-response relationship (i.e., patients receiving 15 mg/day had worse outcomes than did patients receiving 5 mg/day), suggesting that higher doses may be toxic in these patients (see discussion later in this subsection).

The efficacy and tolerability of olanzapine in the treatment of late-life schizophrenia have been confirmed in two randomized comparisons with haloperidol (Barak et al. 2002; Kennedy et al. 2003) and two randomized comparisons with risperidone (Harvey et al. 2003; Jeste et al. 2003; Ritchie et al. 2003, 2006). In one randomized controlled trial in patients with delirium, olanzapine and haloperidol were found to have comparable efficacy (Skrobik et al. 2004). However, caution is needed when using olanzapine in patients with delirium because some controlled trials have reported some cognitive worsening in patients with dementia taking olanzapine (Kennedy et al. 2005; Mulsant et al. 2004), and several case reports of delirium induced by olanzapine have been published. Similarly, the need for caution when olanzapine is used to treat psychosis in patients with Parkinson's disease or Lewy body dementia is reinforced by two comparative trials (Breier et al. 2002; Goetz et al. 2000) and several open trials or case series (e.g., Marsh et al. 2001; Molho and Factor 1999; Parkinson Study Group 1999; Walker et al. 1999) that have reported a significant worsening of motor symptoms in these patients.

The evidence supporting the efficacy and safety of olanzapine in younger patients with bipolar disorder and other mood disorders (Andreescu et al. 2006; Shelton et al. 2001; Thase 2002) is strong. However, there is a paucity of data relevant to older patients with mood disorders (Meyers et al. 2009; Sajatovic et al. 2005a, 2005b; Young et al. 2004). Similarly, very few geriatric data are available on the rapidly dissolving or the intramuscular preparations of olanzapine (Belgamwar and Fenton 2005).

On review of all evidence available in 2004, a consensus conference concluded that among the atypical antipsychotics, clozapine and olanzapine were associated with the highest risk for diabetes and caused the greatest weight gain and dyslipidemia (American Diabetes Association et al. 2004). Limited geriatric data show a similar higher risk of metabolic problems in older patients (Feldman et al. 2004; Micca et al. 2006; Zheng et al. 2009). Other common side effects include sedation and gait disturbance. Extrapyramidal symptoms appear to be dose dependent and are rare at the lower dosages typically used in older patients (5–10 mg/day). Olanzapine also has been associated with electroencephalographic abnormalities (Centorrino et al. 2002), and its strong blocking of the muscarinic receptor (Chew et al. 2005, 2006; Mulsant et al. 2003) (Table 2–6) may explain why it has been associated with the following: constipation, in a large series of long-term-care patients (Martin et al. 2003); decreased efficacy at higher dosages, in a randomized trial in older agitated or psychotic patients with dementia (Street et al. 2000); a differential cognitive effect from risperidone, in randomized trials involving older patients with schizophrenia (Harvey et al. 2003) or dementia (Mulsant et al. 2004); worsening of cognition, in a large placebo-controlled trial in older nonagitated, nonpsychotic patients with Alzheimer's disease (Kennedy et al. 2005); and frank delirium, in some clinical cases. Patients who are older, female, or nonsmokers or who are taking a drug that inhibits CYP1A2 (e.g., fluvoxamine or ciprofloxacin) have higher concentrations of olanzapine and may be at higher risk for adverse effects (Gex-Fabry et al. 2003). Because of its adverse-effect profile, experts do not recommend olanzapine as a first-line antipsychotic in older patients at special risk for anticholinergic or metabolic adverse effects (Bell et al. 2010).

Quetiapine

Results of randomized placebo-controlled trials of quetiapine in older patients with behavioral and psychological symptoms of dementia—both published and unpublished—are inconclusive (Schneider et al. 2006a). For instance, in a large trial of 333 institutionalized participants, quetiapine 200 mg/day (but not 100 mg/day) differed from placebo on global impressions and positive symptom ratings but not on the important primary outcome measures of agitation and psychosis (Zhong et al. 2007). However, several published but uncontrolled or unblinded studies in older patients with primary psychotic disorders (e.g., Madhusoodanan et al. 2000; Tariot et al. 2000; Yang et al. 2005), dementia, or delirium (e.g., Kim et al. 2003; Pae et al. 2004; Sasaki et al. 2003) suggested that quetiapine may be effective for these disorders. The good tolerability of quetiapine observed clinically in patients at high risk for extrapyramidal symptoms suggests that quetiapine should be the first-line antipsychotic for older patients with Parkinson's disease, dementia with Lewy

Table 2–6. Receptor blockade of atypical antipsychotics

	D_2	$5\text{-}HT_2$	M_1	α_1
Aripiprazole	*	++	0	+
Asenapine	+++	+++	0	+++
Clozapine	+	++	+++	+
Iloperidone	+++	++++	0	++++
Lurasidone	+++	++	0	++
Olanzapine	++	+++	++	+
Paliperidone	+++	+++	0	++
Quetiapine	+	++	+	+
Risperidone	+++	++++	0	+++
Ziprasidone	++	++	0	+

Note. Receptor types: α_1 = alpha-adrenergic type 1; D_2 = dopamine type 2; $5\text{-}HT_2$ = 5-hydroxytryptamine (serotonin) type 2; M_1 = muscarinic type 1. 0 = none; + = minimal; ++ = intermediate; +++ = high; ++++ = very high.
*High-affinity partial agonist.

bodies, or tardive dyskinesia (Fernandez et al. 2002; Poewe 2005). However, quetiapine was not found to be efficacious in these patients in two double-blind trials (Kurlan et al. 2007; Rabey et al. 2007).

Quetiapine is approved by the FDA for the treatment of acute mania and depression associated with bipolar disorder in adults. However, relevant published data in geriatric populations are limited (Carta et al. 2007; Tadger et al. 2011). There have been several case reports of inappropriate antidiuretic and serotonin syndromes in these patients (e.g., Atalay et al. 2007; Kohen et al. 2007). Like other antipsychotics, quetiapine also can cause somnolence or dizziness (Jaskiw et al. 2004; Yang et al. 2005), but the incidence of these adverse effects can be minimized by a slower dose titration. The risk for weight gain, diabetes, or dyslipidemia associated with quetiapine appears similar to the risk associated with the use of risperidone but lower than the risk associated with the use of clozapine or olanzapine (American Diabetes Association et al. 2004; Feldman et al. 2004).

Clozapine

Clozapine is still considered the drug of choice for younger patients with treatment-refractory schizophrenia, and one small case series suggested that it can be similarly helpful in older patients for the treatment of primary psychotic disorders refractory to other treatments (Sajatovic et al. 1997). A randomized controlled trial comparing clozapine and chlorpromazine in older patients with schizophrenia (Howanitz et al. 1999) and one large case series (Barak et al. 1999) also supported the use of clozapine in moderate dosages (i.e., approximately 50–200 mg/day) in older patients with primary psychotic disorders. The strongest published geriatric studies of clozapine are focused on the treatment of drug-induced psychosis in patients with Parkinson's disease (Ellis et al. 2000; Goetz et al. 2000; Parkinson Study Group 1999). The results of these studies suggest that clozapine at low dosages (12.5–50 mg/day) could be the preferred treatment for this condition (Parkinson Study Group 1999). However, the use of clozapine in older patients is severely limited because of its significant hematological, neurological, cognitive, metabolic, and cardiac adverse effects (Alvir et al. 1993; Centorrino et al. 2002; Chew et al. 2006; Koller et al. 2001; O'Connor et al. 2010; Rajji et al. 2010).

Aripiprazole

Aripiprazole has partial dopamine type 2 (D_2) receptor agonist properties (i.e., in high dopaminergic states, it acts as an antagonist, and in low dopaminergic states, it acts as an agonist). This may explain why it is unlikely to cause extrapyramidal side effects or prolactin elevation (associated with osteoporosis), even at high D_2 receptor occupancy (Mamo et al. 2007). It has only moderate affinity to the adrenergic α_1 receptor and histamine H_1 receptor and negligible affinity to the muscarinic receptor (Chew et al. 2006). As a result, orthostatic hypotension and antihistaminergic and anticholinergic adverse effects are less likely to occur than with other atypical agents. However, akathisia may be a common side effect in older patients (Coley et al. 2009; Sheffrin et al. 2009). Three randomized placebo-controlled trials of aripiprazole in older patients with behavioral and psychological symptoms of dementia have been published (De Deyn et al. 2005a; Mintzer et al. 2007; Streim et al. 2008), and a meta-analysis of these trials concluded that "efficacy on rating scales was observed by meta-analysis for aripiprazole" (Schneider et al. 2006a, p. 191).

Aripiprazole is approved by the FDA for the treatment of manic or mixed episodes associated with bipolar disorder and as an adjunctive treatment for major depressive disorder. Although no relevant controlled trials have been done in older patients, some prospective open studies (Sajatovic et al. 2008; Sheffrin et al. 2009) and analyses of pooled geriatric data (Steffens et al. 2011; Suppes et al. 2008) have been published.

Ziprasidone

On the basis of ziprasidone's lower effect on glucose, lipids, and weight (American Diabetes Association et al. 2004) and its lack of affinity for the muscarinic receptor (see Table 2–6) (Chew et al. 2006) and thus its low potential to cause cognitive impairment, ziprasidone is an attractive medication for older patients with psychosis. However, geriatric data on oral ziprasidone remain very limited (Berkowitz 2003; Wilner et al. 2000). Three published studies on the use of intramuscular ziprasidone found no adverse cardiovascular or electrocardiographic changes in a small number of older patients (Greco et al. 2005; Kohen et al. 2005; Rais et al. 2010). However, in the absence of systematic study, concern about the potential effects of ziprasidone on cardiac conduction persists, and ziprasidone should not be used in older patients with QTc prolongation or congestive heart failure.

Newer Atypical Antipsychotics

Three other atypical antipsychotics were approved by the FDA in 2009 and 2010 for use in schizophrenia: asenapine, iloperidone, and lurasidone. However, as of June 2013, the paucity of geriatric data for these medications precludes making recommendations for their use in older patients.

Mood Stabilizers

As a class, mood stabilizers are high-risk medications for older patients. There is a paucity of controlled studies as well as an abundance of concerns regarding the drugs' potential toxicity, problematic side effects, and drug interactions. Beyond their approved indications, anticonvulsants are also used in the management of agitation accompanying dementia. Currently, no consensus exists as to which drug should be preferred as a first-line mood stabilizer in older patients with bipolar disorder or secondary mania (Sajatovic et al. 2005b; Shulman 2010; Young et al. 2004).

Lithium

Lithium continues to be used in older patients for the treatment of bipolar disorder (Shulman 2010) or, less commonly, as an augmentation agent in treatment-resistant depression (Cooper et al. 2011; Flint and Rifat 2001; Ross 2008) and for the prevention of depressive relapse following electroconvulsive therapy (Sackeim et al. 2001). Data from open and controlled trials suggest that lithium is efficacious in the acute treatment and prophylaxis of mania in older patients (Sajatovic et al. 2005a; Shulman 2010). However, age-related reductions in renal clearance and decreased total body water significantly affect the pharmacokinetics of lithium in older patients, increasing the risk of toxicity. Medical comorbidities common in late life—such as impaired renal function, hyponatremia, dehydration, and heart failure—exacerbate further the risk of toxicity (Sajatovic et al. 2006). Thiazide diuretics, angiotensin-converting enzyme inhibitors, and NSAIDs may precipitate toxicity by further diminishing the renal clearance of lithium. Lithium toxicity can produce persistent central nervous system impairment or be fatal: it is a medical emergency that requires careful correction of fluid and electrolyte imbalances and that may require administration of mannitol (or even hemodialysis) to increase lithium excretion.

Older patients require lower lithium dosages than do younger patients to produce similar serum lithium levels, and their lithium levels, electrolytes, and thyrotropin concentration should be monitored regularly. Also, older persons are more sensitive to neurological side effects at lower lithium levels. This sensitivity may be a consequence of increased permeability of the blood-brain barrier and subtle changes in sodium-lithium countertransport, resulting in a higher brain-to-serum concentration ratio than in younger patients (Forester et al. 2009). Neurotoxicity may manifest as coarse tremor, slurred speech, ataxia, hyperreflexia, and muscle fasciculations. In vitro, lithium has moderate anticholinergic activity (Chew et al. 2008). This may explain why cognitive impairment has been observed with levels well below 1 mEq/L, and frank delirium has been reported with levels as low as 1.5 mEq/L (Sproule et al. 2000). Consequently, treatment in older patients may require lithium levels to be kept as low as 0.4–0.8 mEq/L. Despite its potential toxicity, lithium remains an important drug in the treatment of bipolar disorder and treatment-resistant depression in late life because of its potential effect on suicidality and neuroprotective properties (Müller-Oerlinghausen and Lewitzka 2010; Shulman 2010).

Anticonvulsants

Anticonvulsants are used as alternatives to lithium in the treatment of bipolar disorder and as alternatives to antipsychotics for the management of agitation associated with dementia. There may be a subgroup of patients with bipolar disorder with dysphoria or rapid cycling who respond poorly to lithium but do well with anticonvulsants (Post et al. 1998).

Divalproex

Divalproex, a compound of sodium valproate and valproic acid in an enteric-coated form, is a broad-spectrum anticonvulsant approved by the FDA for the treatment of acute manic or mixed episodes associated with bipolar disorder, with or without psychotic features. It also may be efficacious in the treatment of bipolar depression (Bond et al. 2010). Small case series have suggested that divalproex is relatively well tolerated by older patients with bipolar disorder (Kando et al. 1996; Noaghiul et al. 1998) and those with agitation in the context of dementia. Nonetheless, in four negative placebo-controlled trials, valproate was not more effective than placebo in treating agitation of dementia (Sink et al. 2005; Tariot et al. 2005). Sedation, nausea, weight gain, and hand tremors are common dose-related side effects. Reversible thrombocytopenia can occur in as many as half of elderly patients taking divalproex and may ensue at lower total drug levels than in younger patients (Fenn et al. 2006). Other dose-related adverse effects include reversible elevations in liver enzymes and transient elevations in blood ammonia levels. However, liver failure and pancreatitis are rare. Divalproex has other metabolic effects of concern to aging patients, such as increases in bone turnover and reductions of serum folate, with concomitant elevations in plasma homocysteine concentrations (Sato et al. 2001; Schwaninger et al. 1999).

The pharmacokinetics of valproate vary according to formulation, and valproic acid, divalproex sodium, and its XR preparation are not interchangeable. Valproate is metabolized principally by mitochondrial β-oxidation and secondarily by the CYP system; typical half-lives are in the range of 5–16 hours and are not affected by aging alone. Concomitant administration of valproate will increase concentrations of carbamazepine, diazepam, lamotrigine, phenobarbital, and primidone. Conversely, concurrent administration of carbamazepine, lamotrigine, phenytoin, and topiramate may decrease levels of valproate. Fluoxetine and erythromycin may potentiate the effects of valproate. Changes in protein binding as a result of drug interactions are no longer considered clinically important beyond causing the misinterpretation of total (i.e., free and bound) drug levels (Benet and Hoener 2002). Because valproate binding to plasma proteins is generally reduced in the elderly, free drug levels correlate better with adverse effects (Fenn et al. 2006).

Lamotrigine

Lamotrigine is approved by the FDA for the maintenance treatment of bipolar I disorder to prevent mood episodes (depressive, manic, or mixed episodes), and it is considered a first-line agent for the treatment of bipolar depression (Fenn et al. 2006). Pooled geriatric data from two randomized placebo-controlled trials support the efficacy of lamotrigine in preventing bipolar depression in older patients (Sajatovic et al. 2005a, 2007). Open studies and case reports suggest a possible role for lamotrigine in the treatment of bipolar depression, bipolar mania, and agitation associated with dementia (Sajatovic et al. 2007). In contrast with many other mood stabilizers and antidepressants, lamotrigine does not seem to be associated with weight gain or to cause significant drug interactions. Typically, it is well tolerated, but somnolence and rashes have been observed in older patients. Rashes are the most common reason for discontinuation, but their incidence is far less frequent with lamotrigine than with carbamazepine (Fenn et al. 2006). Severe rashes, including Stevens-Johnson syndrome and toxic epidermal necrolysis, have been observed in about 0.3% of adult patients (Messenheimer 1998). At the first sign of rash or other evidence of hypersensitivity (e.g., fever, lymphadenopathy), lamotrigine should be discontinued, and the patient should be evaluated. The incidence of rashes can be reduced by using a low initial dose and a slow titration. Because valproate increases lamotrigine concentrations, the initial and target doses need to be halved in patients who are receiving divalproex and the titration of lamotrigine needs to be slowed down. Conversely, carbamazepine approximately halves lamotrigine concentrations, and the initial lamotrigine dose needs to be doubled in patients who are receiving carbamazepine.

Carbamazepine and Oxcarbazepine

The XR formulation of carbamazepine is approved by the FDA for the acute treatment of manic and mixed episodes associated with bipolar disorder. In a placebo-controlled trial in 51 nursing home patients, carbamazepine also was shown to be efficacious in treating agitation and aggression associated with dementia (Tariot et al. 1998). Common side effects in older patients include sedation, nausea, dizziness, rash, ataxia, neutropenia, and hyponatremia. Older patients are also at risk for agranulocytosis, aplastic anemia, hepatitis, and problematic drug interactions (Fenn et al. 2006). Carbamazepine is primarily eliminated by CYP3A4, and its clearance is reduced with aging. Its interactions with other drugs are protean: carbamazepine concentrations are increased to potential toxicity by CYP3A4 inhibitors such as macrolide antibiotics, antifungals, and some antidepressants (see list of antidepressants that inhibit CYP3A4 in Table 2–4). CYP3A4 inducers—such as phenobarbital, phenytoin, and carbamazepine itself—lower the concentration of carbamazepine and the concentrations of many drugs metabolized by this isoenzyme, including lamotrigine, valproate, some antidepressants, and antipsychotics

(Fenn et al. 2006). Oxcarbazepine, the 10-keto analogue of carbamazepine, is a less potent CYP3A4 inducer and is less likely to be involved in drug interactions. Although oxcarbazepine has been studied in a small number of younger patients with bipolar disorder, there is a paucity of data pertaining to older psychiatric patients (Sommer et al. 2007). Thus, its use cannot be recommended in these patients.

Gabapentin and Pregabalin

Although gabapentin has been used in bipolar disorder, trials have not borne out its effectiveness, and only small case series or case reports of its use in dementia are available (Sommer et al. 2007). Nonetheless, it has a generally favorable side-effect profile and modest anxiolytic and analgesic effects, particularly for neuropathic pain. Gabapentin does not bind to plasma proteins and is not metabolized, being eliminated by renal excretion. In patients with renal impairment, neurological adverse effects such as ataxia, involuntary movements, disorganized thinking, excitation, and extreme sedation have been noted. Even in the absence of renal dysfunction, elderly patients may be prone to excessive sedation. Therefore, in the elderly, initial dosages of 100 mg twice daily are more prudent than the 900 mg/day recommended as a starting dosage for younger patients with epilepsy. Pregabalin is a structural congener of gabapentin. It has an improved pharmacokinetic profile and may be helpful for neuropathic pain in elderly patients. No data pertaining to its use are available in older psychiatric patients.

Topiramate

Early reports of the efficacy of topiramate in younger patients with bipolar disorder have not been confirmed by subsequent studies (Sommer et al. 2007). In younger patients, topiramate is one of the few psychotropic medications that has been associated with weight loss. However, it also has been associated with cognitive impairment that can be severe enough to interfere with functioning. Because of the paucity of data pertaining to use of topiramate in older psychiatric patients (Sommer et al. 2007), it cannot be recommended in these patients.

Anxiolytics and Sedative-Hypnotics

Social isolation, financial concerns, and declining intellectual and physical function may predispose elders to anxiety. New-onset anxiety is a frequent accompaniment of physical illness, depression, or medication side effects. The SSRIs and SNRIs have displaced benzodiazepines as first-line pharmacotherapy for anxiety in late life, whereas benzodiazepine receptor agonist hypnotics (i.e., eszopiclone, zaleplon, zolpidem) and the intermediate half-life benzodiazepine lorazepam have become the most commonly used hypnotics.

Benzodiazepines and Benzodiazepine Receptor Agonists

Detrimental effects of benzodiazepines in elderly patients frequently outweigh any short-term symptomatic relief that these medications may provide. Even single small doses of diazepam, nitrazepam, and temazepam cause significant impairment in memory and psychomotor performance in older subjects (Nikaido et al. 1990; Pomara et al. 1989). Even benzodiazepines with shorter half-lives increase the risk of falls and hip fractures in frail elderly patients (Ray et al. 2000). Benzodiazepine receptor agonists also have been associated with falls and hip fractures (Wang et al. 2001) or cognitive impairment and traffic accidents (Glass et al. 2005; Gustavsen et al. 2008; Leufkens et al. 2009).

Nevertheless, adjunctive treatment with a sedative-hypnotic may be indicated for a few weeks in the treatment of anxiety- or depression-related sleep disturbance when the primary pharmacotherapy is an antidepressant. Relative contraindications include heavy snoring (because it suggests sleep apnea), dementia (because such patients are at increased risk for daytime confusion, impairment in activities of daily living, and daytime sleepiness), and the use of other sedating medications or alcohol. Benzodiazepines with long half-lives (chlorazepate, chlordiazepoxide, clonazepam, diazepam, flurazepam, halazepam, and quazepam) should be avoided (Fick et al. 2003; Hemmelgarn et al. 1997). Also, several drugs with shorter half-lives (i.e., alprazolam, triazolam, midazolam, eszopiclone, zaleplon, and zolpidem) undergo phase I hepatic metabolism by CYP3A4 that is subject to specific interactions and age-associated decline (Freudenreich and Menza 2000; Greenblatt et al. 1991). Sedatives with very short half-lives also may increase the likelihood that confused elderly patients will awake in the middle of the night to stagger off to the bathroom. Lorazepam and oxazepam do not undergo phase I hepatic metabolism, have no active metabolites, have acceptable half-lives that do not increase with age, and are not subject to drug interactions. Lorazepam is available in appropriately small doses (0.5-mg pills) and is well absorbed intramuscularly. It is preferred for inducing sleep because oxazepam has a relatively slow and erratic absorption.

Buspirone

The anxiolytic buspirone, a partial 5-HT_{1A} agonist, is rarely used. Nevertheless, it may be beneficial for some patients with generalized anxiety disorder or as an augmentation agent in treatment-resistant depression (Trivedi et al. 2006). It appears to be well tolerated by elderly patients, without the sedation or addiction liability of the benzodiazepines (Steinberg 1994). Thus, it may be helpful for some older patients who are prone to falls, confusion, or chronic lung disease. Nonetheless, buspirone may take several weeks to exert an anxiolytic effect, has no cross-tolerance with benzodiazepines, and may cause dizziness, headache, or nervousness (Strand et al. 1990). It is of limited use for panic or obsessive-compulsive disorders. The pharmacokinetics of buspirone are not affected by age or gender, but coadministration with verapamil, diltiazem, erythromycin, or itraconazole will substantially increase buspirone concentrations, and its combination with serotonergic medications may result in the serotonin syndrome (Mahmood and Sahajwalla 1999).

Cognitive Enhancers

Cholinesterase Inhibitors

In addition to memantine (discussed in the next subsection), four cholinesterase inhibitors have received FDA approval for the symptomatic improvement of Alzheimer's disease. Table 2–7 describes three of these drugs: donepezil, galantamine, and rivastigmine. The fourth, tacrine, is no longer recommended because of its potential hepatotoxic effects. The principal adverse effects of these medications are concentration dependent and result from their peripheral cholinergic actions. With these adverse effects in mind, clinicians should be aware of the drugs' specific pathways of elimination and potential pharmacokinetic drug interactions with CYP2D6 or CYP3A4 inhibitors and CYP3A4 inducers when prescribing donepezil and galantamine (Pilotto et al. 2009; Seritan 2008). Rivastigmine is affected by renal function, and FDA warnings have emphasized the need for careful dose titration (and retitration if restarting) to prevent severe vomiting (Birks et al. 2009). Drugs with potent anticholinergic effects directly antagonize cholinesterase inhibitors (Chew et al. 2008; Modi et al. 2009) and should be avoided in patients with dementia.

Cognitive enhancers produce modest improvements in cognition and function in patients with Alzheimer's disease (Hansen et al. 2008), including those with severe Alzheimer's disease (Winblad et al. 2006). A modest benefit of uncertain clinical significance is also observed in vascular dementia (Kavirajan and Schneider 2007). Cognitive enhancers may also have a role in the management of other dementias, such as Lewy body dementia (Gustavsson et al. 2009) or dementia with Parkinson's disease, mild cognitive impairment (Diniz et al. 2009; Doody et al. 2009), cognitive impairment associated with late-life depression (Reynolds et al. 2011), and behavioral and psychological symptoms of dementia (Gauthier et al. 2010; Rodda et al. 2009; Sink et al. 2005), but more research is needed.

A rapid symptomatic deterioration may occur when cholinesterase inhibitors are discontinued, and no evidence suggests that they alter the underlying neuropathology of Alzheimer's disease or its eventual progression. Before anticholinesterase therapy is initiated, it is imperative that unnecessary anticholinergic medications be discontinued (Lu and Tune 2003; Modi et al. 2009). In patients with diminished cognitive reserve, even small anticholinergic effects can substantially impair cognition (Mulsant et al. 2003; Nebes et al. 2005). Adverse effects, including nausea, diarrhea, weight loss, bradycardia, syncope, and nightmares, are associated with all of the cholinesterase inhibitors and may lead to discontinuation (see Table 2–7; Gill et al. 2009; Hernandez et al. 2009; Park-Wyllie et al. 2009); gastrointestinal adverse effects may be less frequent with donepezil (Mayeux 2010).

NMDA Receptor Antagonist

Memantine, an *N*-methyl-D-aspartate (NMDA) receptor antagonist, has FDA approval for the treatment of moderate to severe Alzheimer's disease. As an uncompetitive antagonist with moderate affinity for NMDA receptors, memantine may attenuate neurotoxicity without interfering with glutamate's normal

Table 2–7.   Cholinesterase inhibitors

	Clearance	Dosing	Significant adverse effects	Pharmacodynamics
Donepezil	Half-life = 70–80 hours; CYP3A4, CYP2D6	5–10 mg/day in one dose; start at 5 mg at bedtime	Mild nausea, diarrhea, bradycardia	Reversible acetylcholinesterase inhibition
Galantamine, galantamine ER	Half-life = 7 hours; CYP2D6, CYP3A4	8–24 mg/day divided into two doses; start at 4 mg twice daily	Moderate nausea, vomiting, diarrhea, anorexia, tremor, insomnia	Reversible acetylcholinesterase inhibition; nicotinic modulation may increase acetylcholine release
Rivastigmine, rivastigmine patch	Half-life = 1.25 hours; renal	6–12 mg/day divided into two doses; start at 1.5 mg twice daily. For patch, start at 4.6 mg/day and increase after 4 weeks to 9.5 mg/day. Retitrate if drug is stopped.	Severe nausea, vomiting, anorexia, weight loss, sweating, dizziness	Pseudoirreversible acetylcholinesterase inhibition; also butylcholinesterase inhibition

Note.   CYP = cytochrome P450; ER = extended-release.

physiological actions. In placebo-controlled clinical trials in patients with Alzheimer's disease, memantine was associated with modest delay in deterioration of cognition and activities of daily living either alone (Reisberg et al. 2003) or in combination with donepezil (Tariot et al. 2004). Memantine also may have a role in the treatment of Parkinson's disease dementia and Lewy body dementia (Aarsland et al. 2009). It is well tolerated, although it may cause confusion in some patients (Kavirajan 2009). It does not appear to be implicated in drug-drug interactions, but it is excreted by the kidneys, and its dosage needs to be reduced in patients with significant impairment in renal function. In a recent study of patients with moderate or severe Alzheimer's disease, memantine and donepezil were found to have similar efficacy with respect to cognitive outcomes and activities of daily living. Further, there were no significant benefits of the combination of donepezil and memantine over donepezil alone (Howard et al. 2012).

References

Aarsland D, Ballard C, Walker Z, et al: Memantine in patients with Parkinson's disease dementia or dementia with Lewy bodies: a double-blind, placebo-controlled, multicentre trial. Lancet Neurol 8:613–618, 2009

Aichhorn W, Weiss U, Marksteiner J, et al: Influence of age and gender on risperidone plasma concentrations. J Psychopharmacol 19:395–401, 2005

Aiken CB: Pramipexole in psychiatry: a systematic review of the literature. J Clin Psychiatry 68:1230–1236, 2007

Alexopoulos GS, Katz IR, Reynolds CF 3rd, et al: Pharmacotherapy of depression in older patients: a summary of the expert consensus guidelines. J Psychiatr Pract 7:361–376, 2001

Allard P, Gram L, Timdahl K, et al: Efficacy and tolerability of venlafaxine in geriatric outpatients with major depression: a double-blind, randomised 6-month comparative study. Int J Geriatr Psychiatry 19:1123–1130, 2004

Altamura AC, De Novellis F, Guercetti G, et al: Fluoxetine compared with amitriptyline in elderly depression: a controlled clinical trial. Int J Clin Pharmacol Res 9:391–396, 1989

Alvir JJ, Lieberman JA, Safferman AZ, et al: Clozapine-induced agranulocytosis: incidence and risk factors in the United States. N Engl J Med 329:162–167, 1993

American Diabetes Association, American Psychiatric Association, American Association of Clinical Endocrinologists, et al: Consensus development conference on antipsychotic drugs and obesity and diabetes. Diabetes Care 27:596–601, 2004

Andersen G, Vestergaard K, Lauritzen L: Effective treatment of poststroke depression with the selective serotonin reuptake inhibitor citalopram. Stroke 25:1099–1104, 1994

Andreescu C, Mulsant BH, Rothschild AJ, et al: Pharmacotherapy of major depression with psychotic features: what is the evidence? Psychiatr Ann 35:31–38, 2006

Aragona M, Inghilleri M: Increased ocular pressure in two patients with narrow angle glaucoma treated with venlafaxine. Clin Neuropharmacol 21:130–131, 1998

Arranz FJ, Ros S: Effects of comorbidity and polypharmacy on the clinical usefulness of sertraline in elderly depressed patients: an open multicentre study. J Affect Disord 46:285–291, 1997

Atalay A, Turhan N, Aki OE: A challenging case of syndrome of inappropriate secretion of antidiuretic hormone in an elderly patient secondary to quetiapine. South Med J 100:832–833, 2007

Bailer U, Fischer P, Kufferle B, et al: Occurrence of mirtazapine-induced delirium in organic brain disorder. Int Clin Psychopharmacol 15:239–243, 2000

Ballard C, Corbett A: Management of neuropsychiatric symptoms in people with dementia. CNS Drugs 24:729–739, 2010

Ballard C, Hanney ML, Theodoulou M, et al: The Dementia Antipsychotic Withdrawal Trial (DART-AD): long-term follow-up of a randomised placebo-controlled trial. Lancet Neurol 8:151–157, 2009

Banerjee S, Hellier J, Dewey M, et al: Sertraline or mirtazapine for depression in dementia (HTA-SADD): a randomised, multicentre, double-blind, placebo-controlled trial. Lancet 378:403–411, 2011

Barak Y, Wittenberg N, Naor S, et al: Clozapine in elderly psychiatric patients: tolerability, safety, and efficacy. Compr Psychiatry 40:320–325, 1999

Barak Y, Shamir E, Zemishlani H, et al: Olanzapine vs. haloperidol in the treatment of elderly chronic schizophrenia patients. Prog Neuropsychopharmacol Biol Psychiatry 26:1199–1202, 2002

Barbui C, Esposito E, Cipriani A: Selective serotonin reuptake inhibitors and risk of suicide: a systematic review of observational studies. CMAJ 180:291–297, 2009

Barone P, Scarzella L, Marconi R, et al: Pramipexole versus sertraline in the treatment of depression in Parkinson's disease: a national multicenter parallel-group randomized study. J Neurol 253:601–607, 2006

Barone P, Poewe W, Albrecht S, et al: Pramipexole for the treatment of depressive symptoms in patients with Parkinson's disease: a randomised, double-blind, placebo-controlled trial. Lancet Neurol 9:573–580, 2010

Beers MH: Explicit criteria for determining potentially inappropriate medication use by the elderly. Arch Intern Med 157:1531–1536, 1997

Belgamwar RB, Fenton M: Olanzapine IM or velotab for acutely disturbed/agitated people with suspected serious mental illnesses. Cochrane Database of Systematic Reviews 2005, Issue 2. Art. No.: CD003729. DOI: 10.1002/14651858.

Bell JS, Taipale HT, Soini H, et al: Sedative load among long-term care facility residents with and without dementia: a cross-sectional study. Clin Drug Invest 30:63–70, 2010

Benazzi F: Urinary retention with venlafaxine-haloperidol combination. Pharmacopsychiatry 30:27, 1997

Benazzi F: Serotonin syndrome with mirtazapine-fluoxetine combination. Int J Geriatr Psychiatry 13:495–496, 1998

Benet LZ, Hoener B: Changes in plasma protein binding have little clinical relevance. Clin Pharmacol Ther 71:115–121, 2002

Berkowitz A: Ziprasidone for dementia in elderly patients: case review. J Psychiatr Pract 9:469–473, 2003

Bigos KL, Bies RR, Pollock BG: Population pharmacokinetics in geriatric psychiatry. Am J Geriatr Psychiatry 14:993–1003, 2006

Birks J, Grimley Evans J, Iakovidou V, et al: Rivastigmine for Alzheimer's disease. Cochrane Database of Systematic Reviews 2009, Issue 2. Art. No.: CD001191. DOI: 10.1002/14651858. CD001191.pub2.

Bodkin JA, Lasser RA, Wines JD Jr, et al: Combining serotonin reuptake inhibitors and bupropion in partial responders to antidepressant monotherapy. J Clin Psychiatry 58:137–145, 1997

Bond DJ, Lam RW, Yatham LN: Divalproex sodium versus placebo in the treatment of acute bipolar depression: a systematic review and meta-analysis. J Affect Disord 124:228–234, 2010

Bondareff W, Alpert M, Friedhoff AJ, et al: Comparison of sertraline and nortriptyline in the treatment of major depressive disorder in late life. Am J Psychiatry 157:729–736, 2000

Bose A, Li D, Ghandi C: Escitalopram in the acute treatment of depressed patients aged 60 years and older. Am J Geriatr Psychiatry 16:14–20, 2008

Branconnier RJ, Cole JO, Ghazvinian S, et al: Clinical pharmacology of bupropion and imipramine in elderly depressives. J Clin Psychiatry 44:130–133, 1983

Breier A, Sutton VK, Feldman PD, et al: Olanzapine in the treatment of dopamimetic-induced psychosis in patients with Parkinson's disease. Biol Psychiatry 52:438–445, 2002

Brodaty H, Ames D, Snowdon J, et al: A randomized placebo-controlled trial of risperidone for the treatment of aggression, agitation, and psychosis of dementia. J Clin Psychiatry 64:134–143, 2003

Burrows AB, Salzman C, Satlin A, et al: A randomized, placebo-controlled trial of paroxetine in nursing home residents with non-major depression. Depress Anxiety 15:102–110, 2002

Carta MG, Zairo F, Mellino G, et al: Add-on quetiapine in the treatment of major depressive disorder in elderly patients with cerebrovascular damage. Clin Pract Epidemiol Ment Health 3:28, 2007

Carvajal García-Pando A, García del Pozo J, Sánchez AS, et al: Hepatotoxicity associated with the new antidepressants. J Clin Psychiatry 63:135–137, 2002

Centorrino F, Price BH, Tuttle M, et al: EEG abnormalities during treatment with typical and atypical antipsychotics. Am J Psychiatry 159:109–115, 2002

Chalon SA, Granier LA, Vandenhende FR, et al: Duloxetine increases serotonin and norepinephrine availability in healthy subjects: a double-blind, controlled study. Neuropsychopharmacology 28:1685–1693, 2003

Chan WC, Lam LC, Choy CN, et al: A double-blind randomised comparison of risperidone and haloperidol in the treatment of behavioural and psychological symptoms in Chinese dementia patients. Int J Geriatr Psychiatry 16:1156–1162, 2001

Cheah CY, Ladhams B, Fegan PG: Mirtazapine associated with profound hyponatremia: two case reports. Am J Geriatr Pharmacother 6:91–95, 2008

Chen P, Kales HC, Weintraub D, et al: Antidepressant treatment of veterans with Parkinson's disease and depression: analysis of a national sample. J Geriatr Psychiatry Neurol 20:161–165, 2007

Chen Y, Patel NC, Guo JJ, et al: Antidepressant prophylaxis for poststroke depression: a meta-analysis. Int Clin Psychopharmacol 22:159–166, 2007

Chew ML, Mulsant BH, Rosen J, et al: Serum anticholinergic activity and cognition in patients with moderate to severe dementia. Am J Geriatr Psychiatry 13:535–538, 2005

Chew ML, Mulsant BH, Pollock BG, et al: A model of anticholinergic activity of atypical antipsychotic medications. Schizophr Res 88:63–72, 2006

Chew ML, Mulsant BH, Pollock BG, et al: Anticholinergic activity of 107 medications commonly used by older adults. J Am Geriatr Soc 56:1333–1341, 2008

Cipriani A, Furukawa TA, Salanti G, et al: Comparative efficacy and acceptability of 12 new-generation antidepressants: a multiple-treatments meta-analysis. Lancet 373:746–758, 2009

Clark WS, Street JS, Feldman PD, et al: The effects of olanzapine in reducing the emergence of psychosis among nursing home patients with Alzheimer's disease. J Clin Psychiatry 62:34–40, 2001

Clayton AH, Kornstein SG, Rosas G, et al: An integrated analysis of the safety and tolerability of desvenlafaxine compared with placebo in the treatment of major depressive disorder. CNS Spectr 14:183–195, 2009

Cohn CK, Shrivastava R, Mendels J, et al: Double-blind, multicenter comparison of sertraline and amitriptyline in elderly depressed patients. J Clin Psychiatry 51(suppl):28–33, 1990

Coley KC, Scipio TM, Ruby C, et al: Aripiprazole prescribing patterns and side effects in elderly psychiatric inpatients. J Psychiatr Pract 15:150–153, 2009

Cooper C, Katona C, Lyketsos K, et al: A systematic review of treatments for refractory depression in older people. Am J Geriatr Psychiatry 168:681–688, 2011

Culang ME, Sneed JR, Keilp JG, et al: Change in cognitive functioning following acute antidepressant treatment in late-life depression. Am J Geriatr Psychiatry 17:881–888, 2009

Culo S, Mulsant BH, Rosen J, et al: Treating neuropsychiatric symptoms in dementia with Lewy bodies: a randomized controlled trial. Alzheimer Dis Assoc Disord 24:360–364, 2010

Dahmen N, Marx J, Hopf HC, et al: Therapy of early poststroke depression with venlafaxine: safety, tolerability, and efficacy as determined in an open, uncontrolled clinical trial. Stroke 30:691–692, 1999

Dalton SO, Sorensen HT, Johansen C: SSRIs and upper gastrointestinal bleeding: what is known and how should it influence prescribing? CNS Drugs 20:143–151, 2006

Davidson J, Watkins L, Owens M, et al: Effects of paroxetine and venlafaxine XR on heart rate variability in depression. J Clin Psychopharmacol 25:480–484, 2005

Davidson M, Harvey PD, Vervarcke J, et al: A long-term, multicenter, open-label study of risperidone in elderly patients with psychosis. On behalf of the Risperidone Working Group. Int J Geriatr Psychiatry 15:506–514, 2000

Davidson M, Emsley R, Kramer M, et al: Efficacy, safety and early response of paliperidone extended-release tablets (paliperidone ER): results of a 6-week, randomized, placebo-controlled study. Schizophr Res 93:117–130, 2007

de Abajo FJ, Garcia-Rodriguez LA: Risk of upper gastrointestinal tract bleeding associated with selective serotonin reuptake inhibitors and venlafaxine therapy: interaction with nonsteroidal anti-inflammatory drugs and effect of acid-suppressing agents. Arch Gen Psychiatry 65:795–803, 2008

De Deyn PP, Rabheru K, Rasmussen A, et al: A randomized trial of risperidone, placebo, and haloperidol for behavioral symptoms of dementia. Neurology 53:946–955, 1999

De Deyn PP, Carrasco MM, Deberdt W, et al: Olanzapine versus placebo in the treatment of psychosis with or without associated behavioral disturbances in patients with Alzheimer's disease. Int J Geriatr Psychiatry 19:115–126, 2004

De Deyn PP, Jeste DV, Swanik R, et al: Aripiprazole for the treatment of psychosis in patients with Alzheimer's disease: a randomized placebo-controlled study. J Clin Psychopharmacol 25:463–467, 2005a

De Deyn PP, Katz IR, Brodaty H, et al: Management of agitation, aggression, and psychosis associated with dementia: a pooled analysis including three randomized, placebo-controlled double-blind trials in nursing home residents treated with risperidone. Clin Neurol Neurosurg 107:497–508, 2005b

Devanand DP, Pelton GH, Marston K, et al: Sertraline treatment of elderly patients with depression and cognitive impairment. Int J Geriatr Psychiatry 18:123–130, 2003

Devanand DP, Juszczak N, Nobler MS, et al: An open treatment trial of venlafaxine for elderly patients with dysthymic disorder. J Geriatr Psychiatry Neurol 17:219–224, 2004

Devanand DP, Nobler MS, Cheng J, et al: Randomized, double-blind, placebo-controlled trial of fluoxetine treatment for elderly patients with dysthymic disorder. Am J Geriatr Psychiatry 13:59–68, 2005

Devos D, Dujardin K, Poirot I, et al: Comparison of desipramine and citalopram treatments for depression in Parkinson's disease: a double-blind, randomized, placebo-controlled study. Mov Disord 23:850–857, 2008

Diem SJ, Blackwell TL, Stone KL, et al: Use of antidepressants and rates of hip bone loss in older women: the Study of Osteoporotic Fractures. Arch Intern Med 167:1240–1245, 2007

Diniz BS, Pinto JA Jr, Gonzaga ML, et al: To treat or not to treat? A meta-analysis of the use of cholinesterase inhibitors in mild cognitive impairment for delaying progression to Alzheimer's disease. Eur Arch Psychiatry Clin Neurosci 259:248–256, 2009

Dolder C, Nelson M, Stump A: Pharmacological and clinical profile of newer antidepressants: implications for the treatment of elderly patients. Drugs Aging 27:625–640, 2010

Doody RS, Ferris SH, Salloway S, et al: Donepezil treatment of patients with MCI: a 48-week randomized, placebo-controlled trial. Neurology 72:1555–1561, 2009

Doraiswamy PM, Khan ZM, Donahue RM, et al: Quality of life in geriatric depression: a comparison of remitters, partial responders, and nonresponders. Am J Geriatr Psychiatry 9:423–428, 2001

Doraiswamy PM, Krishnan KR, Oxman T, et al: Does antidepressant therapy improve cognition in elderly depressed patients? J Gerontol A Biol Sci Med Sci 58:M1137–M1144, 2003

Dunlop BW, Crits-Christoph P, Evans DL, et al: Coadministration of modafinil and a selective serotonin reuptake inhibitor from the initiation of treatment of major depressive disorder with fatigue and sleepiness: a double-blind, placebo-controlled study. J Clin Psychopharmacol 27:614–619, 2007

Dunner DL, Cohn JB, Walshe TD, et al: Two combined, multicenter double-blind studies of paroxetine and doxepin in geriatric patients with major depression. J Clin Psychiatry 53(suppl):57–60, 1992

Dunner DL, Zisook S, Billow AA, et al: A prospective safety surveillance study for bupropion sustained-release in the treatment of depression. J Clin Psychiatry 59:366–373, 1998

Ellis T, Cudkowicz ME, Sexton PM, et al: Clozapine and risperidone treatment of psychosis in Parkinson's disease. J Neuropsychiatry Clin Neurosci 12:364–369, 2000

Evans M, Hammond M, Wilson K, et al: Treatment of depression in the elderly: effect of physical illness on response. Int J Geriatr Psychiatry 12:1189–1194, 1997

Fabian TJ, Amico JA, Kroboth PD, et al: Paroxetine-induced hyponatremia in older adults: a 12-week prospective study. Arch Intern Med 164:327–332, 2004

Fava M, Thase ME, DeBattista C, et al: Modafinil augmentation of selective serotonin reuptake inhibitor therapy in MDD partial responders with persistent fatigue and sleepiness. Ann Clin Psychiatry 19:153–159, 2007

Feighner JP, Cohn JB: Double-blind comparative trials of fluoxetine and doxepin in geriatric patients with major depressive disorder. J Clin Psychiatry 46:20–25, 1985

Feldman PD, Hay LK, Deberdt W, et al: Retrospective cohort study of diabetes mellitus and antipsychotic treatment in a geriatric population in the United States. J Am Med Dir Assoc 5:38–46, 2004

Fenn HH, Sommer BR, Ketter TA, et al: Safety and tolerability of mood-stabilising anticonvulsants in the elderly. Expert Opin Drug Saf 5:401–416, 2006

Fernandez HH, Trieschmann ME, Burke MA, et al: Quetiapine for psychosis in Parkinson's disease versus dementia with Lewy bodies. J Clin Psychiatry 63:513–515, 2002

Fick DM, Cooper JW, Wade WE, et al: Updating the Beers criteria for potentially inappropriate medication use in older adults: results of a US consensus panel of experts. Arch Intern Med 163:2716–2724, 2003

Finkel SI, Richter EM, Clary CM, et al: Comparative efficacy of sertraline vs. fluoxetine in patients age 70 or over with major depression. Am J Geriatr Psychiatry 7:221–227, 1999

Flint AJ: Generalised anxiety disorder in elderly patients: epidemiology, diagnosis and treatment options. Drugs Aging 22:101–114, 2005

Flint AJ, Rifat SL: Nonresponse to first-line pharmacotherapy may predict relapse and recurrence of remitted geriatric depression. Depress Anxiety 13:125–131, 2001

Fontaine CS, Hynan LS, Koch K, et al: A double-blind comparison of olanzapine versus risperidone in the acute treatment of dementia-related behavioral disturbances in extended care facilities. J Clin Psychiatry 64:726–730, 2003

Forester BP, Streeter CC, Berlow YA, et al: Brain lithium levels and effects on cognition and mood in geriatric bipolar disorder: a lithium-7 magnetic resonance spectroscopy study. Am J Geriatr Psychiatry 17:13–23, 2009

Forlenza OV, Almeida OP, Stoppe A Jr, et al: Antidepressant efficacy and safety of low-dose sertraline and standard-dose imipramine for the treatment of depression in older adults: results from a double-blind, randomized, controlled clinical trial. Int Psychogeriatr 13:75–84, 2001

Freudenreich O, Menza M: Zolpidem-related delirium: a case report. J Clin Psychiatry 61:449–450, 2000

Friedman RA, Leon AC: Expanding the black box: depression, antidepressants, and the risk of suicide. N Engl J Med 356:2343–2346, 2007

Furlan PM, Kallan MJ, Ten Have T, et al: Cognitive and psychomotor effects of paroxetine and sertraline on healthy elderly volunteers. Am J Geriatr Psychiatry 9:429–438, 2001

Gareri P, Cotroneo A, Lacava R, et al: Comparison of the efficacy of new and conventional antipsychotic drugs in the treatment of behavioral and psychological symptoms of dementia (BPSD). Arch Gerontol Geriatr Suppl 9:207–215, 2004

Gasto C, Navarro V, Marcos T, et al: Single-blind comparison of venlafaxine and nortriptyline in elderly major depression. J Clin Psychopharmacol 23:21–26, 2003

Gauthier S, Cummings J, Ballard C, et al: Management of behavioral problems in Alzheimer's disease. Int Psychogeriatr 22:346–372, 2010

Gelenberg AJ, Laukes C, McGahuey C, et al: Mirtazapine substitution in SSRI-induced sexual dysfunction. J Clin Psychiatry 61:356–360, 2000

Georgotas A, McCue RE, Hapworth W, et al: Comparative efficacy and safety of MAOIs versus TCAs in treating depression in the elderly. Biol Psychiatry 21:1155–1166, 1986

Geretsegger C, Stuppaeck CH, Mair M, et al: Multicenter double blind study of paroxetine and amitriptyline in elderly depressed inpatients. Psychopharmacology (Berl) 119:277–281, 1995

Gex-Fabry M, Balant-Gorgia AE, Balant LP: Therapeutic drug monitoring of olanzapine: the combined effect of age, gender, smoking, and comedication. Ther Drug Monit 25:46–53, 2003

Gill SS, Rochon PA, Herrmann N, et al: Atypical antipsychotic drugs and risk of ischaemic stroke: population based retrospective cohort study. BMJ 330:445, 2005

Gill SS, Anderson GM, Fischer HD, et al: Syncope and its consequences in patients with dementia receiving cholinesterase inhibitors: a population-based cohort study. Arch Int Med 169:867–873, 2009

Glass J, Lanctôt KL, Herrmann N, et al: Sedative hypnotics in older people with insomnia: meta-analysis of risks and benefits. BMJ 331:1169, 2005

Glassman AH, O'Connor CM, Califf RM, et al: Sertraline treatment of major depression in patients with acute MI or unstable angina [published erratum appears in JAMA 288:1720, 2002]. JAMA 288:701–709, 2002

Goetz CG, Blasucci LM, Leurgans S, et al: Olanzapine and clozapine: comparative effects on motor function in hallucinating PD patients. Neurology 55:789–794, 2000

Goodnick PJ, Hernandez M: Treatment of depression in comorbid medical illness. Expert Opin Pharmacother 1:1367–1384, 2000

Gorwood P, Weiller E, Lemming O, et al: Escitalopram prevents relapse in older patients with major depressive disorder. Am J Geriatr Psychiatry 15:581–593, 2007

Greco KE, Tune LE, Brown FW, et al: A retrospective study of the safety of intramuscular ziprasidone in agitated elderly patients. J Clin Psychiatry 66:928–929, 2005

Greenblatt DJ, Harmatz JS, Shapiro L, et al: Sensitivity to triazolam in the elderly. N Engl J Med 324:1691–1698, 1991

Grothe DR, Scheckner B, Albano D: Treatment of pain syndromes with venlafaxine. Pharmacotherapy 24:621–629, 2004

Guillibert E, Pelicier Y, Archambault JC, et al: A double-blind, multicentre study of paroxetine versus clomipramine in depressed elderly patients. Acta Psychiatr Scand Suppl 350:132–134, 1989

Gustavsen I, Bramness JG, Skurtveit S, et al: Road traffic accident risk related to prescriptions of the hypnotics zopiclone, zolpidem, flunitrazepam and nitrazepam. Sleep Med 9:818–822, 2008

Gustavsson A, Van Der Putt R, Jonsson L, et al: Economic evaluation of cholinesterase inhibitor therapy for dementia: comparison of Alzheimer's disease and dementia with Lewy bodies. Int J Geriatr Psychiatry 24:1072–1078, 2009

Han CS, Kim YK: A double-blind trial of risperidone and haloperidol for the treatment of delirium. Psychosomatics 45:297–301, 2004

Hansen RA, Gartlehner G, Lohr KN, et al: Efficacy and safety of second-generation antidepressants in the treatment of major depressive disorder. Ann Intern Med 143:415–426, 2005

Hansen RA, Gartlehner G, Webb AP, et al: Efficacy and safety of donepezil, galantamine, and rivastigmine for the treatment of Alzheimer's disease: a systematic review and meta-analysis. Clin Interv Aging 3:211–225, 2008

Harvey AT, Rudolph RL, Preskorn SH: Evidence of the dual mechanisms of action of venlafaxine. Arch Gen Psychiatry 57:503–509, 2000

Harvey PD, Napolitano JA, Mao L, et al: Comparative effects of risperidone and olanzapine on cognition in elderly patients with schizophrenia or schizoaffective disorder. Int J Geriatr Psychiatry 18:820–829, 2003

Hemmelgarn B, Suissa S, Huang A, et al: Benzodiazepine use and the risk of motor vehicle crash in the elderly. JAMA 278:27–31, 1997

Hernandez RK, Farwell W, Cantor MD, et al: Cholinesterase inhibitors and incidence of bradycardia in patients with dementia in the Veterans Affairs New England Healthcare System. J Am Geriatr Soc 57:1997–2003, 2009

Herrmann N, Mamdani M, Lanctôt KL: Atypical antipsychotics and risk of cerebrovascular accidents. Am J Psychiatry 161:1113–1115, 2004

Herrmann N, Rothenburg LS, Black SE, et al: Methylphenidate for the treatment of apathy in Alzheimer disease: prediction of response using dextroamphetamine challenge. J Clin Psychopharmacol 28:296–301, 2008

Hesse LM, He P, Krishnaswamy S, et al: Pharmacogenetic determinants of interindividual variability in bupropion hydroxylation by cytochrome P450 2B6 in human liver microsomes. Pharmacogenetics 14:225–238, 2004

Hien le TT, Cumming RG, Cameron ID, et al: Atypical antipsychotic medications and risk of falls in residents of aged care facilities. J Am Geriatr Soc 53:1290–1295, 2005

Howanitz E, Pardo M, Smelson DA, et al: The efficacy and safety of clozapine versus chlorpromazine in geriatric schizophrenia. J Clin Psychiatry 60:41–44, 1999

Howard R, McShane R, Lindesay J, et al: Donepezil and memantine for moderate-to-severe Alzheimer's disease. N Engl J Med 366:893–903, 2012

Howard WT, Warnock JK: Bupropion-induced psychosis. Am J Psychiatry 156:2017–2018, 1999

Hoyberg OJ, Maragakis B, Mullin J, et al: A double-blind multicentre comparison of mirtazapine and amitriptyline in elderly depressed patients. Acta Psychiatr Scand 93:184–190, 1996

Hutchison LC: Mirtazapine and bone marrow suppression: a case report. J Am Geriatr Soc 49:1129–1130, 2001

Jaskiw GE, Thyrum PT, Fuller MA, et al: Pharmacokinetics of quetiapine in elderly patients with selected psychotic disorders. Clin Pharmacokinet 43:1025–1035, 2004

Jeste DV, Barak Y, Madhusoodanan S, et al: International multisite double-blind trial of the atypical antipsychotics risperidone and olanzapine in 175 elderly patients with chronic schizophrenia. Am J Geriatr Psychiatry 11:638–647, 2003

Jin Y, Pollock BG, Frank E, et al: Effect of age, weight and CYP2C19 genotype on escitalopram exposure. J Clin Pharmacol 50:62–72, 2010

Johnson EM, Whyte E, Mulsant BH, et al: Cardiovascular changes associated with venlafaxine in the treatment of late life depression. Am J Geriatr Psychiatry 14:796–802, 2006

Joo JH, Lenze EJ, Mulsant BH, et al: Risk factors for falls during treatment of late-life depression. J Clin Psychiatry 63:936–941, 2002

Jorge RE, Acion L, Moser D, et al: Escitalopram and enhancement of cognitive recovery following stroke. Arch Gen Psychiatry 67:187–196, 2010

Juurlink DN, Mamdani MM, Kopp A, et al: The risk of suicide with selective serotonin reuptake inhibitors in the elderly. Am J Psychiatry 163:813–821, 2006

Kando JC, Tohen M, Castillo J, et al: The use of valproate in an elderly population with affective symptoms. J Clin Psychiatry 57:238–240, 1996

Kane J, Canas F, Kramer M, et al: Treatment of schizophrenia with paliperidone extended-release tablets: a 6-week placebo-controlled trial. Schizophr Res 90:147–161, 2007

Karp JF, Weiner D, Seligman K, et al: Body pain and treatment response in late-life depression. Am J Geriatr Psychiatry 13:188–194, 2005

Karp JF, Whyte EM, Lenze EJ, et al: Rescue pharmacotherapy with duloxetine for selective serotonin reuptake inhibitor nonresponders in late-life depression: outcome and tolerability. J Clin Psychiatry 69:457–463, 2008

Karp JF, Weiner DK, Dew MA, et al: Duloxetine and care management treatment of older adults with comorbid major depressive disorder and chronic low back pain: results of an open-label pilot study. Int J Geriatr Psychiatry 25:633–642, 2010

Kasckow JW, Mohamed S, Thallasinos A, et al: Citalopram augmentation of antipsychotic treatment in older schizophrenia patients. Int J Geriatr Psychiatry 16:1163–1167, 2001

Kasper S, de Swart H, Andersen HF: Escitalopram in the treatment of depressed elderly patients. Am J Geriatr Psychiatry 13:884–891, 2005

Katona CLE, Hunter BN, Bray J: A double-blind comparison of the efficacy and safety of paroxetine and imipramine in the treatment of depression with dementia. Int J Geriatr Psychiatry 13:100–108, 1998

Katz IR, Jeste DV, Mintzer JE, et al: Comparison of risperidone and placebo for psychosis and behavioral disturbances associated with dementia: a randomized, double-blind trial. Risperidone Study Group. J Clin Psychiatry 60:107–115, 1999

Katz IR, Reynolds CF 3rd, Alexopoulos GS, et al: Venlafaxine ER as a treatment for generalized anxiety disorder in older adults: pooled analysis of five randomized placebo-controlled clinical trials. J Am Geriatr Soc 50:18–25, 2002

Kavirajan H: Memantine: a comprehensive review of safety and efficacy. Expert Opin Drug Saf 8:89–109, 2009

Kavirajan H, Schneider LS: Efficacy and adverse effects of cholinesterase inhibitors and memantine in vascular dementia: a meta-analysis of randomised controlled trials. Lancet Neurol 6:782–792, 2007

Kennedy JS, Jeste D, Kaiser CJ, et al: Olanzapine vs. haloperidol in geriatric schizophrenia: analysis of data from a double-blind controlled trial. Int J Geriatr Psychiatry 18:1013–1020, 2003

Kennedy J, Deberdt W, Siegal A, et al: Olanzapine does not enhance cognition in nonagitated and non-psychotic patients with mild to moderate Alzheimer's dementia. Int J Geriatr Psychiatry 20:1020–1027, 2005

Kiev A, Masco HL, Wenger TL, et al: The cardiovascular effects of bupropion and nortriptyline in depressed outpatients. Ann Clin Psychiatry 6:107–115, 1994

Kim KY, Bader GM, Kotlyar V, et al: Treatment of delirium in older adults with quetiapine. J Geriatr Psychiatry Neurol 16:29–31, 2003

Kinon BJ, Stauffer VL, McGuire HC, et al: The effects of antipsychotic drug treatment on prolactin concentrations in elderly patients. J Am Med Dir Assoc 4:189–194, 2003

Kirby D, Harrigan S, Ames D: Hyponatraemia in elderly psychiatric patients treated with selective serotonin reuptake inhibitors and venlafaxine: a retrospective controlled study in an inpatient unit. Int J Geriatr Psychiatry 17:231–237, 2002

Kleijer BC, Heerdink ER, Egberts TC, et al: Antipsychotic drug use and the risk of venous thromboembolism in elderly patients. J Clin Psychopharmacol 30:526–530, 2010

Kohen I, Preval H, Southard R, et al: Naturalistic study of intramuscular ziprasidone versus conventional agents in agitated elderly patients: retrospective findings from a psychiatric emergency service. Am J Geriatr Pharmacother 3:240–245, 2005

Kohen I, Gordon ML, Manu P: Serotonin syndrome in elderly patients treated for psychotic depression with atypical antipsychotics and antidepressants: two case reports. CNS Spectr 12:596–598, 2007

Kok RM, Nolen WA, Heeren TJ: Venlafaxine versus nortriptyline in the treatment of elderly depressed inpatients: a randomised, double-blind, controlled trial. Int J Geriatr Psychiatry 22:1247–1254, 2007

Koller E, Schneider B, Bennett K, et al: Clozapine-associated diabetes. Am J Med 111:716–723, 2001

Koller EA, Cross JT, Doraiswamy PM, et al: Pancreatitis associated with atypical antipsychotics: from the Food and Drug Administration's MedWatch surveillance system and published reports. Pharmacotherapy 23:1123–1130, 2003

Kornstein SG, Clayton AH, Soares CN, et al: Analysis by age and sex of efficacy data from placebo-controlled trials of desvenlafaxine in outpatients with major depressive disorder. J Clin Psychopharmacol 30:294–299, 2010a

Kornstein SG, Jiang Q, Reddy S, et al: Short-term efficacy and safety of desvenlafaxine in a randomized, placebo-controlled study of perimenopausal and postmenopausal women with major depressive disorder. J Clin Psychiatry 71:1088–1096, 2010b

Kotlyar M, Brauer LH, Tracy TS, et al: Inhibition of CYP2D6 activity by bupropion. J Clin Psychopharmacol 25:226–229, 2005

Kuehn BM: FDA warns antipsychotic drugs may be risky for elderly. JAMA 293:2462, 2005

Kurlan R, Cummings J, Raman R, et al: Quetiapine for agitation or psychosis in patients with dementia and parkinsonism. Neurology 68:1356–1363, 2007

Kyle CJ, Petersen HE, Overo KF: Comparison of the tolerability and efficacy of citalopram and amitriptyline in elderly depressed patients treated in general practice. Depress Anxiety 8:147–153, 1998

Lam RW, Lönn SL, Despiégel N: Escitalopram versus serotonin noradrenaline reuptake inhibitors as second step treatment for patients with major depressive disorder: a pooled analysis. Int Clin Psychopharmacol 25:199–203, 2010

Landi F, Onder G, Cesari M, et al: Psychotropic medications and risk for falls among community-dwelling frail older people: an observational study. J Gerontol A Biol Sci Med Sci 60:622–626, 2005

Laroche ML, Charmes JP, Nouaille Y, et al: Is inappropriate medication use a major cause of adverse drug reactions in the elderly? Br J Clin Pharmacol 63:177–186, 2007

Lasser RA, Bossie CA, Zhu Y, et al: Efficacy and safety of long-acting risperidone in elderly patients with schizophrenia and schizoaffective disorder. Int J Geriatr Psychiatry 19:898–905, 2004

Lavretsky H, Park S, Siddarth P, et al: Methylphenidate-enhanced antidepressant response to citalopram in the elderly: a double-blind, placebo-controlled pilot trial. Am J Geriatr Psychiatry 142:181–185, 2006

Lavretsky H, Siddarth P, Irwin MR: Improving depression and enhancing resilience in family dementia caregivers: a pilot randomized placebo-controlled trial of escitalopram. Am J Geriatr Psychiatry 18:154–162, 2010

Lee PE, Gill SS, Freedman M, et al: Atypical antipsychotic drugs in the treatment of behavioural and psychological symptoms of dementia: systematic review. BMJ 329:75, 2004

Lenze EJ, Mulsant BH, Shear MK, et al: Anxiety symptoms in elderly patients with depression: what is the best approach to treatment? Drugs Aging 19:753–760, 2002

Lenze EJ, Mulsant BH, Shear MK, et al: Efficacy and tolerability of citalopram in the treatment of late-life anxiety disorders: results from an 8-week randomized, placebo-controlled trial. Am J Psychiatry 162:146–150, 2005

Lenze EJ, Rollman BL, Shear MK, et al: Escitalopram for older adults with generalized anxiety disorder: a randomized controlled trial. JAMA 301:295–303, 2009

Leopold NA: Risperidone treatment of drug-related psychosis in patients with parkinsonism. Mov Disord 15:301–304, 2000

Lessard E, Yessine MA, Hamelin BA, et al: Influence of CYP2D6 activity on the disposition and cardiovascular toxicity of the antidepressant agent venlafaxine in humans. Pharmacogenetics 9:435–443, 1999

Leufkens TR, Lund JS, Vermeeren A: Highway driving performance and cognitive functioning the morning after bedtime and middle-of-the-night use of gaboxadol, zopiclone and zolpidem. J Sleep Res 18:387–396, 2009

Liebowitz MR, Tourian KA: Efficacy, safety, and tolerability of desvenlafaxine 50 mg/d for the treatment of major depressive disorder: a systematic review of clinical trials. Prim Care Companion J Clin Psychiatry 12(3), 2010

Liperoti R, Pedone C, Lapane KL, et al: Venous thromboembolism among elderly patients treated with atypical and conventional antipsychotic agents. Arch Intern Med 165:2677–2682, 2005

Liperoti R, Onder G, Lapane KL, et al: Conventional or atypical antipsychotics and the risk of femur fracture among elderly patients: results of a case-control study. J Clin Psychiatry 68:929–934, 2007

Lipscombe LL, Levesque L, Gruneir A, et al: Antipsychotic drugs and hyperglycemia in older patients with diabetes. Arch Intern Med 169:1282–1289, 2009

Liu B, Anderson G, Mittmann N, et al: Use of selective serotonin reuptake inhibitors or tricyclic antidepressants and risk of hip fractures in elderly people. Lancet 351:1303–1307, 1998

Looper KJ: Potential medical and surgical complications of serotonergic antidepressants. Psychosomatics 48:1–9, 2007

Lotrich FE, Rabinovitz F, Gironda P, et al: Depression following pegylated interferon-alpha: characteristics and vulnerability. J Psychosom Res 63:131–135, 2007

Lu CJ, Tune LE: Chronic exposure to anticholinergic medications adversely affects the course of Alzheimer disease. Am J Geriatr Psychiatry 14:458–461, 2003

Lyketsos CG, DelCampo L, Steinberg M, et al: Treating depression in Alzheimer disease: efficacy and safety of sertraline therapy, and the benefits of depression reduction: the DIADS. Arch Gen Psychiatry 60:737–746, 2003

Madhusoodanan S, Zaveri D: Paliperidone use in the elderly. Curr Drug Saf 5:149–152, 2010

Madhusoodanan S, Suresh P, Brenner R, et al: Experience with the atypical antipsychotics—risperidone and olanzapine in the elderly. Ann Clin Psychiatry 11:113–118, 1999

Madhusoodanan S, Brenner R, Alcantra A: Clinical experience with quetiapine in elderly patients with psychotic disorders. J Geriatr Psychiatry Neurol 13:28–32, 2000

Mahapatra SN, Hackett D: A randomised, double-blind, parallel-group comparison of venlafaxine and dothiepin in geriatric patients with major depression. Int J Clin Pract 51:209–213, 1997

Mahmood I, Sahajwalla C: Clinical pharmacokinetics and pharmacodynamics of buspirone, an anxiolytic drug. Clin Pharmacokinet 36:277–287, 1999

Mamo DC, Sweet RA, Mulsant BH, et al: The effect of nortriptyline and paroxetine on extrapyramidal signs and symptoms: a prospective double-blind study in depressed elderly patients. Am J Geriatr Psychiatry 8:226–231, 2000

Mamo D, Graff A, Mizrahi R, et al: Differential effects of aripiprazole on D_2, $5\text{-}HT_2$, and $5\text{-}HT_{1A}$ receptor occupancy in patients with schizophrenia: a triple tracer PET study. Am J Psychiatry 164:1411–1417, 2007

Mariappan P, Alhasso AA, Grant A, et al: Serotonin and noradrenaline reuptake inhibitors (SNRI) for stress urinary incontinence in adults. Cochrane Database of Systematic Reviews 2005, Issue 3. Art. No. CD004742. DOI: 10.1002/14651858. CD004742.pub2.

Marsh L, Lyketsos C, Reich SG: Olanzapine for the treatment of psychosis in patients with Parkinson's disease and dementia. Psychosomatics 42:477–481, 2001

Martin H, Slyk MP, Deymann S, et al: Safety profile assessment of risperidone and olanzapine in long-term care patients with dementia. J Am Med Dir Assoc 4:183–188, 2003

Mayeux R: Early Alzheimer's disease. N Engl J Med 362:2194–2201, 2010

Mazeh D, Shahal B, Aviv A, et al: A randomized, single-blind, comparison of venlafaxine with paroxetine in elderly patients suffering from resistant depression. Int Clin Psychopharmacol 22:371–375, 2007

McCue RE, Joseph M: Venlafaxine- and trazodone-induced serotonin syndrome. Am J Psychiatry 158:2088–2089, 2001

Messenheimer JA: Rash in adult and pediatric patients treated with lamotrigine. Can J Neurol Sci 25:S14–S18, 1998

Meyers BS, Flint AJ, Rothschild AJ, et al: A double-blind randomized controlled trial of olanzapine plus sertraline versus olanzapine plus placebo for psychotic depression: the STOP-PD Study. Arch Gen Psychiatry 66:838–847, 2009

Micca JL, Hoffmann VP, Lipkovich I, et al: Retrospective analysis of diabetes risk in elderly patients with dementia in olanzapine clinical trials. Am J Geriatr Psychiatry 14:62–70, 2006

Mintzer JE, Tune LE, Breder CD, et al: Aripiprazole for the treatment of psychoses in institutionalized patients with Alzheimer dementia: a multicenter, randomized, double-blind, placebo-controlled assessment of three fixed doses. Am J Geriatr Psychiatry 15:918–931, 2007

Mittal D, Jimerson NA, Neely EP, et al: Risperidone in the treatment of delirium: results from a prospective open-label trial. J Clin Psychiatry 65:662–667, 2004

Modi A, Weiner M, Craig BA, et al: Concomitant use of anticholinergics with acetylcholinesterase inhibitors in Medicaid recipients with dementia and residing in nursing homes. J Am Geriatr Soc 57:1238–1244, 2009

Molho ES, Factor SA: Worsening of motor features of parkinsonism with olanzapine. Mov Disord 14:1014–1016, 1999

Montejo AL, Llorca G, Izquierdo JA, et al: Incidence of sexual dysfunction associated with antidepressant agents: a prospective multicenter study of 1022 outpatients. Spanish Working Group for the Study of Psychotropic-Related Sexual Dysfunction. J Clin Psychiatry 62(suppl):10–21, 2001

Montgomery SA, Fava M, Padmanabhan SK, et al: Discontinuation symptoms and taper/poststudy-emergent adverse events with desvenlafaxine treatment for major depressive disorder. Int Clin Psychopharmacol 24:296–305, 2009

Mottram PG, Wilson K, Strobl JJ: Antidepressants for depressed elderly. Cochrane Database of Systematic Reviews 2006, Issue 1. Art. No.: CD003491. DOI: 10.1002/14651858.CD003491.pub2.

Mukai Y, Tampi RR: Treatment of depression in the elderly: a review of the recent literature on the efficacy of single- versus dual-action antidepressants. Clin Ther 31:945–961, 2009

Müller-Oerlinghausen B, Lewitzka U: Lithium reduces pathological aggression and suicidality: a mini-review. Neuropsychobiology 62:43–49, 2010

Mulsant BH, Alexopoulos GS, Reynolds CF 3rd, et al: Pharmacological treatment of depression in older primary care patients: the PROSPECT algorithm. Int J Geriatr Psychiatry 16:585–592, 2001a

Mulsant BH, Pollock BG, Nebes R, et al: A twelve-week, double-blind, randomized comparison of nortriptyline and paroxetine in older depressed inpatients and outpatients. Am J Geriatr Psychiatry 9:406–414, 2001b

Mulsant BH, Pollock BG, Kirshner M, et al: Serum anticholinergic activity in a community-based sample of older adults: relationship with cognitive performance. Arch Gen Psychiatry 60:198–203, 2003

Mulsant BH, Gharabawi GM, Bossie CA, et al: Correlates of anticholinergic activity in patients with dementia and psychosis treated with risperidone or olanzapine. J Clin Psychiatry 65:1708–1714, 2004

Murray V, von Arbin M, Bartfai A, et al: Double-blind comparison of sertraline and placebo in stroke patients with minor depression and less severe major depression. J Clin Psychiatry 66:708–716, 2005

Nagaraja D, Jayashree S: Randomized study of the dopamine receptor agonist piribedil in the treatment of mild cognitive impairment. Am J Psychiatry 158:1517–1519, 2001

Nandagopal JJ, DelBello MP: Selegiline transdermal system: a novel treatment option for major depressive disorder. Expert Opin Pharmacother 10:1665–1673, 2009

National Collaborating Centre for Mental Health: Management of Depression in Primary and Secondary Care (Clinical Guideline 23). London, National Institute for Clinical Excellence, 2004

Navarro V, Gasto C, Torres X, et al: Citalopram versus nortriptyline in late-life depression: a 12-week randomized single-blind study. Acta Psychiatr Scand 103:435–440, 2001

Nebes RD, Pollock BG, Meltzer CC, et al: Cognitive effects of serum anticholinergic activity and white matter hyperintensities. Neurology 65:1487–1489, 2005

Nelson JC, Wohlreich MM, Mallinckrodt CH, et al: Duloxetine for the treatment of major depressive disorder in older patients. Am J Geriatr Psychiatry 13:227–235, 2005

Nelson JC, Delucchi K, Schneider L: Suicidal thinking and behavior during treatment with sertraline in late-life depression. Am J Geriatr Psychiatry 15:573–580, 2007

Nelson JC, Delucchi K, Schneider LS: Efficacy of second generation antidepressants in late-life depression: a meta-analysis of the evidence. Am J Geriatr Psychiatry 16:558–567, 2008

Newhouse PA, Krishnan KR, Doraiswamy PM, et al: A double-blind comparison of sertraline and fluoxetine in depressed elderly outpatients. J Clin Psychiatry 61:559–568, 2000

Nicholas LM, Ford AL, Esposito SM, et al: The effects of mirtazapine on plasma lipid profiles in healthy subjects. J Clin Psychiatry 64:883–889, 2003

Nieuwstraten CE, Dolovich LR: Bupropion versus selective serotonin-reuptake inhibitors for treatment of depression. Ann Pharmacother 35:1608–1613, 2001

Nikaido AM, Ellinwood EH Jr, Heatherly DG, et al: Age-related increase in CNS sensitivity to benzodiazepines as assessed by task difficulty. Psychopharmacology (Berl) 100:90–97, 1990

Noaghiul S, Narayan M, Nelson JC: Divalproex treatment of mania in elderly patients. Am J Geriatr Psychiatry 6:257–262, 1998

Nyth AL, Gottfries CG: The clinical efficacy of citalopram in treatment of emotional disturbances in dementia disorders: a Nordic multicentre study. Br J Psychiatry 157:894–901, 1990

Nyth AL, Gottfries CG, Lyby K, et al: A controlled multicenter clinical study of citalopram and placebo in elderly depressed patients with and without concomitant dementia. Acta Psychiatr Scand 86:138–145, 1992

O'Connor DW, Sierakowski C, Chin LF, et al: The safety and tolerability of clozapine in aged patients: a retrospective clinical file review. World J Biol Psychiatry 11:788–791, 2010

Oganesian A, Shilling AD, Young-Sciame R, et al: Desvenlafaxine and venlafaxine exert minimal in vitro inhibition of human cytochrome p450 and p-glycoprotein activities. Psychopharmacol Bull 42:47–63, 2009

Olafsson K, Jorgensen S, Jensen HV, et al: Fluvoxamine in the treatment of demented elderly patients: a double-blind, placebo-controlled study. Acta Psychiatr Scand 85:453–456, 1992

Oslin DW, Streim JE, Katz IR, et al: Heuristic comparison of sertraline with nortriptyline for the treatment of depression in frail elderly patients. Am J Geriatr Psychiatry 8:141–149, 2000

Oslin DW, Ten Have TR, Streim JE, et al: Probing the safety of medications in the frail elderly: evidence from a randomized clinical trial of sertraline and venlafaxine in depressed nursing home residents. J Clin Psychiatry 64:875–882, 2003

Pact V, Giduz T: Mirtazapine treats resting tremor, essential tremor, and levodopa-induced dyskinesias. Neurology 53:1154, 1999

Pae CU, Lee SJ, Lee CU, et al: A pilot trial of quetiapine for the treatment of patients with delirium. Hum Psychopharmacol 19:125–127, 2004

Papakostas GI, Thase ME, Fava M, et al: Are antidepressant drugs that combine serotonergic and noradrenergic mechanisms of action more effective than the selective serotonin reuptake inhibitors in treating major depressive disorder? A meta-analysis of studies of newer agents. Biol Psychiatry 62:1217–1227, 2007

Parellada E, Baeza I, de Pablo J, et al: Risperidone in the treatment of patients with delirium. J Clin Psychiatry 65:348–353, 2004

Parkinson Study Group: Low-dose clozapine for the treatment of drug-induced psychosis in Parkinson's disease. N Engl J Med 340:757–763, 1999

Park-Wyllie LY, Mamdani MM, Li P, et al: Cholinesterase inhibitors and hospitalization for bradycardia: a population-based study. PLoS Med 6:e1000157, 2009

Pedersen L, Klysner R: Antagonism of selective serotonin reuptake inhibitor–induced nausea by mirtazapine. Int Clin Psychopharmacol 12:59–60, 1997

Percudani M, Barbui C, Fortino I, et al: Second-generation antipsychotics and risk of cerebrovascular accidents in the elderly. J Clin Psychopharmacol 25:468–470, 2005

Perry NK: Venlafaxine-induced serotonin syndrome with relapse following amitriptyline. Postgrad Med J 76:254–256, 2000

Petracca GM, Chemerinski E, Starkstein SE: A double-blind, placebo-controlled study of fluoxetine in depressed patients with Alzheimer's disease. Int Psychogeriatr 13:233–240, 2001

Phanjoo AL, Wonnacott S, Hodgson A: Double-blind comparative multicentre study of fluvoxamine and mianserin in the treatment of major depressive episode in elderly people. Acta Psychiatr Scand 83:476–479, 1991

Pilotto A, Franceschi M, D'Onofrio G, et al: Effect of a CYP2D6 polymorphism on the efficacy of donepezil in patients with Alzheimer disease. Neurology 73:761–767, 2009

Pinquart M, Duberstein PR, Lyness JM: Treatments for later-life depressive conditions: a meta-analytic comparison of pharmacotherapy and psychotherapy. Am J Psychiatry 163:1493–1501, 2006

Poewe W: Treatment of dementia with Lewy bodies and Parkinson's disease dementia. Mov Disord 20(suppl):S77–S82, 2005

Pollock BG, Mulsant BH, Sweet R, et al: An open pilot study of citalopram for behavioral disturbances of dementia. Am J Geriatr Psychiatry 5:70–78, 1997

Pollock BG, Laghrissi-Thode F, Wagner WR: Evaluation of platelet activation in depressed patients with ischemic heart disease after paroxetine or nortriptyline treatment. J Clin Psychopharmacol 20:137–140, 2000

Pollock BG, Mulsant BH, Rosen J, et al: Comparison of citalopram, perphenazine, and placebo for the acute treatment of psychosis and behavioral disturbances in hospitalized, demented patients. Am J Psychiatry 159:460–465, 2002

Pollock BG, Mulsant BH, Rosen J, et al: A double-blind comparison of citalopram and risperidone for the treatment of behavioral and psychotic symptoms associated with dementia. Am J Geriatr Psychiatry 15:942–952, 2007

Pollock BG, Forsyth CE, Bies RR: The critical role of clinical pharmacology in geriatric psychopharmacology. Clin Pharmacol Ther 85:89–93, 2009

Pomara N, Deptula D, Medel M, et al: Effects of diazepam on recall memory: relationship to aging, dose, and duration of treatment. Psychopharmacol Bull 25:144–148, 1989

Post RM, Frye MA, Denicoff KD, et al: Beyond lithium in the treatment of bipolar illness. Neuropsychopharmacology 19:206–219, 1998

Rabey JM, Prokhorov T, Miniovitz A, et al: Effect of quetiapine in psychotic Parkinson's disease patients: a double-blind labeled study of 3 months' duration. Mov Disord 22:313–318, 2007

Rabins PV, Lyketsos CG: Antipsychotic drugs in dementia: what should be made of the risks? JAMA 294:1963–1965, 2005

Rahman MK, Akhtar MJ, Savla NC, et al: A double-blind, randomised comparison of fluvoxamine with dothiepin in the treatment of depression in elderly patients. Br J Clin Pract 45:255–258, 1991

Rais AR, Williams K, Rais T, et al: Use of intramuscular ziprasidone for the control of acute psychosis or agitation in an inpatient geriatric population: an open-label study. Psychiatry (Edgmont) 7:17–24, 2010

Raji MA, Brady SR: Mirtazapine for treatment of depression and comorbidities in Alzheimer disease. Ann Pharmacother 35:1024–1027, 2001

Rajji TK, Mulsant BH, Lotrich FE, et al: Use of antidepressants in late-life depression. Drugs Aging 25:841–853, 2008

Rajji TK, Uchida H, Ismail Z, et al: Clozapine and global cognition in schizophrenia. J Clin Psychopharmacol 30:431–436, 2010

Rampello L, Chiechio S, Nicoletti G, et al: Prediction of the response to citalopram and reboxetine in post-stroke depressed patients. Psychopharmacology (Berl) 173:73–78, 2004

Rapaport MH, Schneider LS, Dunner DL, et al: Efficacy of controlled-release paroxetine in the treatment of late-life depression. J Clin Psychiatry 64:1065–1074, 2003

Raskin J, Wiltse CG, Siegal A, et al: Efficacy of duloxetine on cognition, depression, and pain in elderly patients with major depressive disorder: an 8-week, double-blind, placebo-controlled trial. Am J Psychiatry 164:900–909, 2007

Rasmussen A, Lunde M, Poulsen DL, et al: A double-blind, placebo-controlled study of sertraline in the prevention of depression in stroke patients. Psychosomatics 44:216–221, 2003

Ray WA, Thapa PB, Gideon P: Benzodiazepines and the risk of falls in nursing home residents. J Am Geriatr Soc 48:682–685, 2000

Ray WA, Chung CP, Murray KT, et al: Atypical antipsychotic drugs and the risk of sudden cardiac death. N Engl J Med 360:225–235, 2009

Reifler BV, Teri L, Raskind M: Double-blind trial of imipramine in Alzheimer's disease in patients with and without depression. Am J Psychiatry 146:45–49, 1989

Reisberg B, Doody R, Stöffler A, et al: Memantine in moderate-to-severe Alzheimer's disease. N Engl J Med 348:1333–1341, 2003

Rektorová I, Rektor I, Bares M, et al: Pramipexole and pergolide in the treatment of depression in Parkinson's disease: a national multicentre prospective randomized study. Eur J Neurol 10:399–406, 2003

Reynolds CF 3rd, Dew MA, Pollock BG, et al: Maintenance treatment of major depression in old age. N Engl J Med 354:1130–1138, 2006

Reynolds CF 3rd, Butters MA, Lopez O, et al: Maintenance treatment of depression in old age: a randomized, double-blind, placebo-controlled evaluation of the efficacy and safety of donepezil combined with antidepressant pharmacotherapy. Arch Gen Psychiatry 68:51–60, 2011

Reznik I, Rosen Y, Rosen B: An acute ischaemic event associated with the use of venlafaxine: a case report and proposed pathophysiological mechanisms. J Psychopharmacol 13:193–195, 1999

Richards JB, Papaioannou A, Adachi JD, et al; for the Canadian Multicentre Osteoporosis Study Research Group: Effect of selective serotonin reuptake inhibitors on the risk of fracture. Arch Intern Med 167:188–194, 2007

Ridout F, Meadows R, Johnsen S, et al: A placebo controlled investigation into the effects of paroxetine and mirtazapine on measures related to car driving performance. Hum Psychopharmacol 18:261–269, 2003

Ritchie CW, Chiu E, Harrigan S, et al: The impact upon extrapyramidal side effects, clinical symptoms and quality of life of a switch from conventional to atypical antipsychotics (risperidone or olanzapine) in elderly patients with schizophrenia. Int J Geriatr Psychiatry 18:432–440, 2003

Ritchie CW, Chiu E, Harrigan S, et al: A comparison of the efficacy and safety of olanzapine and risperidone in the treatment of elderly patients with schizophrenia: an open study of six months duration. Int J Geriatr Psychiatry 21:171–179, 2006

Robinson DS, Amsterdam JD: The selegiline transdermal system in major depressive disorder: a systematic review of safety and tolerability. J Affect Disord 105:15–23, 2008

Robinson R, Schultz S, Castillo C, et al: Nortriptyline versus fluoxetine in the treatment of depression and in short-term recovery after stroke: a placebo-controlled, double-blind study. Am J Psychiatry 157:351–359, 2000

Robinson RG, Jorge RE, Moser DJ, et al: Escitalopram and problem-solving therapy for prevention of poststroke depression: a randomized controlled trial. JAMA 299:2391–2400, 2008

Rocca P, Calvarese P, Faggiano F, et al: Citalopram versus sertraline in late-life nonmajor clinically significant depression: a 1-year follow-up clinical trial. J Clin Psychiatry 66:360–369, 2005

Rochon PA, Stukel TA, Sykora K, et al: Atypical antipsychotics and parkinsonism. Arch Intern Med 165:1882–1888, 2005

Rodda J, Morgan S, Walker Z: Are cholinesterase inhibitors effective in the management of the behavioral and psychological symptoms of dementia in Alzheimer's disease? A systematic review of randomized, placebo-controlled trials of donepezil, rivastigmine and galantamine. Int Psychogeriatr 21:813–824, 2009

Roose SP, Dalack GW, Glassman AH, et al: Cardiovascular effects of bupropion in depressed patients with heart disease. Am J Psychiatry 148:512–516, 1991

Roose SP, Nelson JC, Salzman C, et al: Open-label study of mirtazapine orally disintegrating tablets in depressed patients in the nursing home. Mirtazapine in the Nursing Home Study Group. Curr Med Res Opin 19:737–746, 2003

Roose SP, Miyazaki M, Devanand D, et al: An open trial of venlafaxine for the treatment of late-life atypical depression. Int J Geriatr Psychiatry 19:989–994, 2004a

Roose SP, Sackeim HA, Krishnan KR, et al: Antidepressant pharmacotherapy in the treatment of depression in the very old: a randomized, placebo-controlled trial. Am J Psychiatry 161:2050–2059, 2004b

Rosen J, Sweet R, Pollock BG, et al: Nortriptyline in the hospitalized elderly: tolerance and side effect reduction. Psychopharmacol Bull 29:327–331, 1993

Rosenberg C, Lauritzen L, Brix J, et al: Citalopram versus amitriptyline in elderly depressed patients with or without mild cognitive dysfunction: a Danish multicentre trial in general practice. Psychopharmacol Bull 40:63–73, 2007

Rosenberg PB, Drye LT, Martin BK, et al: Sertraline for the treatment of depression in Alzheimer disease. Am J Geriatr Psychiatry 18:136–145, 2010

Ross J: Discontinuation of lithium augmentation in geriatric patients with unipolar depression: a systematic review. Can J Psychiatry 53:117–120, 2008

Rossini D, Serretti A, Franchini L, et al: Sertraline versus fluvoxamine in the treatment of elderly patients with major depression: a double-blind, randomized trial. J Clin Psychopharmacol 25:471–475, 2005

Rush AJ, Trivedi MH, Wisniewski SR, et al: Acute and longer-term outcomes in depressed outpatients requiring one or several treatment steps: a STAR*D report. Am J Psychiatry 163:1905–1917, 2006

Sackeim HA, Haskett RF, Mulsant BH, et al: Continuation pharmacotherapy in the prevention of relapse following electroconvulsive therapy: a randomized controlled trial. JAMA 285:1299–1307, 2001

Saiz-Ruiz J, Ibanez A, Diaz-Marsa M, et al: Nefazodone in the treatment of elderly patients with depressive disorders: a prospective, observational study. CNS Drugs 16:635–643, 2002

Sajatovic M, Jaskiw G, Konicki PE, et al: Outcome of clozapine therapy for elderly patients with refractory primary psychosis. Int J Geriatr Psychiatry 12:553–558, 1997

Sajatovic M, Gyulai L, Calabrese JR, et al: Maintenance treatment outcomes in older patients with bipolar I disorder. Am J Geriatr Psychiatry 13:305–311, 2005a

Sajatovic M, Madhusoodanan S, Coconcea N: Managing bipolar disorder in the elderly: defining the role of the newer agents. Drugs Aging 22:39–54, 2005b

Sajatovic M, Blow FC, Ignacio RV: Psychiatric comorbidity in older adults with bipolar disorder. Int J Geriatr Psychiatry 21:582–587, 2006

Sajatovic M, Ramsay E, Nanry K, et al: Lamotrigine therapy in elderly patients with epilepsy, bipolar disorder or dementia. Int J Geriatr Psychiatry 22:945–950, 2007

Sajatovic M, Coconcea N, Ignacio RV, et al: Aripiprazole therapy in 20 older adults with bipolar disorder: a 12-week, open-label trial. J Clin Psychiatry 69:41–46, 2008

Salzman C, Jeste DV, Meyer RE, et al: Elderly patients with dementia-related symptoms of severe agitation and aggression: consensus statement on treatment options, clinical trials methodology, and policy. J Clin Psychiatry 69:889–898, 2008

Sasaki Y, Matsuyama T, Inoue S, et al: A prospective, open-label, flexible-dose study of quetiapine in the treatment of delirium. J Clin Psychiatry 64:1316–1321, 2003

Satel SL, Nelson JC: Stimulants in the treatment of depression: a critical overview. J Clin Psychiatry 50:241–249, 1989

Sato Y, Kondo I, Ishida S, et al: Decreased bone mass and increased bone turnover with valproate therapy in adults with epilepsy. Neurology 57:445–449, 2001

Savaskan E, Muller SE, Bohringer A, et al: Antidepressive therapy with escitalopram improves mood, cognitive symptoms, and identity memory for angry faces in elderly depressed patients. Int J Neuropsychopharmacol 11:381–388, 2008

Schatzberg A, Roose S: A double-blind, placebo-controlled study of venlafaxine and fluoxetine in geriatric outpatients with major depression. Am J Geriatr Psychiatry 14:361–370, 2006

Schatzberg AF, Kremer C, Rodrigues HE, et al: Double-blind, randomized comparison of mirtazapine and paroxetine in elderly depressed patients. Am J Geriatr Psychiatry 10:541–550, 2002

Schneider LS, Nelson JC, Clary CM, et al: An 8-week multicenter, parallel-group, double-blind, placebo-controlled study of sertraline in elderly outpatients with major depression. Am J Psychiatry 160:1277–1285, 2003

Schneider LS, Dagerman KS, Insel P: Risk of death with atypical antipsychotic drug treatment for dementia: meta-analysis of randomized placebo-controlled trials. JAMA 294:1934–1943, 2005

Schneider LS, Dagerman K, Insel PS: Efficacy and adverse effects of atypical antipsychotics for dementia: meta-analysis of randomized placebo-controlled trials. Am J Geriatr Psychiatry 14:191–210, 2006a

Schneider LS, Tariot PN, Dagerman KS, et al: Effectiveness of atypical antipsychotic drugs in patients with Alzheimer's disease. N Engl J Med 355:1525–1538, 2006b

Schone W, Ludwig M: A double-blind study of paroxetine compared with fluoxetine in geriatric patients with major depression. J Clin Psychopharmacol 13(suppl):34S–39S, 1993

Schwaninger M, Ringleb P, Winter R, et al: Elevated plasma concentrations of homocysteine in antiepileptic drug treatment. Epilepsia 40:345–350, 1999

Scott J, Greenwald BS, Kramer E, et al: Atypical (second generation) antipsychotic treatment response in very late-onset schizophrenia-like psychosis. Int Psychogeriatr 23:742–748, 2011

Semenchuk MR, Sherman S, Davis B: Double-blind, randomized trial of bupropion SR for the treatment of neuropathic pain. Neurology 57:1583–1588, 2001

Serebruany VL, Glassman AH, Malinin AI, et al: Platelet/endothelial biomarkers in depressed patients treated with the selective serotonin reuptake inhibitor sertraline after acute coronary events: the Sertraline AntiDepressant Heart Attack Randomized Trial (SADHART) Platelet Substudy. Circulation 108:939–944, 2003

Seritan AL: Prevent drug-drug interactions with cholinesterase inhibitors: avoid adverse events when prescribing medications for patients with dementia. Curr Psychiatry 7:57–67, 2008

Sheffrin M, Driscoll HC, Lenze EJ, et al: Pilot study of augmentation with aripiprazole for incomplete response in late-life depression: getting to remission. J Clin Psychiatry 70:208–213, 2009

Sheikh JI, Cassidy EL, Doraiswamy PM, et al: Efficacy, safety, and tolerability of sertraline in patients with late-life depression and comorbid medical illness. J Am Geriatr Soc 52:86–92, 2004a

Sheikh JI, Lauderdale SA, Cassidy EL: Efficacy of sertraline for panic disorder in older adults: a preliminary open-label trial (letter). Am J Geriatr Psychiatry 12:230, 2004b

Shelton C, Entsuah R, Padmanabhan SK, et al: Venlafaxine XR demonstrates higher rates of sustained remission compared to fluoxetine, paroxetine or placebo. Int Clin Psychopharmacol 20:233–238, 2005

Shelton RC, Tollefson GD, Tohen M, et al: A novel augmentation strategy for treating resistant major depression. Am J Psychiatry 158:131–134, 2001

Shulman KI: Lithium for older adults with bipolar disorder: should it still be considered a first-line agent? Drugs Aging 27:607–615, 2010

Shulman KI, Walker SE: A reevaluation of dietary restrictions for irreversible monoamine oxidase inhibitors. Psychiatr Ann 31:378–384, 2001

Shulman KI, Fischer HD, Herrmann N, et al: Current prescription patterns and safety profile of irreversible monoamine oxidase inhibitors: a population-based cohort study of older adults. J Clin Psychiatry 70:1681–1686, 2009

Siddiqi N, Holt R, Britton AM, et al: Interventions for preventing delirium in hospitalised patients. Cochrane Database of Systematic Reviews 2007, Issue 2. Art. No. CD005563. DOI: 10.1002/14651858. CD005563.pub2.

Sink KM, Holden KF, Yaffe K: Pharmacological treatment of neuropsychiatric symptoms of dementia: a review of the evidence. JAMA 293:596–608, 2005

Skrobik YK, Bergeron N, Dumont M, et al: Olanzapine vs. haloperidol: treating delirium in a critical care setting. Intensive Care Med 30:444–449, 2004

Smeraldi E, Rizzo F, Crespi G: Double-blind, randomized study of venlafaxine, clomipramine and trazodone in geriatric patients with major depression. Primary Care Psychiatry 4:189–195, 1998

Smith D, Dempster C, Glanville J, et al: Efficacy and tolerability of venlafaxine compared with selective serotonin reuptake inhibitors and other antidepressants: a meta-analysis. Br J Psychiatry 180:396–404, 2002

Sneed JR, Culang ME, Keilp JG, et al: Antidepressant medication and executive dysfunction: a deleterious interaction in late-life depression. Am J Geriatr Psychiatry 18:128–135, 2010

Soares CN, Thase ME, Clayton A, et al: Desvenlafaxine and escitalopram for the treatment of postmenopausal women with major depressive disorder. Menopause 17:700–711, 2010

Sommer BR, Fenn HH, Ketter TA: Safety and efficacy of anticonvulsants in elderly patients with psychiatric disorders: oxcarbazepine, topiramate and gabapentin. Expert Opin Drug Saf 6:133–145, 2007

Sonnenberg CM, Deeg DJ, Comijs HC, et al: Trends in antidepressant use in the older population: results from the LASA-study over a period of 10 years. J Affect Disord 111:299–305, 2008

Spier SA: Use of bupropion with SRIs and venlafaxine. Depress Anxiety 7:73–75, 1998

Sproule BA, Hardy BG, Shulman KI: Differential pharmacokinetics of lithium in elderly patients. Drugs Aging 16:165–177, 2000

Stahl SM, Entsuah R, Rudolph RL: Comparative efficacy between venlafaxine and SSRIs: a pooled analysis of patients with depression. Biol Psychiatry 52:1166–1174, 2002

Steffens DC, Doraiswamy PM, McQuoid DR: Bupropion SR in the naturalistic treatment of elderly patients with major depression. Int J Geriatr Psychiatry 16:862–865, 2001

Steffens DC, Nelson JC, Eudicone JM, et al: Efficacy and safety of adjunctive aripiprazole in major depressive disorder in older patients; a pooled subpopulation analysis. Int J Geriatr Psychiatry 26:564–572, 2011

Steinberg JR: Anxiety in elderly patients: a comparison of azapirones and benzodiazepines. Drugs Aging 5:335–345, 1994

Steinmetz K, Coley K, Pollock BG: Assessment of the quantity and quality of geriatric information in the drug label for commonly prescribed drugs in the elderly. J Am Geriatr Soc 53:891–894, 2005

Strand M, Hetta J, Rosen A, et al: A double-blind controlled trial in primary care patients with generalized anxiety: a comparison between buspirone and oxazepam. J Clin Psychiatry 51(suppl):40–45, 1990

Street JS, Clark WS, Gannon KS, et al: Olanzapine treatment of psychotic and behavioral symptoms in patients with Alzheimer disease in nursing care facilities: a double-blind, randomized, placebo-controlled trial. The HGEU Study Group. Arch Gen Psychiatry 57:968–976, 2000

Streim JE, Porsteinsson AP, Breder CD, et al: A randomized, double-blind, placebo-controlled study of aripiprazole for the treatment of psychosis in nursing home patients with Alzheimer disease. Am J Geriatr Psychiatry 16:537–550, 2008

Suh GH, Son HG, Ju YS, et al: A randomized, double-blind, crossover comparison of risperidone and haloperidol in Korean dementia patients with behavioral disturbances. Am J Geriatr Psychiatry 12:509–516, 2004

Suppes T, Eudicone J, McQuade R, et al: Efficacy and safety of aripiprazole in subpopulations with acute manic or mixed episodes of bipolar I disorder. J Affect Disord 107:145–154, 2008

Szuba MP, Leuchter AF: Falling backward in two elderly patients taking bupropion. J Clin Psychiatry 53:157–159, 1992

Tadger S, Paleacu D, Barak Y: Quetiapine augmentation of antidepressant treatment in elderly patients suffering from depressive symptoms: a retrospective chart review. Arch Gerontol Geriatr 53:104–105, 2011

Taragano FE, Lyketsos CG, Mangone CA, et al: A double-blind, randomized, fixed-dose trial of fluoxetine vs. amitriptyline in the treatment of major depression complicating Alzheimer's disease. Psychosomatics 38:246–252, 1997

Tariot PN, Erb R, Podgorski CA, et al: Efficacy and tolerability of carbamazepine for agitation and aggression in dementia. Am J Psychiatry 155:54–61, 1998

Tariot PN, Salzman C, Yeung PP, et al: Long-term use of quetiapine in elderly patients with psychotic disorders. Clin Ther 22:1068–1084, 2000

Tariot PN, Farlow MR, Grossberg GT, et al: Memantine treatment in patients with moderate to severe Alzheimer disease already receiving donepezil: a randomized controlled trial. JAMA 291:317–324, 2004

Tariot PN, Raman R, Jakimovich L, et al: Divalproex sodium in nursing home residents with possible or probable Alzheimer disease complicated by agitation: a randomized, controlled trial. Am J Geriatr Psychiatry 13:942–949, 2005

Tashkin D, Kanner R, Bailey W, et al: Smoking cessation in patients with chronic obstructive pulmonary disease: a double-blind, placebo-controlled, randomised trial. Lancet 357:1571–1575, 2001

Thase ME: Effects of venlafaxine on blood pressure: a meta-analysis of original data from 3744 depressed patients. J Clin Psychiatry 59:502–508, 1998

Thase ME: What role do atypical antipsychotic drugs have in treatment-resistant depression? J Clin Psychiatry 63:95–103, 2002

Thase ME, Entsuah AR, Rudolph RL: Remission rates during treatment with venlafaxine or selective serotonin reuptake inhibitors. Br J Psychiatry 178:234–241, 2001

Thase ME, Entsuah R, Cantillon M, et al: Relative antidepressant efficacy of venlafaxine and SSRIs: sex-age interactions. J Womens Health (Larchmt) 14:609–616, 2005a

Thase ME, Haight BR, Richard N, et al: Remission rates following antidepressant therapy with bupropion or selective serotonin reuptake inhibitors: a meta-analysis of original data from 7 randomized controlled trials. J Clin Psychiatry 66:974–981, 2005b

Thase ME, Tran PV, Wiltse C, et al: Cardiovascular profile of duloxetine, a dual reuptake inhibitor of serotonin and norepinephrine. J Clin Psychopharmacol 25:132–140, 2005c

Thompson DS: Mirtazapine for the treatment of depression and nausea in breast and gynecological oncology. Psychosomatics 41:356–359, 2000

Tollefson GD, Bosomworth JC, Heiligenstein JH, et al: A double-blind, placebo-controlled clinical trial of fluoxetine in geriatric patients with major depression. The Fluoxetine Collaborative Study Group. Int Psychogeriatr 7:89–104, 1995

Trappler B, Cohen CI: Use of SSRIs in "very old" depressed nursing home residents. Am J Geriatr Psychiatry 6:83–89, 1998

Trick L, Stanley N, Rigney U, et al: A double-blind, randomized, 26-week study comparing the cognitive and psychomotor effects and efficacy of 75 mg (37.5 mg b.i.d.) venlafaxine and 75 mg (25 mg mane, 50 mg nocte) dothiepin in elderly patients with moderate major depression being treated in general practice. J Psychopharmacol 18:205–214, 2004

Trivedi MH, Fava M, Wisniewski SR, et al: Medication augmentation after the failure of SSRIs for depression. N Engl J Med 354:1243–1252, 2006

Uchida H, Mamo DC, Mulsant BH, et al: Increased antipsychotic sensitivity in elderly patients: evidence and mechanisms. J Clin Psychiatry 70:397–405, 2009

U.S. Food and Drug Administration: FDA Drug Safety Communication: Revised recommendations for Celexa (citalopram hydrobromide) related to a potential risk of abnormal heart rhythms with high doses. Updated March 2012. Available at: http://www.fda.gov/Drugs/DrugSafety/ucm297391.htm. Accessed June 8, 2013.

van Iersel MB, Zuidema SU, Koopmans RT, et al: Antipsychotics for behavioral and psychological problems in elderly people with dementia: a systematic review of adverse events. Drugs Aging 22:845–858, 2005

Verhey FR, Verkaaik M, Lousberg R: Olanzapine versus haloperidol in the treatment of agitation in elderly patients with dementia: results of a randomized controlled double-blind trial. Dement Geriatr Cogn Disord 21:1–8, 2006

Vis PM, van Baardewijk M, Einarson TR: Duloxetine and venlafaxine-XR in the treatment of major depressive disorder: a meta-analysis of randomized clinical trials. Ann Pharmacother 39:1798–1807, 2005

Wakelin JS: Fluvoxamine in the treatment of the older depressed patient: double-blind, placebo-controlled data. Int Clin Psychopharmacol 1:221–230, 1986

Walker Z, Grace J, Overshot R, et al: Olanzapine in dementia with Lewy bodies: a clinical study. Int J Geriatr Psychiatry 14:459–466, 1999

Wallace AE, Kofoed LL, West AN: Double-blind placebo-controlled trial of methylphenidate in older, depressed, medically ill patients. Am J Psychiatry 152:929–931, 1995

Wang PS, Bohn RL, Glynn RJ, et al: Zolpidem use and hip fractures in older people. J Am Geriatr Soc 49:1685–1690, 2001

Wang PS, Schneeweiss S, Avorn J, et al: Risk of death in elderly users of conventional vs. atypical antipsychotic medications. N Engl J Med 353:2335–2341, 2005

Wehmeier PM, Kluge M, Maras A, et al: Fluoxetine versus trimipramine in the treatment of depression in geriatric patients. Pharmacopsychiatry 38:13–16, 2005

Weihs KL, Settle EC Jr, Batey SR, et al: Bupropion sustained release versus paroxetine for the treatment of depression in the elderly. J Clin Psychiatry 61:196–202, 2000

Weintraub D, Rosenberg PB, Drye LT, et al: Sertraline for the treatment of depression in Alzheimer disease: week-24 outcomes. Am J Geriatr Psychiatry 18:332–340, 2010

Whyte EM, Basinski J, Farhi P, et al: Geriatric depression treatment in nonresponders to selective serotonin reuptake inhibitors. J Clin Psychiatry 65:1634–1641, 2004

Whyte E, Romkes M, Mulsant BH, et al: CYP2D6 genotype and venlafaxine-XR concentrations in depressed elderly. Int J Geriatr Psychiatry 21:1–8, 2006

Wilner KD, Tensfeldt TG, Baris B, et al: Single- and multiple-dose pharmacokinetics of ziprasidone in healthy young and elderly volunteers. Br J Clin Pharmacol 49(suppl):15S–20S, 2000

Wilson K, Mottram P: A comparison of side effects of selective serotonin reuptake inhibitors and tricyclic antidepressants in older depressed patients: a meta-analysis. Int J Geriatr Psychiatry 19:754–762, 2004

Winblad B, Kilander L, Eriksson S, et al: Donepezil in patients with severe Alzheimer's disease: double-blind, parallel-group, placebo-controlled study. Lancet 367:1057–1065, 2006

Wingen M, Bothmer J, Langer S, et al: Actual driving performance and psychomotor function in healthy subjects after acute and subchronic treatment with escitalopram, mirtazapine, and placebo: a crossover trial. J Clin Psychiatry 66:436–443, 2005

Wohlreich MM, Sullivan MD, Mallinckrodt CH, et al: Duloxetine for the treatment of recurrent major depressive disorder in elderly patients: treatment outcomes in patients with comorbid arthritis. Psychosomatics 50:402–412, 2009

Wu E, Greenberg PE, Yang E, et al: Comparison of escitalopram versus citalopram for the treatment of major depressive disorder in a geriatric population. Curr Med Res Opin 24:2587–2595, 2008a

Wu E, Greenberg P, Yang E, et al: Comparison of treatment persistence, hospital utilization and costs among major depressive disorder geriatric patients treated with escitalopram versus other SSRI/SNRI antidepressants. Curr Med Res Opin 24:2805–2813, 2008b

Wylie ME, Miller MD, Shear MK, et al: Fluvoxamine pharmacotherapy of anxiety disorders in late life: preliminary open-trial data. J Geriatr Psychiatry Neurol 13:43–48, 2000

Yang CH, Tsai SJ, Hwang JP: The efficacy and safety of quetiapine for treatment of geriatric psychosis. J Psychopharmacol 19:661–666, 2005

Young RC, Gyulai L, Mulsant BH, et al: Pharmacotherapy of bipolar disorder in old age: review and recommendations. Am J Geriatr Psychiatry 12:342–357, 2004

Yuan Y, Tsoi K, Hunt RH: Selective serotonin reuptake inhibitors and risk of upper GI bleeding: confusion or confounding? Am J Med 119:719–727, 2006

Zheng L, Mack WJ, Dagerman KS, et al: Metabolic changes associated with second-generation antipsychotic use in Alzheimer's disease patients: the CATIE-AD study. Am J Psychiatry 166:583–590, 2009

Zhong KX, Tariot PN, Mintzer J, et al: Quetiapine to treat agitation in dementia: a randomized, double-blind, placebo-controlled study. Curr Alzheimer Res 4:81–93, 2007

Zimmer B, Kant R, Zeiler D, et al: Antidepressant efficacy and cardiovascular safety of venlafaxine in young vs. old patients with comorbid medical disorders. Int J Psychiatry Med 27:353–364, 1997

Suggested Readings

Alexopoulos GS, Katz IR, Reynolds CF 3rd, et al: Pharmacotherapy of depression in older patients: a summary of the expert consensus guidelines. J Psychiatr Pract 7:361–376, 2001

Gauthier S, Cummings J, Ballard C, et al: Management of behavioral problems in Alzheimer's disease. Int Psychogeriatr 22:346–372, 2010

Pinquart M, Duberstein PR, Lyness JM: Treatments for later-life depressive conditions: a meta-analytic comparison of pharmacotherapy and psychotherapy. Am J Psychiatry 163:1493–1501, 2006

Rabins PV, Lyketsos CG: Antipsychotic drugs in dementia: what should be made of the risks? JAMA 294:1963–1965, 2005

Schneider LS, Dagerman KS, Insel P: Efficacy and adverse effects of atypical antipsychotics for dementia: meta-analysis of randomized placebo-controlled trials. Am J Geriatr Psychiatry 14:191–210, 2006

Sink KM, Holden KF, Yaffe K: Pharmacological treatment of neuropsychiatric symptoms of dementia: a review of the evidence. JAMA 293:596–608, 2005

Young RC, Gyulai L, Mulsant BH, et al: Pharmacotherapy of bipolar disorder in old age: review and recommendations. Am J Geriatr Psychiatry 12:342–357, 2004

3

Delirium

Li-Wen Huang, M.D.
Sharon K. Inouye, M.D., M.P.H.

Delirium, defined as an acute change in attention and overall cognitive function, is a common, morbid, yet potentially preventable medical problem for older persons. Patients age 65 years and older account for almost half (49%) of all days of hospital care, and although delirium is the most frequent complication affecting this population, it often goes unrecognized (Inouye 2006; U.S. Department of Health and Human Services 2004). Delirium is independently associated with an increased risk of mortality, institutionalization, long-term cognitive decline and dementia, and functional decline (Inouye 2006; MacLullich et al. 2009; Saczynski et al. 2012; Witlox et al. 2010). Total health care costs related to delirium are estimated at $45 billion to $181 billion (2013 USD) annually (Leslie et al. 2008).

Definition and Assessment Tools

The DSM-5 (American Psychiatric Association 2013) diagnostic criteria for delirium are generally accepted as the diagnostic standard. Compared with DSM-IV-TR, DSM-5 has shifted away from using "disturbance of consciousness" in favor of "disturbance of attention and awareness" as a core symptom of delirium, given the difficulty of operationalizing the term "consciousness." DSM-5 also introduced the categorization of delirium into different motoric subtypes, which may be clinically useful given differences in their prognoses and associated symptoms.

The Confusion Assessment Method (CAM; Inouye et al. 1990) provides a simple yet highly sensitive and specific diagnostic algorithm and has become widely used for the identification of delirium (Table 3–1). The CAM also has been adapted for use in the intensive care unit (CAM-ICU; Ely et al. 2001) and nursing home (Minimum Data Set Version 3.0; Centers for Medicare & Medicaid Services 2010).

DSM-5 Diagnostic Criteria for Delirium

A. A disturbance in attention (i.e., reduced ability to direct, focus, sustain, and shift attention) and awareness (reduced orientation to the environment).

B. The disturbance develops over a short period of time (usually hours to a few days), represents a change from baseline attention and awareness, and tends to fluctuate in severity during the course of a day.

C. An additional disturbance in cognition (e.g., memory deficit, disorientation, language, visuospatial ability, or perception).

D. The disturbances in Criteria A and C are not better explained by another preexisting, established, or evolving neurocognitive disorder and do not occur in the context of a severely reduced level of arousal, such as coma.

E. There is evidence from the history, physical examination, or laboratory findings that the disturbance is a direct physiological consequence of another medical condition, substance intoxication or withdrawal (i.e., due to a drug of abuse or to a medication), or exposure to a toxin, or is due to multiple etiologies.

Specify whether:

Substance intoxication delirium: This diagnosis should be made instead of substance intoxication when the symptoms in Criteria A and C predominate in the clinical picture and when they are sufficiently severe to warrant clinical attention.

Substance withdrawal delirium: This diagnosis should be made instead of substance withdrawal when the symptoms in Criteria A and C predominate in the clinical picture and when they are sufficiently severe to warrant clinical attention.

Medication-induced delirium: This diagnosis applies when the symptoms in Criteria A and C arise as a side effect of a medication taken as prescribed.

Delirium due to another medical condition: There is evidence from the history, physical examination, or laboratory findings that the disturbance is attributable to the physiological consequences of another medical condition.

Delirium due to multiple etiologies: There is evidence from the history, physical examination, or laboratory findings that the delirium has more than one etiology (e.g., more than one etiological medical condition; another medical condition plus substance intoxication or medication side effect).

Specify if:

Acute: Lasting a few hours or days.

Persistent: Lasting weeks or months.

Specify if:

Hyperactive: The individual has a hyperactive level of psychomotor activity that may be accompanied by mood lability, agitation, and/or refusal to cooperate with medical care.

Hypoactive: The individual has a hypoactive level of psychomotor activity that may be accompanied by sluggishness and lethargy that approaches stupor.

Mixed level of activity: The individual has a normal level of psychomotor activity even though attention and awareness are disturbed. Also includes individuals whose activity level rapidly fluctuates.

Note. Details on coding not included. See DSM-5 for full criteria, including coding information.

Table 3–1.   Confusion Assessment Method (CAM) diagnostic algorithm

Feature 1. Acute onset and fluctuating course

This feature is usually obtained from a reliable reporter, such as a family member, caregiver, or nurse, and is shown by positive responses to these questions: Is there evidence of an acute change in mental status from the patient's baseline? Did the (abnormal) behavior fluctuate during the day, that is, tend to come and go, or did it increase and decrease in severity?

Feature 2. Inattention

This feature is shown by a positive response to this question: Did the patient have difficulty focusing attention, for example, being easily distractible, or have difficulty keeping track of what was being said?

Feature 3. Disorganized thinking

This feature is shown by a positive response to this question: Was the patient's thinking disorganized or incoherent, such as rambling or irrelevant conversation, unclear or illogical flow of ideas, or unpredictable switching from subject to subject?

Feature 4. Altered level of consciousness

This feature is shown by any answer other than "alert" to this question: Overall, how would you rate this patient's level of consciousness (alert [normal], vigilant [hyperalert], lethargic [drowsy, easily aroused], stupor [difficult to arouse], or coma [unarousable])?

Note.   The CAM ratings should be completed following brief cognitive assessment of the patient, for example, with the Mini-Mental State Examination. The diagnosis of delirium by CAM requires the presence of features 1 and 2 and of either 3 or 4.
Source.   Adapted from Inouye SK, Vandyck CH, Alessi CA, et al.: "Clarifying Confusion: The Confusion Assessment Method—A New Method for Detection of Delirium." *Annals of Internal Medicine* 113:941–948, 1990. Used with permission.

Epidemiology

Delirium is often the only sign of an acute and serious medical condition affecting a patient, and it most commonly occurs in frail older persons with an underlying disease process. Delirium affects 11%–42% of hospitalized older adults (Siddiqi et al. 2006), up to 30% of older patients in the emergency department, up to 60% of those in nursing home or post–acute care settings (Inouye 2006), and 2%–73% of older patients postoperatively (Sieber 2009).

Incidence rates increase to 70%–87% of older patients in intensive care units and in palliative care settings (Inouye 2006).

Clinical Features

Acute onset, fluctuating course, and alteration in attention are the core features of delirium. Establishing a patient's level of baseline cognitive function and the course of cognitive change is critical. Cognitive changes that occur abruptly over days are indicative of delirium, whereas changes that progress gradually over months to years are indicative of dementia. The cognitive evaluation for delirium should examine for evidence of global cognitive changes, impairment in attention, disorganized thought process, and altered level of consciousness. Other clinical features commonly associated with delirium are psychomotor agitation, paranoid delusions, sleep-wake cycle disruption, emotional lability, and perceptual disturbances or hallucinations.

Clinically, delirium can present as different psychomotor subtypes. Hypoactive delirium, more common in older patients, is characterized by lethargy and reduced psychomotor functioning, which is often misattributed to depression or fatigue. Although the hypoactive form of delirium is associated with a poorer prognosis, it is often unrecognized or misdiagnosed (Yang et al. 2009). Hyperactive delirium, characterized by agitation, increased vigilance, and often hallucinations, rarely goes unnoticed. Mixed delirium, in which patients fluctuate between hypoactive and hyperactive delirium, is difficult to distinguish from symptoms of other psychotic or mood disorders.

Pathophysiology

The fundamental pathophysiological mechanisms of delirium remain unclear. Several cerebral blood flow studies using positron emission tomography or single-photon emission computed tomography have found that delirium is associated with localized hypoperfusion. Other neuroimaging studies, using computed tomography or magnetic resonance imaging, have detected structural abnormalities, such as cortical atrophy, in the brains of patients with delirium (Fong et al. 2009b). Currently, delirium is viewed as the final common pathway of many different pathogenic mechanisms, including imbalances in neurotransmission, inflammation, and chronic stress. The most frequently considered mechanism of delirium is cholinergic dysfunction. Acetylcholine plays a key role in mediating consciousness and attentional processes. Anticholinergic drugs can induce delirium, and serum anticholinergic activity is increased in patients with delirium (Marcantonio et al. 2006). An excess of dopaminergic neurotransmission, which regulates the release of acetylcholine, also has been linked with delirium (Trzepacz and van der Mast 2002). Elevated serotonin is another proposed mechanism of delirium (Marcantonio et al. 2006).

Chronic stress induced by severe illness, trauma, or surgery involves sympathetic and immune system activation that may lead to delirium. This activation may include increased activity of the hypothalamic-pituitary-adrenal axis with hypercortisolism, release of cerebral cytokines that alter neurotransmitter systems, alterations in the thyroid axis, and modification of blood-brain barrier permeability.

Risk Factors

Delirium usually has multifactorial causes. Although it can be caused by a single factor, delirium more typically develops as a result of the interrelation between patient vulnerability and noxious insults or precipitating factors (Inouye and Charpentier 1996). Existing cognitive impairment and dementia are the leading risk factors for the development of delirium (Trzepacz and van der Mast 2002). Other predisposing and precipitating factors for delirium are listed in Table 3–2.

The role of medications in the development of delirium deserves special attention (Table 3–3). Medication use contributes to delirium in more than 40% of cases (Inouye and Charpentier 1996). The clinician must conduct a complete review of all prescription and over-the-counter medications. Medications with known psychoactive effects should be minimized or discontinued. The medications most strongly associated with delirium include sedative-hypnotics such as benzodiazepines, narcotics such as opioids, and histamine H_1 receptor antagonists. Drugs with anticholinergic effects have also been associated with delirium (Alagiakrishnan and Wiens 2004; Clegg and Young 2011). Given the role of medications in contributing to the devel-

Table 3–2. Predisposing and precipitating factors for delirium

Predisposing factors

Demographic characteristics
  Age 65 years or older
  Male gender
Coexisting medical conditions
  Severe illness
  Multiple coexisting conditions
  Chronic renal or hepatic disease
  History of stroke
  Infection with HIV
  Metabolic derangements
  Neurological disease
  Terminal illness
  Fracture or trauma
Cognitive status
  Dementia
  Cognitive impairment
  History of delirium
  Depression

Decreased oral intake
  Dehydration
  Malnutrition
Drugs
  Treatment with psychoactive drugs
  Treatment with many drugs
  Alcohol abuse
Functional status
  Functional dependence
  Immobility
  Low level of activity
  History of falls
Sensory impairment
  Visual impairment
  Hearing impairment

Precipitating factors

Drugs
  Sedative-hypnotics
  Narcotics
  Anticholinergic drugs
  Treatment with multiple drugs
  Alcohol or drug withdrawal
Environment
  Admission to intensive care unit
  Use of physical restraints
  Use of bladder catheter
  Use of multiple procedures
  Pain
  Emotional stress
Primary neurological disease
  Stroke, particularly nondominant
    hemispheric
  Intracranial bleeding
  Meningitis or encephalitis

Intercurrent illnesses
  Infections
  Iatrogenic complications
  Severe acute illness
  Hypoxia
  Shock
  Fever or hypothermia
  Anemia
  Dehydration
  Poor nutritional status
  Low serum albumin level
  Metabolic derangements (e.g., electrolytes)
Sensory impairment
  Visual impairment
  Hearing impairment
Surgery
  Orthopedic surgery
  Cardiac surgery
  Prolonged cardiopulmonary bypass
  Noncardiac surgery

Source. From NEJM, Inouye SK: "Current Concepts: Delirium in Older Persons." 354, 1157–1165. Copyright 2006. Massachusetts Medical Society. Reprinted with permission.

Table 3–3. Medications associated with delirium

Sedative-hypnotics
  Benzodiazepines (especially long-acting agents such as chlordiazepoxide, diazepam, flurazepam)
  Barbiturates (phenobarbital)

Analgesics
  Opioids (especially meperidine)
  Nonsteroidal anti-inflammatory drugs

Psychoactive medications
  Tricyclic antidepressants (amitriptyline, imipramine, doxepin)
  Antipsychotics (chlorpromazine, haloperidol, thioridazine)
  Antiparkinsonian agents (trihexyphenidyl, benztropine, levodopa)

Cardiovascular medications
  Digitalis glycosides (digoxin)
  Antiarrhythmics (quinidine, procainamide, lidocaine, disopyramide)
  Antihypertensives (β-blockers, methyldopa)

Gastrointestinal medications
  Histamine H_2 receptor antagonists (cimetidine, ranitidine, famotidine)
  Antiemetics (scopolamine, metoclopramide)
  Antidiarrheals (diphenoxylate/atropine, loperamide)

Other
  Incontinence medications (oxybutynin, hyoscyamine)
  Histamine H_1 receptor antagonists (especially first-generation, such as diphenhydramine, hydroxyzine)
  Steroids (prednisone)
  Alternative medicines (*Atropa belladonna*, jimsonweed, henbane, mandrake)

opment of delirium, the clinician must conduct a complete review of all prescription and over-the-counter medications. Medications with known psychoactive effects should be minimized or discontinued.

Diagnosis and Differential Diagnosis

The diagnosis of delirium is based on clinical observation and relies on a thorough cognitive assessment, a detailed history from a reliable informant, and a comprehensive physical and neurological examination. The goal of a thorough history is to establish that a change has occurred from the patient's baseline cognitive functioning. To facilitate early diagnosis and treatment of delirium, clinicians must identify all multifactorial contributors.

The clinician's most important and difficult task is to differentiate delirium from dementia. Nearly two-thirds of cases of delirium occur in patients with dementia (Inouye 2006). Patients with dementia who develop a superimposed delirium experience a more rapid progression of cognitive dysfunction and worse long-term prognosis (Fick and Foreman 2000; Fong et al. 2009a). The key diagnostic feature that aids in distinguishing these two conditions is the acute onset of delirium, which contrasts with the more gradual progression of dementia. Changes in attention and level of consciousness also point to delirium. However, establishing the occurrence of those changes can be difficult in the face of missing baseline cognitive assessment data or preexisting cognitive deficits. If the differentiation cannot be made with certainty, then given the life-threatening nature of delirium, the patient should receive treatment for delirium until proven otherwise.

Other important diagnoses that must be differentiated from delirium include psychiatric conditions such as depression, mania, and schizophrenia. Differentiating among diagnoses is critical because delirium carries a more serious prognosis without proper evaluation and management. Treatment for certain conditions such as depression or mood disorders may involve the use of drugs with anticholinergic activity, which could exacerbate an unrecognized case of delirium.

No specific laboratory tests currently exist for the definitive identification of delirium. The laboratory evaluation for delirium is intended to identify contributing factors that need to be addressed, and the approach should be guided by clinical judgment and tailored to the individual situation. Laboratory tests that should be considered include complete blood count, electrolytes, kidney and liver function, oxygen saturation, and glucose levels. Evaluation of occult infection can be performed through blood cultures, urinalysis, and urine culture. Other laboratory tests, such as thyroid function, arterial blood gas, vitamin B_{12} level, cortisol level, drug levels, toxicology screen, and ammonia levels, are also helpful in identifying factors that contribute to delirium. Overall, the routine use of neuroimaging in delirium is not recommended because the overall diagnostic yield is low, and the findings change the management of patients in less than 10% of cases (Hirano et al. 2006).

Prevention and Management

Prevention

Primary prevention is the most effective strategy to decrease delirium and its complications. The Hospital Elder Life Program (HELP; www.hospitalelder-lifeprogram.org) uses a targeted risk factor reduction approach for prevention of delirium (Inouye et al. 1999, 2000). HELP is a hospital-wide program that is cost-effective and contributes to overall improvement in geriatric care in the hospital setting. Several multicomponent interventions, including staff education, individually tailored treatments, and proactive geriatric consultation, have been shown to be effective in reducing delirium incidence, duration, or severity (Marcantonio et al. 2001; Milisen et al. 2005; Naughton et al. 2005). Overall, these trials suggest that 40% of cases of delirium may be preventable and that prevention strategies should begin as soon as possible after hospital admission.

Studies have explored the potential of pharmacological prevention of delirium. Some studies suggest that risperidone, olanzapine, and haloperidol may be effective for decreasing delirium incidence or duration and severity, but these trials remain inconclusive. Cholinesterase inhibitors have not been found to be effective for prevention. There has been interest in the effect of α_2-adrenergic agonist dexmedetomidine instead of other sedative agents in perioperative delirium, but results thus far have been contradictory (Campbell et al. 2009; Steiner 2011).

Management

In general, nonpharmacological approaches should be implemented as the first-line treatment of delirium. Nonpharmacological treatment approaches include reorientation, behavioral interventions, increased supervision, correcting sensory deficits, and minimizing use of physical restraints (Inouye et al. 2007). Strategies that increase the patient's mobility, self-care, and independence should be promoted. Other environmental interventions include limiting room and staff changes, providing a quiet patient care setting with low-level lighting at night, and implementing a nonpharmacological sleep protocol (McDowell et al. 1998), allowing for an uninterrupted period for sleep.

Pharmacological management of delirium (Table 3–4; Campbell et al. 2009; Grover et al. 2011; Steiner 2011) should be used only in patients who have severe agitation that interferes with the application of medical treatments (e.g., intubation) or in patients who pose a danger to themselves, other patients, or staff. The lowest dose of medication should be prescribed for the shortest time possible, because drugs used to treat delirium can also lead to an increase in acute confusion. The goal for drug management should be an alert and manageable patient, not one who is lethargic and sedated. Data on pharmacological treatment of delirium have been limited by small sample sizes and a lack of placebo-controlled trials (Campbell et al. 2009; Grover et al. 2011). If required, haloperidol remains the first-line pharmacological treatment for delirium. Haloperidol is the most widely used agent, with documented efficacy for decreasing delirium symptoms (Breitbart et al. 1996), although no placebo-controlled trials exist.

Compared with haloperidol, atypical antipsychotics have been found to have roughly similar efficacy and a lower rate of extrapyramidal side effects in small trials (Lonergan et al. 2007). Benzodiazepines are not recommended for treating non-alcohol-related delirium because they typically lead to oversedation, exacerbation of confusion, and prolonged delirium (Breitbart et al. 1996; Lonergan et al. 2009). However, they remain the treatment of choice for alcohol or sedative-hypnotic drug withdrawal. The cholinesterase inhibitor rivastigmine has been found to increase mortality among patients with delirium in intensive care units, and thus cholinesterase inhibitors are not recommended for the treatment of delirium (van Eijk et al. 2010).

References

Alagiakrishnan K, Wiens CA: An approach to drug induced delirium in the elderly. Postgrad Med J 80:388–393, 2004

American Psychiatric Association: Diagnostic and Statistical Manual of Mental Disorders, 5th Edition. Washington, DC, American Psychiatric Association, 2013

Table 3–4.   Pharmacological management of delirium

Medication	Geriatric dosing and route of administration	Adverse effects	Evidence
First-generation (typical) antipsychotic *Haloperidol is the recommended first-line agent.*			
Haloperidol	0.25–0.50 mg twice daily orally, repeat every 4 hours as needed (peak effect, 4–6 hours). 0.25–0.50 mg intramuscularly; observe after 30–60 minutes and repeat as needed (peak effect, 20–40 minutes). Total daily dose not to exceed 3 mg. Intravenous use not FDA approved and should be avoided due to increased risk of hypotension and QTc prolongation.	Extrapyramidal symptoms, especially if dosage is >3 mg/day. QTc prolongation, torsades de pointes, hypotension. Use with caution in patients with hepatic impairment, Parkinson's disease, or neuroleptic malignant syndrome.	Decreased delirium symptoms in randomized, non-placebo-controlled trial.

Table 3–4. Pharmacological management of delirium *(continued)*

Medication	Geriatric dosing and route of administration	Adverse effects	Evidence
Second-generation (atypical) antipsychotics			
Effective alternatives to haloperidol, associated with fewer extrapyramidal effects. Possible increased mortality in dementia patients.			
Risperidone	0.5 mg twice daily orally as needed.	Extrapyramidal side effects at higher dosages; QTc prolongation, torsades de pointes, hypotension, neuroleptic malignant syndrome, diabetes. Use with caution in patients with renal or hepatic impairment.	Efficacy similar to that of haloperidol in small or isolated randomized trials.
Olanzapine	2.5–5.0 mg once daily orally as needed.		
Quetiapine	25 mg twice daily orally as needed.		
Benzodiazepines			
Second-line agents for delirium; reserve for use in sedative and alcohol withdrawal, Parkinson's disease, or neuroleptic malignant syndrome.			
Lorazepam	0.5–1.0 mg orally, repeat every 4 hours as needed. Intravenous use of lorazepam should be reserved for emergencies only.	Increased confusion, paradoxical excitation, respiratory depression, oversedation.	

Note. FDA = U.S. Food and Drug Administration.

Breitbart W, Marotta R, Platt MM, et al: A double-blind trial of haloperidol, chlorpromazine, and lorazepam in the treatment of delirium in hospitalized AIDS patients. Am J Psychiatry 153:231–237, 1996

Campbell N, Boustani MA, Ayub A, et al: Pharmacological management of delirium in hospitalized adults: a systematic evidence review. J Gen Intern Med 24:848–853, 2009

Centers for Medicare & Medicaid Services: MDS 3.0 for Nursing Homes and Swing Bed Providers. Available at: http://www.cms.gov/Medicare/Quality-Initiatives-Patient-Assessment-Instruments/NursingHomeQualityInits/NHQIMDS30.html. Accessed December 8, 2010.

Clegg A, Young JB: Which medications to avoid in people at risk of delirium: a systematic review. Age Ageing 40:23–29, 2011

Ely EW, Margolin R, Francis J, et al: Evaluation of delirium in critically ill patients: validation of the Confusion Assessment Method for the Intensive Care Unit (CAM-ICU). Crit Care Med 29:1370–1379, 2001

Fick D, Foreman M: Consequences of not recognizing delirium superimposed on dementia in hospitalized elderly individuals. J Gerontol Nurs 26:30–40, 2000

Fong TG, Jones RN, Shi P, et al: Delirium accelerates cognitive decline in Alzheimer disease. Neurology 72:1570–1575, 2009a

Fong TG, Tulebaev SR, Inouye SK: Delirium in elderly adults: diagnosis, prevention and treatment. Nat Rev Neurol 5:210–220, 2009b

Grover S, Mattoo SK, Gupta N: Usefulness of atypical antipsychotics and choline esterase inhibitors in delirium: a review. Pharmacopsychiatry 44:43–54, 2011

Hirano LA, Bogardus ST, Saluja S, et al: Clinical yield of computed tomography brain scans in older general medical patients. J Am Geriatr Soc 54:587–592, 2006

Inouye SK: Current concepts: delirium in older persons. N Engl J Med 354:1157–1165, 2006. Available at: www.nejm.org/doi/full/10.1056/NEJMra052321.

Inouye SK, Charpentier PA: Precipitating factors for delirium in hospitalized elderly persons: predictive model and interrelationship with baseline vulnerability. JAMA 275:852–857, 1996

Inouye SK, Vandyck CH, Alessi CA, et al: Clarifying confusion: the Confusion Assessment Method—a new method for detection of delirium. Ann Intern Med 113:941–948, 1990

Inouye SK, Bogardus ST, Charpentier PA, et al: A multicomponent intervention to prevent delirium in hospitalized older patients. N Engl J Med 340:669–676, 1999

Inouye SK, Bogardus ST, Baker DI, et al: The Hospital Elder Life Program: a model of care to prevent cognitive and functional decline in hospitalized older patients. J Am Geriatr Soc 48:1697–1706, 2000

Inouye SK, Zhang Y, Jones RN, et al: Risk factors for delirium at discharge: development and validation of a predictive model. Arch Intern Med 167:1406–1413, 2007

Leslie DL, Marcantonio ER, Zhang Y, et al: One-year health care costs associated with delirium in the elderly population. Arch Intern Med 168:27–32, 2008

Lonergan E, Britton AM, Luxenberg J: Antipsychotics for delirium. Cochrane Database of Systematic Reviews 2007, Issue 2. Art. No. CD005594. DOI: 10.1002/14651858. CD005594.pub2.

Lonergan E, Luxenberg J, Areosa Sastre A: Benzodiazepines for delirium. Cochrane Database of Systematic Reviews 2009, Issue 4. Art. No.: CD006379. DOI: 10.1002/14651858. CD006379. pub3.

MacLullich AM, Beaglehole A, Hall RJ, et al: Delirium and long-term cognitive impairment. Int Rev Psychiatry 21:30–42, 2009

Marcantonio ER, Flacker JM, Wright RJ, et al: Reducing delirium after hip fracture: a randomized trial. J Am Geriatr Soc 49:516–522, 2001

Marcantonio ER, Rudolph JL, Culley D, et al: Serum biomarkers for delirium. J Gerontol A Biol Sci Med Sci 61:1281–1286, 2006

McDowell JA, Mion LC, Lydon TJ, et al: A nonpharmacologic sleep protocol for hospitalized older patients. J Am Geriatr Soc 46:700–705, 1998

Milisen K, Lemiengre J, Braes T, et al: Multicomponent intervention strategies for managing delirium in hospitalized older people: systematic review. J Adv Nurs 52:79–90, 2005

Naughton BJ, Saltzman S, Ramadan F, et al: A multifactorial intervention to reduce prevalence of delirium and shorten hospital length of stay. J Am Geriatr Soc 53:18–23, 2005

Saczynski JS, Marcantonio ER, Quach L, et al: Cognitive trajectories after postoperative delirium. N Engl J Med 367:30–39, 2012

Siddiqi N, House AO, Holmes JD: Occurrence and outcome of delirium in medical in-patients: a systematic literature review. Age Ageing 35:350–364, 2006

Sieber FE: Postoperative delirium in the elderly surgical patient. Anesthesiol Clin 27:451–464, 2009

Steiner LA: Postoperative delirium, part 2: detection, prevention and treatment. Eur J Anaesthesiol 28:723–732, 2011

Trzepacz PT, van der Mast R: The neuropathophysiology of delirium, in Delirium in Old Age. Edited by Lindesay J, Rockwood K, MacDonald AJ. New York, Oxford University Press, 2002, pp 51–90

U.S. Department of Health and Human Services: 2004 CMS statistics. Washington, DC, Centers for Medicare and Medicaid Services, 2004 van Eijk MM, Roes KC, Honing ML, et al: Effect of rivastigmine as an adjunct to usual care with haloperidol on duration of delirium and mortality in critically ill patients: a multicentre, double-blind, placebo-controlled randomised trial. Lancet 376:1829–1837, 2010

Witlox J, Eurelings LS, de Jonghe JF, et al: Delirium in elderly patients and the risk of postdischarge mortality, institutionalization, and dementia: a meta-analysis. JAMA 304:443–451, 2010

Yang FM, Marcantonio ER, Inouye SK, et al: Phenomenological subtypes of delirium in older persons: patterns, prevalence, and prognosis. Psychosomatics 50:248–254, 2009

4

Dementia and Milder Cognitive Syndromes

Constantine G. Lyketsos, M.D., M.H.S.

Dementia is a clinical syndrome that can be caused by a range of diseases or injuries to the brain. Given that dementia is a chronic disease, with estimates of its duration ranging from 3 to 4 years in community settings (Graham et al. 1997) and from 10 to 12 years in clinical settings (Rabins et al. 2006), it poses a unique public health problem with serious effects on its victims, their families, and society at large. In the United States alone, it is estimated that by 2050, the annual cost of heath care, long-term care, and hospice care for patients with dementia will be close to $1.2 trillion (in 2013 dollars) (Alzheimer's Association 2013).

In this chapter, I discuss definitions, clinical presentation, and evaluation, including differential diagnosis, of dementia and related cognitive disorders; describe specific dementia syndromes according to their etiology; and discuss how to approach treatment. For an in-depth discussion of the clinical management of dementia, the reader is referred to *Practical Dementia Care* by Rabins et al. (2006).

Definitions

Definitions related to dementia, as espoused by the American Association for Geriatric Psychiatry (Lyketsos et al. 2006), are presented below.

- **Cognitive impairment not dementia (CIND):** A clinical syndrome consisting of a measurable or evident decline in memory or other cognitive abilities, with little effect on day-to-day functioning; does not meet criteria for dementia.
- **Mild cognitive impairment:** A clinical subsyndrome of CIND, most likely the prodrome to Alzheimer's dementia. Can be amnestic (having memory deficits) or nonamnestic.
- **Dementia:** A clinical syndrome not entirely due to delirium, consisting of global cognitive decline, with several areas of cognition affected, and significant effect on day-to-day functioning.
- **Alzheimer's dementia:** A dementia syndrome that has gradual onset and slow progression and is best explained as caused by Alzheimer's disease.
- **Alzheimer's disease:** A brain disease characterized by plaques, tangles, and neuronal loss.

Although these definitions are important to the clinical world, one should recognize that uncertainty remains about linking cognitive syndromes to brain pathology. For example, in community settings, most patients with dementia have mixed brain pathologies, including Alzheimer's disease, microinfarcts, lacunar infarcts, and Lewy bodies (Neuropathology Group, Medical Research Council Cognitive Function and Aging Study 2001; White and Launer 2006).

Clinical Presentation

Patients With the Dementia Syndrome

One of the most important changes in DSM-5 (American Psychiatric Association 2013) is the new category of neurocognitive disorders (NCDs) that replaces the category of "Dementia, Delirium, Amnestic, and Other Cognitive Disorders" in DSM-IV-TR (American Psychiatric Association 2000). The term "dementia" is replaced with the term "major neurocognitive disorder." The term dementia is however retained in DSM-5 for continuity any may be used by physicians and patients accustomed to this term. The term neurocognitive disorder is thought to better describe conditions affecting younger adults, such as impairment secondary to traumatic brain injury or HIV infection, whereas dementia has customarily been used for degenerative disorders typically seen in older adults. For the purpose of this chapter, we will continue to use the term "dementia" rather than "major neurocognitive disorder" and will clarify any additional terms that are updated in DSM-5.

Dementia is defined entirely on clinical grounds. Table 4–1 lists the four critical elements of the definition. Dementia is a condition that affects *cognition*. For the dementia syndrome to be present, several areas of cognition must be affected (*global*). To differentiate dementia from mental retardation, the cognitive symptoms must represent a cognitive *decline* for the individual. The decline must be significant, typically sufficient to affect the person's daily functioning. Finally, because delirium can cause the full range of cognitive symptoms associated with dementia, it is critical that the cognitive syndrome be present in the *absence of delirium*. This broad definition has been operationalized in several criteria, with those of DSM-IV-TR (American Psychiatric Association 2000) being the most commonly used.

Table 4–1.   Four key elements of the dementia syndrome

Cognitive

Global

Decline

Absence of delirium

Although dementia is defined around cognitive disturbances, patients with dementia have a wider range of impairments. These include functional, neuropsychiatric (behavioral), and neurological impairments. In the functional realm, patients have problems in their social and interpersonal functioning and in their ability to live independently. Patients with milder dementia have difficulties with instrumental abilities, whereas patients with more severe dementia develop impairments in their basic abilities to perform activities of daily living.

Dementia also has been associated with several neuropsychiatric symptoms, such as apathy, depression, agitation, psychosis, and disinhibited behaviors. Over the course of a progressive dementia, essentially all patients develop one or more of these symptoms (Steinberg et al. 2008).

Finally, patients with dementia develop a range of neurological findings. Most common are gait disorders, especially unstable, ataxic, or labored gait. Other neurological symptoms include incontinence, focal findings, seizures, and, less commonly, cranial nerve findings.

Patients With Milder Cognitive Syndromes

Large numbers of older people have cognitive impairments that are troubling to them or family members but not sufficiently severe or broad to meet criteria for dementia. The prevalence of these impairments might be as high as 18% after age 65 (Lopez et al. 2003). Most patients who develop progressive dementia do so in stages and typically go through a prodromal period of cognitive impairment, most often with memory symptoms, that is characteristic of the specific cause of the dementia. Thus, for example, it appears that mild cognitive impairment (MCI) is a prodrome to Alzheimer's disease because many patients who meet MCI criteria have Alzheimer's disease pathology. The term *vascular cognitive impairment* (Hachinski 2007) refers to nondementia disturbances associated with brain vascular disease, likely the prodrome of vascular dementia. Whereas the prodrome of Alzheimer's disease, MCI, appears to have primarily cortical features, the prodrome of vascular dementia, vascular cognitive impairment, typically affects executive functions (Hayden et al. 2006).

DSM-5 formally introduces these milder cognitive syndromes under the category of "Mild Neurocognitive Disorder," which, like MCI, is characterized by evidence of mild cognitive decline in one or more cognitive domains that does not interfere with capacity for independence in everyday activities. The diagnosis is further subtyped based on presumed etiology (e.g., Alzheimer's disease, vascular disease). Mild neurocognitive disorder is thought to be on a continuum with major neurocognitive disorder, and the precise threshold for making the diagnoses depends on careful history, collateral information and observation while taking into account other findings of relevance to cognition.

Conducting an Evaluation

History Taking

The patient's medical history is critical to a good dementia evaluation. The inclusion of an informant is critical. Because informants themselves can be influenced by their own mental states, it is often useful to have additional informants to confirm or disconfirm discrepancies between the history and the evaluation of the patient. Dating the onset of cognitive symptoms is critical. It is important to spend a lot of time trying to determine when the patient was last well as opposed to when the first symptom started. The history should survey for cognitive symptoms; functional losses in social, interpersonal, and daily functioning; the full range of neuropsychiatric symptoms; and neurological deficits.

Communication With Dementia Patients[1]

It is important to highlight that optimally communicating with dementia patients, beginning with the history taking, requires extra care on the clinician's part. Initially, the clinician must get the person's attention and ensure that vision and hearing are "tuned up." The clinician should use eye contact, call the person by name in a clear adult tone, approach slowly from the side or front or crouch down to his or her level, and offer his or her hand, palm up. The clinician should listen but not feel compelled to talk constantly. Words are not as important as a calm tone, pleasant expression, and nondistracting environment (e.g., the television or radio should be turned off or down). Clinicians should use familiar

---

[1]I wish to thank Lisa Gwyther, M.S.W., and Harold Goforth, M.D., for providing this subsection on communication with dementia patients.

words and speak in a normal tone and tempo but give the person time to process and respond. Words should be repeated exactly, if necessary. The clinician who is unsure of the patient's meaning should ask clarifying questions and be patient—repetition of their words can be reassuring to patients.

If frustration mounts, the clinician should suggest a better time to talk or another topic. He or she should avoid ambiguous or vague expressions such as "Don't go there," "NOT," or "bottom line" and use concrete subjects, names, and references. He or she should demonstrate or model so that the patient can follow the clinician's lead. Complex multistep directions must be avoided. The clinician should use appropriate respectful humor or the patient's favorite phrases ("See ya later, alligator") and smile, nod, gesture, or touch gently when words fail.

Cognitive Assessment

Conducting a cognitive assessment is the central aspect of the evaluation. Many specialists use the Mini-Mental State Examination (MMSE; Folstein et al. 1975) as their primary tool. The MMSE is inefficient in evaluating milder cognitive symptoms or mild dementia. The Modified Mini-Mental State provides a broader assessment (Teng and Chui 1987) and has many advantages. For closer assessments of executive functioning, clinicians should consider incorporating the Clock Drawing Test (van der Burg et al. 2004), the Frontal Assessment Battery (Dubois et al. 2000), and the Mental Alternation Test (Jones et al. 1993).

Differential Diagnosis and Diagnostic Testing

The establishment of a careful differential diagnosis is a key aspect of the dementia evaluation. The first step is to develop a differential diagnosis of the syndrome. Figure 4–1 provides a useful flowchart for this purpose.

Neuropsychological testing, although not needed in every case, is often useful in differentiating dementia from milder cognitive syndromes or normal aging, especially in investigating profiles of cognitive impairment that suggest specific etiologies. Further workup using laboratory studies is needed in most cases. Blood tests and brain imaging are typically used in all cases. The American Academy of Neurology (Knopman et al. 2001) recommends thyroid studies, liver tests, metabolic panel, complete blood count, and vitamin B_{12} and

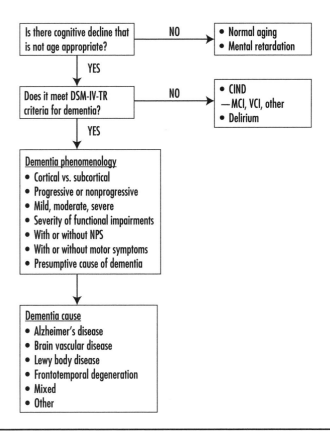

Figure 4–1.   Flowchart for the diagnosis of dementia.

CIND = cognitive impairment not dementia; MCI = mild cognitive impairment; NPS = neuropsychiatric symptoms; VCI = vascular cognitive impairment.

folate levels. Additional tests, such as heavy metal screen, syphilis serology, toxicology, electrocardiogram, and chest X ray, should be considered to determine possible underlying causes. Computed tomography of the head is usually adequate, but some believe it is important to perform magnetic resonance imaging (MRI), especially when brain vascular disease may be involved. Functional brain imaging with positron emission tomography (fluorodeoxyglucose [^{18}FDG]-PET) has come into broader use (Kulasingam et al. 2003). This is most useful in the differential diagnosis of dementia caused by Alzheimer's disease or by frontotemporal degeneration (FTD). In the past, reference was made to treatable and nontreatable dementias. This differentiation is no longer useful for two reasons. First, reversibility of a "treatable dementia" depends on the severity of brain damage that has occurred, not its cause. Second, the implication that Alzheimer's disease, vascular dementia, and other dementias are not treatable is also incorrect. Although these cases tend to be progressive, the application of available treatments makes a big difference to patients, caregivers, and families.

Specific Dementias

Dementia Due to Alzheimer's Disease

Alzheimer's dementia is the most common form of dementia. Depending on the population series, 50%–70% of people with dementia are diagnosed clinically as having dementia due to Alzheimer's disease (McKhann et al. 1984; Ranginwala et al. 2008).

The prevalence of Alzheimer's dementia is closely tied to age, which is the primary risk factor. Other risk factors include traumatic brain injury, reduced reserve capacity of the brain, limited educational or occupational attainment, brain vascular disease, hyperlipidemia, hypertension, atherosclerosis, coronary heart disease, atrial fibrillation, smoking, obesity, and diabetes.

A major risk factor is genetic (Blennow et al. 2006). Alzheimer's disease is a heterogeneous genetic disorder with some familial forms (mutations in genes associated with the amyloid precursor protein (APP) on chromosome 21, as well as the presenilin 1 and 2 genes on chromosomes 14 and 1, respectively) and mostly polygenic forms. Several genes, most unknown, likely increase risk but do not absolutely determine the occurrence of the disease. The most well-known is the apolipoprotein E gene (*APOE*), whose ε4 allele is a risk factor for Alzheimer's dementia.

Neuropsychiatric symptoms are nearly universal. Affective, psychotic, and sleep symptoms relapse and remit through the course of Alzheimer's dementia, whereas apathy appears to be a steadily accumulating symptom in that many but not all patients gradually develop persistent and pervasive apathy (Onyike et al. 2007; Steinberg et al. 2008).

The brain changes seen in Alzheimer's dementia are well known. Even in early disease, atrophy in the hippocampus occurs bilaterally and progresses throughout the brain. Pathologically, the characteristic lesions of Alzheimer's disease include senile or neuritic plaques and neurofibrillary tangles, with associated loss of neurons in several neurotransmitter systems: cholinergic, serotonergic, and dopaminergic. The current hypothesis about etiopathogenesis suggests a cascade (Blennow et al. 2006). Genetic and environmental risk factors interact to increase the production or to decrease the clearance of amyloid derived from APP. APP may be processed through cleavage by β-secretase preferentially over α-secretase, leading to the formation of a form of amyloid beta (Aβ1–42). The latter is prone to dimerization, oligomerization, and deposition in the extracellular space. The deposition of this toxic form of Aβ accumulates close to the synaptic cleft and is thought to lead over time to synaptic disconnection, the loss of neurotransmitter systems, and the emergence of symptoms.

Dementia Due to Brain Vascular Disease (Vascular Dementia)

Vascular dementia is a controversial nosological entity. It is difficult to differentiate on clinical grounds those patients who have Alzheimer's dementia from those who have vascular dementia (Groves et al. 2000). Further complicating the differentiation, subsequent evidence suggests that cerebrovascular risk factors and diseases influence the progression of Alzheimer's dementia (Mielke et al. 2007) and the emergence of Alzheimer's pathology in the brain (Beach et al. 2007; Roher et al. 2006). Most patients with vascular dementia who come to autopsy have mixed pathology, often with significant Alzheimer's disease pathology (Jellinger and Attems 2006).

Vascular dementia, therefore, is best understood as a heterogeneous group of dementias. On one end are patients with pure genetic forms, such as 1) cerebral autosomal dominant arteriopathy with subcortical infarcts and leukoencephalopathy and 2) mitochondrial encephalopathy with lactic acidosis and strokelike episodes. At the other end are patients who develop dementia after multiple strokes in which significant portions of the brain are damaged. Between those two end points are patients with mixtures of pathologies and clinical presentations that affect one another.

The following are some of the risk factors for cerebrovascular disease that are also risk factors for vascular dementia: disease of the large and small vessels of the brain, diabetes, hypertension, and atrial fibrillation and other cardiac disease.

The clinical presentation of vascular dementia is variable. Typically, it presents in fits and spurts, often with acute or subacute onset after a cerebrovascular event. A mix of symptoms usually presents, often including apathy, depression, and motor symptoms. Of patients with vascular dementia or Alzheimer's dementia who have similar MMSE scores, those with vascular dementia are usually more functionally impaired. Gait disorders, parkinsonism, and incontinence are early features.

The diagnosis of vascular dementia is based on a typical clinical history and associated physical examination findings. The diagnosis requires brain imaging that shows completed infarcts or lacunes in brain areas associated with the cognitive changes. A temporal relation between the brain vascular disease and the cognitive changes should be demonstrable, but this might be difficult. Radiological findings of white matter change alone, with no evidence of completed strokes or associated examination findings (e.g., motor focality or gait disorder), are not supportive of a diagnosis of vascular dementia.

Dementias Due to Lewy Body Disease

A consensus panel (Lippa et al. 2007) proposed the term *Lewy body disorders* as an umbrella term for Parkinson's disease (PD), Parkinson's disease dementia (PDD), and dementia with Lewy bodies (DLB). The hypothesis is that these three conditions, which can also be termed *synucleinopathies,* represent brain diseases in which abnormal synuclein metabolism leads to dementia. The sequence of events involved is poorly known. One of the complicating factors in determining a diagnosis is that many patients with Lewy body pathologies have coexisting pathologies, in particular Alzheimer's and vascular pathology. Additionally, the clinical presentations of PDD and DLB can be similar, with motor parkinsonism, gait imbalance, visual hallucinations, and dementia being the unifying clinical features.

Parkinson's Disease Dementia

With the advent of the use of L-dopa to help control Parkinson's motor symptoms, it has become apparent that some of the most common and impairing symptoms of PD are in the cognitive realm. Patients with PD typically show impairments in executive functioning. They also have memory impairments, which affect working memory and the organization of explicit memory. In early to mid-stage PD, 16%–20% of patients develop dementia, with as many as 80% in later PD. In early stages, a further 15%–30% have milder cognitive symptoms (Aarsland et al. 2005). *Parkinson's disease dementia* refers to dementia that develops in patients who have had PD for many years, and this dementia is most likely caused by the PD itself.

Dementia With Lewy Bodies

The most recent DLB diagnostic criteria (McKeith et al. 2005) include central, core, suggestive, and supportive features. The central feature is a progressive dementia with primary persistent memory impairment and deficits in attention and executive and visuospatial abilities. Core features, at least one of which is necessary for the diagnosis of DLB, include fluctuating cognition with pronounced variations in attention and alertness, visual hallucinations, and spontaneous parkinsonism. Suggestive features include rapid eye movement sleep behavior disorder, severe neuroleptic sensitivity, and low dopamine transporter uptake in the basal ganglia demonstrated on PET or single-photon emission computed tomography imaging. The long list of supportive features includes falls and syncope, unexplained loss of consciousness, autonomic dysfunction, nonvisual hallucinations, delusions, depression, and brain imaging or electroencephalographic findings consistent with the diagnosis.

The early presence of dementia in a patient with motor parkinsonism supports a diagnosis of DLB.

Because the dementia in many patients with DLB has a more fulminant course, some experts believe that DLB has a worse prognosis than Alzheimer's dementia (McKeith et al. 2003, 2004). DLB is associated with considerable suffering for patients, particularly because of the very common, persistent, and hard-to-treat neuropsychiatric symptoms, especially hallucinations, delusions, and affective symptomatology (Ballard et al. 1999; McKeith and Cummings 2005). Patients also tend to become affected early with balance, sleep, and motor disorders and to become confined in their mobility.

Dementia Due to Frontotemporal Degeneration

Frontotemporal dementia is in many ways the paradigmatic non-Alzheimer's dementia. FTD has become a major focus of interest because in individuals younger than 65 years, it is the second most common form of dementia (Neary et al. 2005). Previously referred to as *Pick's disease,* FTD is heterogeneous both clinically and pathologically (Kertesz 2005; Neary et al. 2005). The clinical syndrome typically begins with changes in behavior, affect, and personality, which result in disinhibition, hyperorality, social inappropriateness, apathy, and related symptoms of loss of executive control. Cognitive changes leading to difficulties in attention, memory, set shifting, and organization occur early in the disease (Kertesz et al. 2005). The phenotype, however, is variable because many patients develop progressive expressive aphasia, whereas others develop semantic dementia early on (Shinagawa et al. 2006). As the condition progresses, disinhibited behaviors and apathy—often at the same time—worsen, leading to admixtures of productive-type and deficit-type loss of executive control.

Pathologically, FTD is characterized by knife-edge lobar atrophy, typically in the anterior temporal and posterior inferior areas of the frontal lobes. Most of these conditions appear to be tauopathies and include the pathologies of FTD with Pick bodies, corticobasal degeneration, progressive supranuclear palsy, hippocampal sclerosis, and other less common pathologies. TDP-43 proteinopathy appears to be the most frequent histological finding in FTD. FTD is familial in a considerable number of patients; mutations in the tau, progranulin, and ubiquitin genes have been associated with the condition. FTD is almost invariably progressive, especially if language symptoms occur early on. In clinical settings, the time from an FTD diagnosis to death is on the order of 3–5 years, shorter than the periods associated with Alzheimer's dementia (Chow et al. 2006).

Treatment

Treatment for Milder Cognitive Syndromes

Given the increased public awareness of dementia, memory clinics and primary care physicians anecdotally report that patients are presenting with increasingly milder cognitive symptoms to request diagnosis and treatment. At present, little empirical knowledge exists about how to manage these patients clinically; most experts recommend continued observation, the use of nonpharmacological therapies such as exercise and mental activity, and possibly cognitive rehabilitation. The results of at least one randomized trial suggest that the cholinesterase inhibitor donepezil may delay progression to dementia, especially in patients who are *APOE*E4* carriers (Petersen et al. 2005), but this has not been replicated or supported by other trials (Rosenberg et al. 2006). Initiation of pharmacological therapy is reserved for cases for which there is strong evidence of likely benefit—for example, when the patient appears to be about to transition to Alzheimer's dementia.

The Four Pillars of Dementia Care

Dementia care has four basic elements or pillars (Lyketsos et al. 2006), as described in the following subsections.

Disease Therapies: Alzheimer's Dementia

Probably the most effective therapy for Alzheimer's disease is management of associated vascular risk factors—blood pressure in particular—and treatment with the glutamatergic antagonist memantine. Reduction of blood pressure, weight loss, exercise, management of diabetes, and a healthy diet all probably constitute effective therapy for Alzheimer's disease. For patients with moderate or more severe Alzheimer's dementia, memantine titrated to 10 mg twice daily has very small but measurable effects, especially in patients with more severe disease.

Therapies for Cognitive Symptoms

The cholinesterase inhibitors donepezil, rivastigmine, and galantamine are all approved by the U.S. Food and Drug Administration (FDA) for treatment of the cognitive symptoms of Alzheimer's dementia. Most of these medications have been approved for the treatment of mild to moderate Alzheimer's dementia; donepezil has been approved for the treatment of severe Alzheimer's dementia. They are available in a variety of formulations, as pills, delayed-release pills, and (for rivastigmine only) patches. Although clinical trials have suggested that these medications may be of value in treating vascular dementia, none of them has been approved by the FDA for that purpose. The results of one study suggested that donepezil is associated with increased mortality in vascular dementia relative to placebo (Roman et al. 2010). Rivastigmine has been approved for the treatment of PDD and also has been found in randomized trials to be effective in DLB.

In primary care settings in the United States, most patients with dementia or milder cognitive symptoms who start a prescription do not continue it for more than a few months. Nevertheless, many experts recommend continuation of therapy once it is started because discontinuation studies suggest that patients may get worse when a cholinesterase inhibitor is stopped. However, other experts point out that some patients do well after a discontinuation trial and that many benefit from switching to another agent when they do not respond to an earlier one (Tariot et al. 2006). In a recent study of patients with moderate or severe Alzheimer's disease, memantine and donepezil were found to have similar efficacy with respect to cognitive outcomes and activities of daily living. Further, there were no significant benefits from the combination of donepezil and memantine over donepezil alone (Howard et al. 2012).

Therapies for Neuropsychiatric Symptoms

A useful approach to the management of neuropsychiatric symptoms uses a mnemonic of four D's: define, decode, devise, and determine. *Define* refers to an evaluation phase in which the patient, caregivers, and other relevant informants (e.g., charts and professional caregivers in long-term-care facilities and hospitals) provide the history, which is used to describe in detail the phenomenology of the patient's disturbance. Then, the patient undergoes an examination, which sometimes involves laboratory studies. This information is used to decide what type of disturbance is present: delirium, mood disorder, psychotic disorder, sleep disturbance, apathy, executive dysfunction, and so on (Lyketsos 2007).

Subsequently, the clinician, working as part of a team, seeks contributing factors to the disorder; this is the *decode* phase. Contributing causes to neuropsychiatric symptoms are listed in Table 4–2. In general, most disturbances are multifactorial; therefore, it is best to address several factors at once. The *devise* phase, which derives from the decoding process, consists of pharmacological, behavioral, environmental, and educational approaches that target the causes identified and are often delivered through the patient's caregiver. Finally, the *determine* phase refers to setting reasonable goals for assessing the

Table 4–2. Contributing causes of neuropsychiatric symptoms

Biological stress or delirium that accompanies a recurrent or new medical condition (e.g., constipation, urinary or upper respiratory infection, pain, poor dentition, headaches, hunger, thirst)

Identifiable psychiatric syndrome that is either recurrent or associated with the dementia

Aspects of the cognitive disturbance itself (catastrophic reaction due to inability to express oneself vocally)

Environmental stressor (e.g., too much noise, not enough heat)

Unmet needs (e.g., hunger, thirst, feeling lonely)

Unsophisticated or intrusive caregiving (e.g., poor communication, being rushed)

Medication side effects, whether from new medications or previously prescribed medications

effect of the intervention and readjusting the plan if the intervention is not successful.

Nonpharmacological strategies for management of dementia[1]. Nonpharmacological strategies can be taught effectively to family and nonprofessional caregivers (Belle et al. 2006; Cohen-Mansfield et al. 2007; Doody et al. 2001; Hepburn et al. 2007; Logsdon et al. 2007; Teri et al. 2005). These strategies focus on changing the patient's activity, routines, and/or human, physical, and social environment to provide reassurance, appropriate stimulation, and security. Behavioral approaches generally include person-specific problem solving, enriched cues, adapted work or expressive activities, exercise, communication strategies, and caregiver skills training. Agitated persons with dementia generally respond well to calm, familiar settings with predictable routines and to requests tailored to their capacities, retained strengths, and energy levels. Although persons with dementia may appear to do less as a result of apathy, they can become fatigued from just trying to make sense of what is expected. Late-day fatigue may explain some agitated behavior or exaggerated reactions to minor incidents associated with "sundowning" (i.e., becoming more con-

---

[1] I wish to thank Lisa Gwyther, M.S.W., and Harold Goforth, M.D., for providing this subsection on nonpharmacological strategies for management of dementia.

fused, agitated, or psychotic in the late afternoon or early evening). Furthermore, people with mild to moderate Alzheimer's disease may actively resist activities they perceive as too difficult or too demeaning, to limit embarrassment or failure. The nonpharmacological interventions with the best evidence to support their use are outlined in Table 4–3.

Table 4–3. Evidence-based nonpharmacological treatments for neuropsychiatric symptoms

Cognitive stimulation and behavioral management techniques centered on patient behavior or caregiver behavior are effective treatments whose benefits last for months.

Music therapy and controlled multisensory stimulation (Snoezelen) are useful during the treatment session but have no longer-term effects.

Specific education for caregiving staff about managing neuropsychiatric symptoms is very beneficial, but other educational interventions are not.

Changing the visual environment (e.g., painting doors to disguise them) is promising, but more research is needed.

Pharmacological treatment for neuropsychiatric symptoms of dementia[1].
Sometimes behavioral symptoms may be severe enough to endanger the safety of the patient or the caregivers, or to interfere with care, or to cause persistent distress to the patient. In such situations, nonpharmacological treatments may prove inadequate or ineffective. If medication treatments are indicated, it is important to follow an approach similar to the one outlined in Table 4–4.

Several different classes of medications have been studied, but for some of them, safety concerns exist and efficacy remains uncertain. The use of antipsychotics is controversial because their efficacy is modest (Schneider et al. 2005, 2006), and they have been associated with a higher risk of cerebrovascular or cardiovascular conditions and mortality in patients with dementia (Schneider et al. 2005). Both conventional and atypical antipsychotics carry this risk in patients with dementia. FDA black box warnings were issued in

---

[1]I wish to thank Mugdha E. Thakur, M.D., for providing this subsection on pharmacologic treatment for neuropsychiatric symptoms of dementia.

Table 4–4. Guidelines for use of medications to treat neuropsychiatric symptoms

Differentiate which disturbance is present; they are not all the same.

Consider possible contributing causes and the need for medical workup.

Implement nonpharmacological interventions.

Decide whether to treat with medications.

Use medications cautiously, with defined targets and close monitoring.

Be mindful that select *isolated* disturbances are unlikely to respond to medications.

Have in place a backup plan and a plan to deal with after-hours crises.

2004 for atypical antipsychotics and in 2008 for typical antipsychotics, indicating increased risk of mortality in patients with dementia. In 10-week trials, all-cause mortality was found to be 1.6–1.7 times greater in patients with dementia treated with atypical antipsychotics than in patients given placebo (Jeste et al. 2008). Although antipsychotics are not contraindicated in dementia, the risk-benefit threshold has been raised, and they should be used with caution (Rabins and Lyketsos 2005).

Cholinesterase inhibitors have shown modest efficacy in treating behavioral symptoms in general, but they may be particularly helpful in treating behavioral symptoms in patients with Lewy body dementia (Howard et al. 2007; McKeith et al. 2000; Rodda et al. 2009). Memantine showed modest benefit in improving behaviors in a pooled retrospective analysis of three trials, but no prospective studies exist (Wilcock et al. 2008). In general, although cholinesterase inhibitors and memantine may delay the emergence of neuropsychiatric symptoms or treat very mild symptoms, they should not be considered first-line agents in managing acute neuropsychiatric symptoms of moderate or greater severity until better evidence of their efficacy emerges.

Similarly, evidence suggests that the selective serotonin reuptake inhibitor citalopram (Pollock et al. 2002) has efficacy for the treatment of agitation in patients with Alzheimer's dementia. Unfortunately, two multicenter studies of sertraline and one of mirtazapine did not show benefit in treatment of depression symptoms in dementia (Banerjee et al. 2011; Rosenberg et al. 2010).

The anticonvulsant carbamazepine has been noted to be effective in treating agitation and aggression in dementia in a double-blind study (Tariot et al. 1998). The drug was well tolerated in spite of its complex pharmacology. Factors that may limit its use include potential for drug interactions, as well as the risk of suppression of blood cell lines that calls for periodic blood monitoring. Most studies comparing valproic acid or divalproex to placebo for behavioral symptoms of dementia have been of poor quality or have shown no benefit of valproic acid in treating neuropsychiatric symptoms of dementia when compared with placebo (Porsteinsson et al. 2001; Sival et al. 2002; Tariot et al. 2001, 2005). Recent studies have reported no benefit of valproic acid in prophylaxis for behavioral symptoms of dementia (Tariot et al. 2011) and evidence of increased brain atrophy and hippocampal atrophy on MRI scans of these patients as well as more rapid cognitive decline over a 1-year period (Fleisher et al. 2011).

Trazodone has shown benefit for treating behavioral symptoms in a small study of patients with frontotemporal dementia (Lebert et al. 2004), but data on this drug in treating other dementias are lacking. The β-blocker propranolol hydrochloride (average dose 106 mg) has shown efficacy in treating agitation and aggression in dementia, but gains were lost at 6 months (Peskind et al. 2005). A small study of prazosin (mean dose 5.7 mg) has also shown benefit in treating behavioral symptoms (Wang et al. 2009); patients with systolic blood pressure less than 110 mm Hg, and those who were orthostatic, were excluded from this study, which still had a high dropout rate of almost 50%.

A well-done cluster randomization trial of pain management in nursing home residents with moderate to severe dementia and behavioral disturbance showed that 8 weeks of pain management protocol was better than usual care. Surprisingly, the majority of patients in the pain management protocol received only scheduled acetaminophen, and the effect size of pain management was similar to that seen in efficacy studies of antipsychotics for agitation in dementia (Husebo et al. 2011). Given how difficult it is to assess pain in patients with severe dementia, this strategy is recommended as a first step in addressing agitation in dementia.

Finally, there are no randomized controlled studies of benzodiazepines in agitation in dementia, and given their unfavorable side-effect profile, they should be avoided in patients with dementia. They may have a role in managing severe anxiety briefly, and benzodiazepines with short half-lives at the lowest doses are preferred.

Supportive Care for Patients and Caregivers

The provision of systematic supportive care to patients with dementia and their caregivers is critical, as described in Tables 4–5 and 4–6, respectively.

Table 4–5. Supportive care for patients

Comfort and emotional support

Safety in regard to driving, living alone, medications, falls

Proper approach and communication

A safe, predictable place to live, with support for independent activities of daily living and activities of daily living

Structure, activity, and stimulation in day-to-day life

Planning and assistance with decision making

Aggressive management of medical comorbidity

Good nursing care in advanced stages

Table 4–6. Supportive care for the caregiver

Comfort and emotional support

Education about dementia and caregiving

Instruction in the skills of caregiving

Support with problem solving

Availability of an expert clinician, especially for crisis intervention

Respite from caregiving

Attention to general and mental health

Maintenance of a social network

References

Aarsland D, Zaccai J, Brayne C: A systematic review of prevalence studies of dementia in Parkinson's disease. Mov Disord 20:1255–1263, 2005

Alzheimer's Association: 2013 Alzheimer's Disease Facts and Figures. Available at: http://www.alz.org/alzheimers_disease_facts_and_figures.asp. Accessed June 24, 2013.

American Psychiatric Association: Diagnostic and Statistical Manual of Mental Disorders, 4th Edition, Text Revision. Washington, DC, American Psychiatric Association, 2000

American Psychiatric Association: Diagnostic and Statistical Manual of Mental Disorders, 5th Edition. Arlington, VA, American Psychiatric Association, 2013

Ballard C, Holmes C, McKeith I, et al: Psychiatric morbidity in dementia with Lewy bodies: a prospective clinical and neuropathological comparative study with Alzheimer's disease. Am J Psychiatry 156:1039–1045, 1999

Banerjee S, Hellier J, Dewey M, et al: Sertraline or mirtazapine for depression in dementia (HTA-SADD): a randomised, multicentre, double-blind, placebo-controlled trial. Lancet 378:403–411, 2011

Beach TG, Wilson JR, Sue LI, et al: Circle of Willis atherosclerosis: association with Alzheimer's disease, neuritic plaques and neurofibrillary tangles. Acta Neuropathol 113:13–21, 2007

Belle SH, Burgio L, Burns R, et al: Enhancing the quality of life of dementia caregivers from different ethnic and racial groups: a randomized, controlled trial. Ann Intern Med 145:727–738, 2006

Blennow K, de Leon MJ, Zetterberg H: Alzheimer's disease. Lancet 368:387–403, 2006

Chow TW, Hynan LS, Lipton AM: MMSE scores decline at a greater rate in frontotemporal degeneration than in AD. Dement Geriatr Cogn Disord 22:194–199, 2006

Cohen-Mansfield J, Libin A, Marx MS: Nonpharmacological treatment of agitation: a controlled trial of systematic individualized intervention. J Gerontol A Biol Sci Med Sci 62:908–916, 2007

Doody RS, Stevens JC, Beck C, et al: Practice parameter: management of dementia (an evidence-based review): report of the Quality Standards Subcommittee of the American Academy of Neurology. Neurology 56:1154–1166, 2001

Dubois B, Slachevsky A, Litvan I, et al: The FAB: a frontal assessment battery at bedside. Neurology 55:1621–1626, 2000

Fleisher AS, Truran D, Mai JT, et al: Chronic divalproex sodium use and brain atrophy in Alzheimer disease. Neurology 77:1263–1271, 2011

Folstein MF, Folstein SE, McHugh PR: "Mini-mental state": a practical method for grading the cognitive state of patients for the clinician. J Psychiatr Res 12:189–198, 1975

Graham JE, Rockwood K, Beattie BL, et al: Prevalence and severity of cognitive impairment with and without dementia in an elderly population. Lancet 349:1793–1796, 1997

Groves WC, Brandt J, Steinberg M, et al: Vascular dementia and Alzheimer's disease: is there a difference? A comparison of symptoms by disease duration. J Neuropsychiatry Clin Neurosci 12:305–315, 2000

Hachinski V: The 2005 Thomas Willis lecture: stroke and vascular cognitive impairment: a transdisciplinary, translational and transactional approach. Stroke 38:1396, 2007

Hayden KM, Zandi PP, Lyketsos CG, et al: Vascular risk factors for incident Alzheimer disease and vascular dementia: the Cache County study. Alzheimer Dis Assoc Disord 20:93–100, 2006

Hepburn K, Lewis M, Tomatore J, et al: The Savvy Caregiver Program: the effectiveness of a transportable dementia caregiver psychoeducational program. J Gerontol Nurs 33:30–36, 2007

Howard RJ, Juszczak E, Ballard CG, et al: Donepezil for the treatment of agitation in Alzheimer's disease. N Engl J Med 357:1382–1392, 2007

Howard R, McShane R, James Lindesay DM, et al: Donepezil and memantine for moderate-to-severe Alzheimer's disease. N Engl J Med 366:893–903, 2012

Husebo BS, Ballard C, Sandvik R, et al: Efficacy of treating pain to reduce behavioural disturbances in residents of nursing homes with dementia: cluster randomised clinical trial. BMJ 343:d4065, 2011

Jellinger KA, Attems J: Prevalence and impact of cerebrovascular pathology in Alzheimer's disease and parkinsonism. Acta Neurol Scand 114:38–46, 2006

Jeste DV, Blazer D, Casey DE, et al: ACNP White Paper: update on the use of antipsychotic drugs in elderly persons with dementia. Neuropsychopharmacology 33:957–970, 2008

Jones BN, Teng EL, Folstein MF, et al: A new bedside test of cognition for patients with HIV infection. Ann Intern Med 119:1001–1004, 1993

Kertesz A: Frontotemporal dementia: one disease, or many? Probably one, possibly two. Alzheimer Dis Assoc Disord 19(suppl):S19–S24, 2005

Kertesz A, McMonagle P, Blair M, et al: The evolution and pathology of frontotemporal dementia. Brain 128:1996–2005, 2005

Knopman DS, DeKosky ST, Cummings JL, et al: Practice parameter: diagnosis of dementia (an evidence-based review): report of the Quality Standards Subcommittee of the American Academy of Neurology. Neurology 56:1143–1153, 2001

Kulasingam SL, Samsa GP, Zarin DA, et al: When should functional neuroimaging techniques be used in the diagnosis and management of Alzheimer's dementia? A decision analysis. Value Health 6:542–550, 2003

Lebert F, Stekke W, Hasenbroekx C, et al: Frontotemporal dementia: a randomised, controlled trial with trazodone. Dement Geriatr Cogn Disord 17:355–359, 2004

Lippa CF, Duda JE, Grossman M, et al: DLB and PDD boundary issues: diagnosis, treatment, molecular pathology, and biomarkers. Neurology 68:812–819, 2007

Logsdon RG, McCurry SM, Teri L: Evidence-based psychological treatments for disruptive behaviors in individuals with dementia. Psychol Aging 22:28–36, 2007

Lopez OL, Jagust WJ, DeKosky ST, et al: Prevalence and classification of mild cognitive impairment in the Cardiovascular Health Study Cognition Study, part 1. Arch Neurol 60:1385–1389, 2003

Lyketsos CG: Neuropsychiatric symptoms (behavioral and psychological symptoms of dementia) and the development of dementia treatments. Int Psychogeriatr 19:409–420, 2007

Lyketsos CG, Colenda CC, Beck C, et al: Position statement of the American Association for Geriatric Psychiatry regarding principles of care for patients with dementia resulting from Alzheimer disease. Am J Geriatr Psychiatry 14:561–572, 2006

McKeith I, Cummings J: Behavioural changes and psychological symptoms in dementia disorders. Lancet Neurol 4:735–742, 2005

McKeith I, Del Ser T, Spano P, et al: Efficacy of rivastigmine in dementia with Lewy bodies: a randomised, double-blind, placebo-controlled international study. Lancet 356:2031–2036, 2000

McKeith IG, Burn DJ, Ballard CG, et al: Dementia with Lewy bodies. Semin Clin Neuropsychiatry 8:46–57, 2003

McKeith I, Mintzer J, Aarsland D, et al: Dementia with Lewy bodies. Lancet Neurol 3:19–28, 2004

McKeith IG, Dickson DW, Lowe J, et al: Diagnosis and management of dementia with Lewy bodies: third report of the DLB consortium. Neurology 65:1863–1872, 2005

McKhann G, Drachman D, Folstein M, et al: Clinical diagnosis of Alzheimer's disease: report of the NINCDS-ADRDA Work Group under the auspices of Department of Health and Human Services Task Force on Alzheimer's Disease. Neurology 34:939–944, 1984

Mielke MM, Rosenberg PB, Tschanz J, et al: Vascular factors predict rate of progression in Alzheimer disease. Neurology 69:1850–1858, 2007

Neary D, Snowden J, Mann D: Frontotemporal dementia. Lancet Neurol 4:771–780, 2005

Neuropathology Group, Medical Research Council Cognitive Function and Aging Study: Pathological correlates of late-onset dementia in a multicentre, community-based population in England and Wales. Lancet 357:169–175, 2001

Onyike CU, Sheppard JM, Tschanz JT, et al: Epidemiology of apathy in older adults: the Cache County study. Am J Geriatr Psychiatry 15:365–375, 2007

Peskind ER, Tsuang DW, Bonner LT, et al: Propranolol for disruptive behaviors in nursing home residents with probable or possible Alzheimer disease: a placebo-controlled study. Alzheimer Dis Assoc Disord 19:23–28, 2005

Petersen RC, Thomas RG, Grundman M, et al: Vitamin E and donepezil for the treatment of mild cognitive impairment. N Engl J Med 352:2379–2388, 2005

Pollock BG, Mulsant BH, Rosen J, et al: Comparison of citalopram, perphenazine, and placebo for the acute treatment of psychosis and behavioral disturbances in hospitalized, demented patients. Am J Psychiatry 159:460–465, 2002

Porsteinsson AP, Tariot PN, Erb R, et al: Placebo-controlled study of divalproex sodium for agitation in dementia. Am J Geriatr Psychiatry 9:58–66, 2001

Rabins PV, Lyketsos CG: Antipsychotic drugs in dementia: what should be made of the risks? JAMA 294:1963–1965, 2005

Rabins PV, Lyketsos CG, Steele CD: Practical Dementia Care, 2nd Edition. New York, Oxford University Press, 2006

Ranginwala NA, Hynan LS, Weiner MF, et al: Clinical criteria for the diagnosis of Alzheimer disease: still good after all these years. Am J Geriatr Psychiatry 16:384–388, 2008

Rodda J, Morgan S, Walker Z: Are cholinesterase inhibitors effective in the management of the behavioral and psychological symptoms of dementia in Alzheimer's disease? A systematic review of randomized, placebo-controlled trials of donepezil, rivastigmine and galantamine. Int Psychogeriatr 21:813–824, 2009

Roher AE, Kokjohn TA, Beach TG: An association with great implications: vascular pathology and Alzheimer disease. Alzheimer Dis Assoc Disord 20:73–75, 2006

Roman GC, Salloway S, Black SE: Randomized, placebo-controlled, clinical trial of donepezil in vascular dementia: differential effects by hippocampal size. Stroke 41:1213–1221, 2010

Rosenberg PB, Johnston D, Lyketsos CG: A clinical approach to mild cognitive impairment. Am J Psychiatry 163:1884–1890, 2006

Rosenberg PB, Dyre LT, Martin BK, et al: Sertraline for the treatment of depression in Alzheimer's disease. Am J Geriatr Psychiatry 18:136–145, 2010

Schneider LS, Dagerman KS, Insel P: Risk of death with atypical antipsychotic drug treatment for dementia: meta-analysis of randomized placebo-controlled trials. JAMA 294:1934–1943, 2005

Schneider LS, Tariot PN, Dagerman KS, et al: Effectiveness of atypical antipsychotic drugs in patients with Alzheimer's disease. N Engl J Med 355:1525–1538, 2006

Shinagawa S, Ikeda M, Fukuhara R, et al: Initial symptoms in frontotemporal dementia and semantic dementia compared with Alzheimer's disease. Dement Geriatr Cogn Disord 21:74–80, 2006

Sival RC, Haffmans J, Jansen PAF, et al: Sodium valproate in the treatment of aggressive behavior in patients with dementia—a randomized placebo controlled clinical trial. Int J Geriatr Psychiatry 17:579–585, 2002

Steinberg M, Shao H, Zandi P, et al: Point and 5-year period prevalence of neuropsychiatric symptoms in dementia: the Cache County study. Int J Geriatr Psychiatry 23:170–177, 2008

Tariot PN, Erb R, Podgorski CA, et al: Efficacy and tolerability of carbamazepine for agitation and aggression in dementia. Am J Psychiatry 155:54–61, 1998

Tariot PN, Schneider LS, Mintzer JE, et al: Safety and tolerability of divalproex sodium in the treatment of signs and symptoms of mania in elderly patients with dementia: results of a double-blind, placebo-controlled trial. Curr Ther Res Clin Exp 62:51–67, 2001

Tariot PN, Raman R, Jakimovich L, et al: Divalproex sodium in nursing home residents with possible or probable Alzheimer disease complicated by agitation: a randomized, controlled trial. Am J Geriatr Psychiatry 13:942–949, 2005

Tariot P, Cummings J, Ismael S, et al: New paradigms in the treatment of Alzheimer's disease. J Clin Psychiatry 67:2002–2013, 2006

Tariot PN, Schneider LS, Cummings J, et al: Chronic divalproex sodium to attenuate agitation and clinical progression of Alzheimer disease. Arch Gen Psychiatry 68:853–861, 2011

Teng EL, Chui HC: The Modified Mini-Mental State (3MS) examination. J Clin Psychiatry 48:314–318, 1987

Teri L, Huda P, Gibbons L, et al: STAR: a dementia-specific training program for staff in assisted living residences. Gerontologist 45:686–693, 2005

van der Burg M, Bouwen A, Stessens J, et al: Scoring clock tests for dementia screening: a comparison of two scoring methods. Int J Geriatr Psychiatry 19:685–689, 2004

Wang LY, Shofer JB, Rohde K, et al: Prazosin for the treatment of behavioral symptoms in patients with Alzheimer disease with agitation and aggression. Am J Geriatr Psychiatry 17:744–751, 2009

White L, Launer L: Relevance of cardiovascular risk factors and ischemic cerebrovascular disease to the pathogenesis of Alzheimer disease: a review of accrued findings from the Honolulu-Asia Aging Study. Alzheimer Dis Assoc Disord 20(suppl):S79–S83, 2006

Wilcock GK, Ballard CG, Cooper JA, et al: Memantine for agitation/aggression and psychosis in moderately severe to severe Alzheimer's disease: a pooled analysis of 3 studies. J Clin Psychiatry 69:341–348, 2008

Suggested Readings

Blennow K, de Leon MJ, Zetterberg H: Alzheimer's disease. Lancet 368:387–403, 2006

Ferri CP, Prince M, Brayne C, et al: Global prevalence of dementia: a Delphi consensus study. Lancet 366:2112–2117, 2005

Lyketsos CG: Lessons from neuropsychiatry. J Neuropsychiatry Clin Neurosci 18:445–449, 2006

Metzler-Baddeley C: A review of cognitive impairments in dementia with Lewy bodies relative to Alzheimer's disease and Parkinson's disease with dementia. Cortex 43:583–600, 2007

Neary D, Snowden J, Mann D: Frontotemporal dementia. Lancet Neurol 4:771–780, 2005

Rosenberg PB, Johnston D, Lyketsos CG: A clinical approach to mild cognitive impairment. Am J Psychiatry 163:1884–1890, 2006

White L, Launer L: Relevance of cardiovascular risk factors and ischemic cerebrovascular disease to the pathogenesis of Alzheimer disease: a review of accrued findings from the Honolulu-Asia Aging Study. Alzheimer Dis Assoc Disord 20(suppl):S79–S83, 2006

5

Mood Disorders

David C. Steffens, M.D., M.H.S.

Dan G. Blazer, M.D., Ph.D.

John L. Beyer, M.D.

Clinical entities listed as mood disorders in DSM-5 (American Psychiatric Association 2013) relevant to depression in elderly patients include 1) bipolar disorder, 2) major depressive disorder (with or without psychotic features), and 3) persistent depressive disorder (dysthymia). Of note, two key changes in DSM-5 pertinent to older adults are elimination of minor depression from the appendix and elimination of the bereavement exclusion criterion for major depression. In a helpful addition, the DSM-5 major depression criteria now include a "note" on the relationship between depressive symptoms and response to significant loss. Depressive symptoms are likewise present in other DSM-5 disorders, such as adjustment disorder with depressed mood and mood disorder due to a general medical condition (see Table 5–1).

Table 5–1.   Subtypes of depression and bipolar disorder in later life

Depressive disorders

    Major depression, single episode or recurrent episode

    Psychotic depression

    Persistent depressive disorder (dysthymia)

    Adjustment disorder with depressed mood

    Substance/medication-induced depressive disorder

    Depressive disorder due to another medical condition

    Other specified depressive disorder

    Unspecified depressive disorder

Bipolar and related disorders

    Bipolar I disorder

    Bipolar II disorder

    Cyclothymic disorder

    Substance/medication-induced bipolar and related disorder

    Bipolar and related disorder due to another medical condition

    Other specified bipolar and related disorder

    Unspecified bipolar and related disorder

A bipolar I disorder diagnosis describes a condition in which a patient has experienced at least one manic episode with or without history of a depressive episode. A *manic episode* is defined as an alteration in mood that is euphoric, expansive, or irritable; lasts for at least 1 week; and occurs with three other associated symptoms (e.g., decreased need for sleep, increased energy, racing thoughts, pressured speech, increased behaviors that may have high likelihood for bad outcome). Manic episodes in later life also may present with a mixture of manic, dysphoric, and cognitive symptoms, with euphoria being less common (Post 1978). When mania is associated with significant changes in cognitive function—so-called manic delirium—it may be difficult to distinguish from organic conditions or schizophrenia (Shulman 1986). A diagnosis of bipolar II disorder can be made when a patient has experienced one or more depressive episodes accompanied by at least one hypomanic episode. A *hypomanic episode* is defined as at least 4 days of altered mood (expansive, euphoric, irritable) occurring with at least three other associated symptoms (see above). *Bipolar disorder not otherwise specified* is defined as disorders with bipolar features that do not meet the criteria for specific bipolar disorders.

Epidemiology

In a community survey of more than 1,300 older adults living in urban and rural communities, 27% reported depressive symptoms; of these, 19% had mild dysphoria only (Blazer et al. 1987). Persons with symptomatic depression—that is, subjects with more severe depressive symptoms—made up 4% of the population. These individuals were primarily experiencing stressors, such as physical illness and stressful life events. Only 2% had a dysthymic disorder, and 0.8% were experiencing a current major depressive episode. No cases of current manic episode were identified. Finally, 1.2% had a mixed depression and anxiety syndrome. These data suggest that the traditional DSM-5 depression categories do not apply to most depressed older adults in the community. Subsequent surveys confirmed the lower frequency of major depression in the community (Kessler et al. 2005), but a more recent, population-representative study of 851 older community-dwelling adults reported a combined prevalence of major and minor depression of 11.2% (Steffens et al. 2009). White and Hispanic older adults had nearly three times the prevalence of depression found in African American older adults.

In hospital and long-term-care settings, the frequency of major depression among older adults is much higher than in community settings. Up to 21% of hospitalized elders have symptoms that meet criteria for a major depressive episode, and an additional 20%–25% have a minor depression (Koenig et al. 1988). Rates of major depression among elderly nursing home patients are even higher, exceeding 25% in some studies (Parmelee et al. 1989).

The Epidemiologic Catchment Area surveys identified bipolar disorder in 9.7% of nursing home patients (Weissman et al. 1991). In clinical settings, about 10%–25% of geriatric patients with mood disorder have bipolar disorder, and 3%–10% of all older psychiatric patients have this disorder (Wylie et al. 1999; Young and Klerman 1992). About 5% of all individuals admitted as geropsychiatry inpatients present with mania (Yassa et al. 1988).

Clinical Course

Episodes of depression across the life cycle, especially episodes of more severe major depression, almost always remit or at least partially remit. Nevertheless, depression is a chronic and recurrent illness. Studies that have focused on older adults in clinical settings have found a chronic course of depression (Alexopoulos et al. 1996; Baldwin and Jolley 1986; Murphy 1983; Post 1962). The prognosis from clinical studies of depressed older adults with uncomplicated late-life depression, however, is similar to that found among younger adults if the older adult does not have significant comorbid medical illness, functional impairment, or cognitive impairment (Keller et al. 1982a, 1982b). Comorbid depression is associated with a less favorable prognosis. Cognitive impairment is often associated with depressive symptoms. When the depression improves, the cognitive impairment often improves as well. Nevertheless, comorbid depression and cognitive impairment is a risk factor for the later emergence of Alzheimer's disease (Alexopoulos et al. 1993). Therefore, early depressive symptoms associated with mild cognitive impairment may represent a preclinical sign and should be considered a risk factor for impending Alzheimer's disease or vascular dementia (Li et al. 2001). Depression can further complicate Alzheimer's disease over time by increasing disability and physical aggression, thereby contributing to depression among caregivers (Gonzalez-Salvador et al. 1999). Depressive symptoms in patients with Alzheimer's disease resolve spontaneously at a greater frequency without requiring intensive therapy (such as medication therapy) than among older adults experiencing depression and vascular dementia, in which depressive symptoms tend to be persistent and refractory to drug treatment (Li et al. 2001).

Depression and medical problems are frequently comorbid, and the causal pathway may be bidirectional (Blazer and Hybels 2005). Depression, for example, is a frequent and important contributing cause of weight loss in late life (Morley and Kraenzle 1994). Frailty, leading to profound weight loss, can contribute to clinically important depressive symptoms (Fried 1994). Many chronic medical illnesses are associated with depression, including cardiovascular disease, diabetes, osteoporosis, and hip fracture (Blazer et al. 2002b; Lenze et al. 2007; Lyles 2001; Williams et al. 2002).

Perhaps the best-established association between depression and physical problems is the association between depression and functional impairment (Blazer et al. 1991; Bruce 2001). For example, in one study, older adults who were depressed were 67% more likely to experience impairment in activities of daily living and 73% more likely to experience mobility restrictions 6 years following initial evaluation than were those who were not depressed (Penninx et al. 1999). Disability, in turn, can increase the risk for depressive symptoms (Kennedy et al. 1990; Roberts et al. 1997). Most clinicians and clinical investigators report that more than 70% of elderly patients with major depression who receive antidepressant medication (at an adequate dosage for a sufficient time) recover from the index episode of depression if the depression is uncomplicated by comorbid factors. Reynolds et al. (1992) reported that treatment of depression in physically healthy elders with combined interpersonal psychotherapy and nortriptyline was associated with response rates nearing 80%. In a long-term outcome study of treatment-resistant depression in older adults, 47% of patients were clinically improved 15 months after treatment with an antidepressant or electroconvulsive therapy (ECT); by 4-year follow-up, the percentage had increased to 71% (Stoudemire et al. 1993). Once an older patient has experienced one or more moderate to severe episodes of major depression, he or she may need to continue antidepressant therapy permanently to minimize the risk of relapse (Reynolds et al. 2006).

Persons with persistent depressive disorder (dysthymia) experience a more chronic clinical course than do persons with major depression. Among older patients with major depression in one study, those with comorbid dysthymia had a less favorable trajectory of recovery over 3 years (Hybels et al. 2008).

Factors associated with improved outcome in late-life depression include a history of recovery from previous episodes, a family history of depression, female gender, extroverted personality, current or recent employment, absence of substance abuse, no history of major psychiatric disorder, less severe depressive symptomatology, and absence of major life events and serious medical illness (Baldwin and Jolley 1986; Cole et al. 1999; Post 1972). An association between depression and mortality holds in many studies, despite the addition of potentially confounding variables. In studies from North Carolina and New York, however, investigators failed to find an association (Blazer et al. 2001; Thomas et al. 1992). One reason for the lack of association in some studies may be the selection of specific control variables, especially chronic disease and functional impairment. The effect of depression on mortality may vary by sex (Hybels et al. 2002; Takeshita et al. 2002; Whooley and Browner 1998). The outcome of bipolar disorder in elderly patients remains virtually unknown. Shulman and Post (1980) studied elderly patients with bipolar disorder and found that only 8% had had their first episode of mania before age 40. In a review of records of a small number of untreated patients with severe and prolonged bipolar disorder, Cutler and Post (1982) found a tendency toward more rapid recurrences late in the illness, with decreasing periods of remission. Ambelas (1987) emphasized a relation between life events and onset of mania, noting that stressful events were more likely to precede early-onset mania than late-onset mania.

Some literature suggests high rates of medical comorbidity in older patients with bipolar disorder. Shulman et al. (1992) compared 50 geriatric patients hospitalized for mania with 50 age-matched patients hospitalized for unipolar depression. They found that the rates of neurological illness in manic patients were significantly higher (36% vs. 8%), suggesting that neurological disease is a risk factor for the development of mania in late life. Depp and Jeste (2004) reviewed eight studies that reported the presence of neurological illness and noted that despite a wide variety in reporting strategies, the sample-weighted prevalence was 23.1%.

Other comorbid medical disorders of note include diabetes. Regenold et al. (2002) reviewed the inpatient charts of 243 older (ages 50–74 years) psychiatric inpatients and found that type 2 diabetes was present in 26% of those with bipolar disorder, a much higher rate than for unipolar depression or schizophrenia.

Dhingra and Rabins (1991) found that mortality rates among elderly patients with bipolar disorder who had been hospitalized 5–7 years previously were higher than expected compared with population norms. Shulman et al. (1992) found that the mortality rate over a 10- to 15-year follow-up for hospitalized elderly bipolar patients was significantly higher than that for hospitalized elderly patients with unipolar depression (50% vs. 20%).

Controversy exists over whether age at onset of first manic episode affects response to treatment. Glasser and Rabins (1984) described no significant age-related differences in presentation or treatment response. Young and Falk (1989) reported that late-onset mania was associated with lower activity level, lower sexual drive, and less-disturbed thought processes; however, they also found that older age was associated with longer hospitalization, greater residual psychopathology, and poorer response to pharmacotherapy. Eastham et al. (1998) suggested that elderly patients with bipolar disorder often require lithium dosages that are 25%–50% lower than those used in younger patients. Data on the use of valproic acid in elderly patients with this disorder are limited but encouraging. Almost no information is available on the use of carbamazepine or other drugs in late-life bipolar disorder. ECT has been reported to be well tolerated and effective in the treatment of these patients (Eastham et al. 1998).

Etiology

The etiology of mood disorders in late life is undoubtedly multifactorial. Although a detailed discussion of the topic is beyond the scope of this chapter, Table 5–2 lists several factors that may be implicated in late-life mood disorders. For a more detailed discussion of this topic, the reader is referred to an article by Blazer and Hybels (2005).

Biological Origins

Genetics

Evidence from studies of unipolar depression in late life suggests that the genetic contribution is weaker in late-life depression than in depression at earlier stages of the life cycle. In a study of elderly twins in Sweden, genetic influences accounted for 16% of the variance in total depression scores on the Center for Epidemiologic Studies Depression Scale (CES-D) and 19% of the somatic symptoms. In contrast, genetic influences minimally contributed to the variance of symptoms of depressed mood and positive affect (Gatz et al. 1992).

Some pharmacological studies with depressed elders have shown associations between the serotonin transporter promoter polymorphism and both speed of response and antidepressant side effects (Pollock 2000). Polymorphisms in genes coding for brain-derived neurotrophic factor (Taylor et al. 2007) and for the enzymes methylenetetrahydrofolate reductase (Hickie et al. 2001) and tryptophan hydroxylase–2 (Zhang et al. 2005) have been associated with geriatric depression. Despite many studies of the ε4 allele of the apo-

Table 5–2.   Origins of late-life depression

Biological risks

Genetics (e.g., abnormalities in the serotonin transporter gene)

Female sex

Neurotransmitter dysfunction (e.g., underactivity of serotonergic neurotransmission)

Endocrine changes (e.g., long-standing elevated blood levels of cortisol)

Vascular changes (e.g., vascular depression secondary to subcortical vascular changes)

Medical illness (e.g., cardiovascular disease)

Other psychiatric disorders (e.g., long-standing anxiety disorder)

Psychological risks

Personality attributes (e.g., hopelessness and ambivalence)

Neuroticism

Cognitive distortions (e.g., feelings of abandonment when left alone for short periods)

Social origins

Stressful life events (e.g., the death of a close friend or a change of residence)

Chronic stress or strain (e.g., residence in an unsafe neighborhood)

Low socioeconomic status

lipoprotein E gene, no association was found in a community sample between the ε4 allele and depressive symptoms (Blazer et al. 2002a).

Neurotransmitter Dysfunction

Serotonin activity, specifically serotonin type 2A (5-HT$_{2A}$) receptor binding, decreases dramatically in a variety of brain regions through midlife, yet less decrease occurs from midlife to late life. 5-HT$_{2A}$ receptors in nondepressed subjects decreased markedly from young adulthood to midlife (70% from the levels at age 20 years through the fifth decade) and then leveled off as age advanced (Sheline et al. 2002). Activity of these receptors, however, may vary with age.

Endocrine Changes

Hypersecretion of corticotropin-releasing factor (CRF) has been associated with depression for many years across the life cycle. CRF is thought to mediate sleep and appetite disturbances, reduced libido, and psychomotor changes (Arborelius et al. 1999) and is diminished with normal aging (Gottfries 1990).

Serum testosterone levels decline with aging (Liverman and Blazer 2004) and have been found to be even lower in elderly men with dysthymic disorder than in men without depressive symptoms (Seidman et al. 2002). The efficacy of testosterone treatment for major depression in men, however, has not been established (Liverman and Blazer 2004). In women, improvement of mood has resulted from hormone replacement (Sherwin and Gelfand 1985).

Depressive symptoms have been hypothesized to cause atrophy of the hippocampus (Sapolsky 1996, 2001; Sheline et al. 1996; Steffens et al. 2002). Stress that accumulates over the life cycle may lead to a sustained increase in secretion of cortisol, leading to loss of preexisting hippocampal neurons (Sapolsky 1996). This loss of neurons may be prevented in part by use of antidepressant medications (Czéh et al. 2001).

Vascular Depression

Because major depression is a frequent outcome of stroke (Robinson and Price 1982) and hypertension (Rabkin et al. 1983), investigators have proposed a vascular-based depression among elderly individuals (Coffey et al. 1990; Krishnan et al. 1988; Kumar et al. 2002; Olin et al. 2002; Post 1962). In a study of 139 depressed older adults, neuroimaging criteria for subcortical ischemic vascular depression were met in 54% of the individuals. Age was most strongly associated with the increased prevalence of subcortical changes; also associated were lassitude, a history of hypertension, and poorer outcome (Krishnan et al. 2004; Taylor et al. 2003). Vascular depression is associated with white matter hyperintensities (Guttmann et al. 1998; Krishnan et al. 1997). These lesions probably contribute to the disruption of neural circuits associated with depression (Taylor et al. 2003).

These studies linking cerebrovascular disease and late-life depression have led investigators to examine genes associated with vascular risk and development of depression. For example, polymorphisms in the angiotensin II type 1 receptor gene have been associated with depression outcome (Kondo et al. 2007) and with change in vascular brain lesions (Taylor et al. 2010).

Medical and Psychiatric Comorbidity

Poor functional status secondary to physical illness and dementing disorders are the most important causes of depressive symptoms in older adults (Bruce 2001; Hays et al. 1997). Depressive symptoms are consistently associated with health status in cross-sectional studies of older adults (Kraaij et al. 2002); however, the association is not always clear-cut (Fiske et al. 2003).

Psychological Origins

Psychological factors, such as personality attributes, neuroticism, cognitive distortions, and emotional control, may contribute to the onset of late-life depression, yet are not specific to the origins of depression in older adults. In a study comparing older patients with and without personality disorder, Morse and Lynch (2004) found that those with a personality disorder were four times more likely to continue with or experience a reemergence of depressive symptoms. Cognitive distortions (Beck 1987) are among the most studied psychological origins of depression across the life cycle. For example, in a study of the experience and effect of adverse life events, older patients with major depression reported more adverse life events in the recent past and a greater negative effect of these events than did comparison groups of elderly patients with dysthymia and healthy control subjects (Devanand et al. 2002). It is not clear whether the reported effect reflects an increased vulnerability to events or a bias in reporting because of current depressed mood.

Beekman et al. (1995), in the Longitudinal Aging Study Amsterdam, found that major and minor depression, as well as the persistence and emergence of depressive symptoms over 3 years (Beekman et al. 2001), were predicted by external locus of control. Higher levels of mastery—that is, a perception of being able to accomplish tasks and having control over one's life—have been shown to have a direct association with fewer depressive symptoms in older adults and to buffer the adverse effect of disability on depression (Jang et al. 2002).

Social Origins

In addition to having biological and psychological origins, late-life depression derives from social origins, including stressful life events, bereavement, chronic stress or strain, low socioeconomic status, and impaired social support. The relative contribution of these factors appears to vary across the life cycle.

Murphy (1982) found that both severe life events (e.g., bereavement, life-threatening illness of someone else, major personal illness) and social difficulties (e.g., health difficulties of someone close to subject, housing issues, difficulties in marital and family relationships) were strongly associated with the onset of late-life depression. Elders lacking a confidant were especially vulnerable to the effects of life stress. Compared with younger adults, older adults are at greater risk for depressive symptoms secondary to stressful life events. Bereavement is a common cause of depressive symptoms in late life (Clayton 1990; de Beurs et al. 2001; Prigerson et al. 1994). In a study of 1,810 community-dwelling older adults, onset of clinically significant depressive symptoms over a 3-year follow-up was predicted by death of a partner or other relatives (Prigerson et al. 1994). Although some studies have found bereavement to predict depressive symptoms, others have not (Prince et al. 1998).

Lower socioeconomic status has been associated with depression across the life cycle. Both the frequency of depressive symptoms and their persistence over 2–4 years were associated with socioeconomic disadvantage in a sample of community-dwelling adults age 50 years or older who originally met criteria for major depression (Mojtabai and Olfson 2004). Perceived social support has proved to be a most consistent predictor of late-life depressive symptoms (Bruce 2002). The clinician must not assume that older adults in general experience a deficit in social support. Social support is perceived to be adequate in older adults, even among clinical samples (Blazer 1982). Old social networks thin out, but new ones emerge for many people. Most older people believe that they have enough contact with both family and friends and assess the relationships that they have with their social networks as positive (Cornoni-Huntley et al. 1990). Even so, when the social network is depleted suddenly, either through loss of someone close to the older adult (such as a spouse or child) or through a change in the quality of the relationship (such as a dispute within the family), impaired social support may emerge as a most important contributor to late-life depression.

The major mood disorders in older adults include the following:

- *Bipolar disorder,* characterized by inflated self-esteem or grandiosity, decreased need for sleep, more talkativeness than usual, flight of ideas, distractibility, psychomotor agitation, and excessive involvement in pleasurable activities (such as unrestricted buying episodes).

- *Major depressive disorder,* for which a diagnosis is made when the older adult has one or both of two core symptoms—depressed mood and lack of interest—as well as four or more of the following symptoms for at least 2 weeks: feelings of worthlessness or inappropriate guilt, diminished ability to concentrate or make decisions, fatigue, psychomotor agitation or retardation, insomnia or hypersomnia, significant decrease or increase in appetite, and recurrent thoughts of death or suicidal ideation.

- *Major depressive episode with psychotic features,* which deserves special attention because patients with onset after age 60 have a higher risk of psychotic depression and may have somatic, nihilistic, or guilty delusions.

- *Persistent depressive disorder,* with fewer criterion symptoms than major depressive disorder, but with symptoms that must last 2 years or more.

- *Adjustment disorder with depressed mood,* reserved for those individuals who show a maladaptive mood reaction to an identifiable stressor.

- *Depression associated with a medical illness,* because depressive disorders have been associated with a variety of physical illnesses, including cardiovascular disease (Glassman and Shapiro 1998; Musselman et al. 1998), endocrine disturbances (Blazer et al. 2002b), Parkinson's disease (Zesiewicz et al. 1999), stroke (Robinson and Price 1982), and cancer (Spiegel 1996).

Diagnostic Workup of Mood Disorders in an Older Adult

The diagnosis of a mood disorder in older adults is made on the basis of a history, augmented with a physical examination and fine-tuned by laboratory studies (Blazer 2003) (see Table 5–3). No biological markers or tests are available to confirm the diagnosis of depression, yet some tests may assist in identifying subtypes of depression; for example, magnetic resonance imaging (MRI) scans for subcortical white matter hyperintensities may help in confirming the presence of vascular depression (Krishnan et al. 1988) and polysomnography may help explain sleep disturbances. Of special importance in evaluating the depressed elder are the following: the duration of the current depressive episode; the history of previous episodes; the history of drug and alcohol abuse; the response to previous therapeutic interventions for the depressive illness; a family history of depression, suicide, and/or alcohol abuse; and the severity of the depressive symptoms. Establishing some indication of the risk of suicide is essential, because suicide risk may determine where the patient is treated.

Screening for depression with standardized scales such as the Geriatric Depression Scale (Yesavage et al. 1983) and the CES-D (Radloff 1977) is helpful. Assessment of cognitive status is critical to the evaluation of depressed older patients. Use of a screening scale such as the Mini-Mental State Examination (Folstein et al. 1975) or the Montreal Cognitive Assessment (Nasreddine et al. 2005) is a good adjunct to the diagnostic workup.

The physical examination must include a thorough neurological examination to determine whether soft neurological signs (e.g., frontal release signs) or laterality is present. The laboratory workup of the depressed older adult is important. It should include a thyroid panel (triiodothyronine, thyroxine, and radioactive iodine uptake) and determination of thyrotropin levels. A blood screen enables the clinician to detect the presence of anemia. However, at least one study has shown that red blood cell enlargement and abnormalities are not good predictors of deficits in vitamin B_{12} or folate (Mischoulon et al. 2000). Because both depressive and cognitive symptoms can result from deficits in vitamin B_{12} or folate, it is important to obtain levels of these vitamins.

The onset of bipolar disorder in late life is relatively uncommon; therefore, every patient who presents with a new onset of mania should have a complete medical evaluation, with special emphasis on the neurological examination. Because older adults often are prescribed medications, these should be reviewed for possible temporal association. A laboratory workup consisting of a thyroid panel and basic tests also should be completed. Finally, neuroimaging should be considered, especially if the presentation is associated with psychosis.

Table 5–3.   Diagnostic workup of late-life depression

Routine studies

Screening (especially in a primary care setting, use standard symptom checklists such as the Geriatric Depression Scale [Yesavage et al. 1983] or the Center for Epidemiologic Studies Depression Scale [Radloff 1977])

Thorough history and assessment, including present and past history of depressive episodes, family history, medication history, and assessment of psychological functioning and of social stressors; medical history, including assessment of nutritional status, current medications, past and current medical history, and functional status

Screening for cognitive impairment with an instrument such as the Mini-Mental State Examination (Folstein et al. 1975)

Physical examination

Laboratory tests, such as a chemistry screen and electrocardiogram if antidepressants are prescribed (previous medical records may provide these data)

Elective studies

Magnetic resonance imaging to establish the diagnosis of vascular depression

Blood screens for evidence of vitamin deficiency such as a deficiency of B_{12} or folate

Polysomnography when sleep abnormalities persist and cannot be explained

Screen for thyroid dysfunction (triiodothyronine, thyroxine, radioactive iodine uptake, thyrotropin levels)

Treatment

Treatment of mood disorders in late life is four-pronged, involving psycho-therapy, pharmacotherapy, ECT, and family therapy. These four approaches are discussed in this section.

Psychotherapy

Please refer to Chapter 10, "Individual and Group Psychotherapy," for an over-view of evidence-based psychotherapeutic treatments of depression.

Pharmacotherapy

Depression

The use of selective serotonin reuptake inhibitors (SSRIs) has been growing in elderly patients (with or without medical illness). Citalopram (Nyth and Gottfries 1990), escitalopram (Gorwood et al. 2007), fluoxetine (Heiligenstein et al. 1995), paroxetine (Bump et al. 2001), and sertraline (Cohn et al. 1990) have been shown to be effective in geriatric depression. SSRIs also have proved effective in depressed older adults who have had a stroke (Cole et al. 2001) or who have vascular disease in general (Krishnan et al. 2001) or Alzheimer's disease (Lyketsos et al. 2000). These agents have become the drugs of first choice for treating mild to moderate forms of depression. Important advantages of the use of these drugs in treating elderly patients are the lack of anticholinergic, orthostatic, and cardiac side effects; the lack of sedation; and safety in overdose. Nevertheless, for a significant number of older adults, these newer antidepressants cause other unacceptable effects, including excessive activation and disturbance of sleep, tremor, headache, significant gastrointestinal side effects, hyponatremia, and weight loss.

Serotonin-norepinephrine reuptake inhibitors (SNRIs) are often considered the best second-line therapy if the patient's response to an SSRI is not adequate. Duloxetine (Raskin et al. 2008) and venlafaxine (Staab and Evans 2000) have been shown to be effective in geriatric depression.

Tricyclic antidepressants (TCAs) are the agents of choice for some patients with more severe forms of major depression who can tolerate the side effects and do not respond to SSRIs or SNRIs. Medications that are effective yet relatively free of side effects (especially cardiovascular effects) are preferred. Nortriptyline, desipramine, and doxepin are the more popular TCAs for treating endogenous or melancholic major depression in older adults. It is recommended that all elderly patients have an electrocardiogram (ECG) before initiation of treatment and again after therapeutic blood levels have been achieved. If the ECG shows a second-degree (or higher) block, a bifascicular bundle branch block, a left bundle branch block, or a QTc interval greater than 480 milliseconds, treatment with TCAs should not be initiated or should be stopped in patients already taking these medications.

Antidepressant dosages administered to persons in late life should be case specific but are generally lower than those given to persons in midlife (see

Table 5–4). Starting therapeutic daily dosages of antidepressants are as follows: citalopram, 10–20 mg; fluoxetine, 5–20 mg; paroxetine, 10–30 mg; sertraline, 12.5–50 mg; mirtazapine, 7.5–30 mg; and venlafaxine, 37.5–200 mg (in divided doses). In 2011, the U.S. Food and Drug Administration (FDA) issued a warning for citalopram in dosages above 20 mg in the elderly for risk of QT prolongation and torsades de pointes (FDA Drug Safety Communication 2012). Citalopram should be prescribed with caution, even at a 20-mg daily dose, in patients who are taking concomitant medications that inhibit hepatic cytochrome P450 2C19, resulting in increased citalopram levels, or in patients who are otherwise at risk for QT prolongation. Bupropion therapy should be initiated at 75 mg twice daily, with an increase to 150 mg twice daily (not to exceed 150 mg in a single dose). With regard to TCAs, 25 mg of desipramine orally twice a day or 25–50 mg of nortriptyline orally at bedtime is frequently adequate for relieving depressive symptoms. Plasma levels of tricyclic medications can be helpful in determining dosing: desipramine levels greater than 125 ng/mL and nortriptyline levels between 50 and 150 ng/mL have been found to be therapeutic.

Trazodone and bupropion (Steffens et al. 2001; Weihs et al. 2000) are alternatives in patients who cannot tolerate TCAs or one of the newer antidepressants. Trazodone has advantages over TCAs in that it is virtually free of anticholinergic effects, and it has advantages over the newer antidepressants in that it has strong sedative effects. Nevertheless, the drug is not without side effects, including excessive daytime sedation, priapism (occasionally), and significant orthostatic hypotension. The therapeutic daily dose of trazodone is 300 mg or more, an amount that many older patients cannot tolerate because of sedation. Bupropion can be effective in treating depression in the elderly but generally is used once other medications have proved ineffective. Agitation is the most common side effect that troubles older adults.

Monoamine oxidase inhibitors (MAOIs) are another alternative to TCAs and the newer antidepressants. However, if MAOIs are being considered because of intolerance of side effects of other antidepressants, older adults usually do not tolerate MAOIs any better. If treatment with an MAOI is to follow treatment with an SSRI, a minimum of 1–2 weeks (or 2–4 weeks following fluoxetine) must elapse after discontinuation of SSRI therapy before initiation of MAOI therapy to avoid a serotonergic syndrome. If a patient's depression is

Table 5–4. Pharmacological treatment of late-life depression

Medication	Dosage
Selective serotonin reuptake inhibitors	
Citalopram	10–20 mg daily
Escitalopram	5–10 mg daily
Fluoxetine	5–20 mg daily
Paroxetine	10–30 mg daily
Sertraline	12.5–50 mg daily
Serotonin-norepinephrine reuptake inhibitors	
Desvenlafaxine	50–100 mg daily
Duloxetine	40–60 mg daily
Mirtazapine	7.5–30 mg daily
Venlafaxine	37.5–200 mg tid
Tricyclic antidepressants	
Desipramine	25 mg bid
Doxepin	100 mg daily
Nortriptyline	25–50 mg daily
Other agents	
Bupropion	75–150 mg bid
Trazodone	300 mg daily

Note. bid = twice daily; tid = three times daily.

severe and ECT is contemplated, use of an MAOI also precludes initiation of ECT until 10–14 days after the drug is discontinued. Such a delay may seriously impede clinical management of the suicidal elder.

Some clinicians prescribe low morning doses of stimulant medications, such as 5 mg of methylphenidate, to improve mood in the apathetic older adult. Although the effectiveness of stimulants has not been conclusively established, these agents are generally safe at low dosages, and rarely does the clinician encounter an elder with a propensity to abuse stimulants or to become addicted when these drugs are given once daily. Another recent addition to the pharmacological armamentarium is use of adjunctive atypical antipsychotics such as aripiprazole, which has shown effectiveness among depressed patients up to age 67 (Steffens et al. 2011).

For further details on psychopharmacological treatment in the older adult, see Chapter 2, "Psychopharmacology."

Bipolar Disorder

Lithium traditionally has been identified as the gold standard for treatment of bipolar disorder; however, no placebo-controlled efficacy trials have been done in geriatric patients. Case series have suggested that elderly patients may respond to lower lithium levels (0.5–0.8 mEq/L) than those recommended for younger adults (Chen et al. 1999; Prien et al. 1972; Roose et al. 1979), whereas other reports have not found a difference (DeBattista and Schatzberg 2006; Young et al. 1992).

Similar to the published research on lithium, only retrospective and open-label studies of valproate in the geriatric population have been published. The recommended blood concentration for valproate in the general population is 50–120 µg/mL (Bowden et al. 2002), and Chen et al. (1999) found that among manic elderly patients, those who had blood concentrations of 65–90 µg/mL improved more than patients with lower concentrations. As patients age, the elimination half-life of valproate may be prolonged and the free fraction of plasma valproate increases. The clinical significance of these changes is unknown, although it should be noted that usual laboratory tests measure the total valproate level. Thus, the reported level may underrepresent the actual dose in geriatric patients (Sajatovic et al. 2005b; Young et al. 2004). Common medications taken concurrently also may influence the level of valproate: aspirin can increase the valproate free fraction, and phenytoin and carbamazepine may decrease the valproate level.

Carbamazepine is even less studied in the older population. In elderly patients, carbamazepine may be started at 100 mg either once or twice daily and gradually increased every 3–5 days to 400–800 mg/day (McDonald 2000). Target serum levels are between 6 and 12 µg/L.

Lamotrigine was studied by Sajatovic et al. (2005a) in a retrospective analysis of two placebo-controlled, double-blind clinical trials for maintenance therapy in bipolar disorder focusing on subjects who were age 55 years or older. Lamotrigine was found to significantly delay the time to intervention for any mood episode, whereas lithium and placebo did not. In a subanalysis, the authors found that lamotrigine was significantly more effective than lithium and placebo at increasing time to intervention for depressive recurrences, but lithium performed much better in increasing time to intervention for manic episodes (Sajatovic et al. 2007).

Although antidepressants are used to treat bipolar disorder, their use is controversial and not well supported by data. The American Psychiatric Association (2005) has maintained its recommendations that primary treatment of bipolar depression be with a mood stabilizer and that antidepressant augmentation of the mood stabilizer be considered if the symptoms have limited or no response.

Although antipsychotics have been studied and have received FDA approval in the treatment of bipolar disorders in younger adults, data in the elderly are lacking. Beyer et al. (2001) reported on a pooled subanalysis of three double-blind, placebo-controlled acute bipolar mania clinical trials with olanzapine, focusing on subjects older than 50 years. Compared with placebo, olanzapine was found to be efficacious for the treatment of acute mania without any significant change in the side-effect profile. Case reports and open-label studies in geriatric bipolar treatment have been published for quetiapine (Madhusoodanan et al. 2000), risperidone (Madhusoodanan et al. 1995, 1999), aripiprazole (Bharadwaj et al. 2011) and clozapine (Frye et al. 1996; Shulman et al. 1997). No published reports are currently available for ziprasidone or aripiprazole.

Electroconvulsive Therapy

ECT continues to be the most effective form of treatment for patients with more severe major depressive episodes (O'Conner et al. 2001). The induction of a seizure via ECT appears to be effective in reversing a major depression. Despite its effectiveness, ECT is not the first-line treatment of choice for a patient with major depression and should be prescribed only because other therapeutic modalities have been ineffective. ECT has been shown to be effective in selected individuals, primarily those who have major depression with melancholia, and especially those who have major depression with psychotic symptoms associated with agitation or withdrawal. The presence of self-destructive behavior, such as a suicide attempt or refusal to eat, increases the necessity for intervening effectively; in such situations, ECT may be the treatment of choice. ECT has long been known to be effective for the treatment of bipolar disorder.

However, data are very limited on the use of ECT in elderly patients with bipolar disorder, especially when compared with the literature on ECT for unipolar depression.

The medical workup before ECT includes acquisition of a complete medical history, a physical examination, and consultation with a cardiologist if any cardiac abnormalities are recognized. Knowledge of any family history of psychiatric disorders, suicide, or treatment with ECT is helpful in predicting a patient's response to treatment. Laboratory examination includes a complete blood count, a urinalysis, routine chemistries, chest and spinal X rays (the latter to document previous compression fractures), an ECG, and a computed tomography (CT) scan or MRI (with CT or MRI available, an electroencephalogram and skull X ray are not routinely required). The presence of some abnormalities seen in MRI scans does not militate against the use of ECT, however. For example, older adults with major depression in one series were found to have subcortical arteriosclerotic encephalopathy, as documented by MRI, but promptly improved after undergoing ECT (Coffey et al. 1987).

ECT treatments are generally administered three times per week, and usually 6–12 treatments are necessary for adequate therapeutic response. A clear improvement is often noted after one of the treatments, with the patient reporting a remarkable improvement in mood and functioning. Two or three treatments are generally given after the ECT administration that leads to improvement.

The risks and side effects of ECT in elderly patients are similar to those in the general population. Cardiovascular effects are of greatest concern and include premature ventricular contractions, ventricular arrhythmias, and transient systolic hypertension. Multiple monitoring during treatment decreases the (infrequent) risk that one of these side effects will lead to permanent problems. Confusion and amnesia often result after a treatment, but the duration of this confusional episode is brief. Even with the use of unilateral nondominant treatment, however, some patients have prolonged memory difficulties. Headaches are a common symptom with ECT; they usually respond to nonnarcotic analgesics. Status epilepticus and vertebral compression fractures are some of the rare but more serious adverse effects. Compression fractures are a particular risk in older women because of the high incidence of osteoporosis in the postmenopausal population.

The overall success rate of ECT in patients who have not responded to drug therapy is usually 80% or greater, and no evidence indicates that effectiveness is lower in older adults (Avery and Lubrano 1979). Wesner and Winokur (1989) examined the influence of age on the natural history of major depressive disorder and found that ECT reduced the rate of chronicity when it was used in patients age 40 or older but, surprisingly, not in those younger than 40 years.

The relapse rate with no prophylactic intervention may exceed 50% in the year after a course of ECT. This relapse rate can be decreased if antidepressants or lithium carbonate is prescribed after the treatment. Maintenance ECT may be necessary for some patients who have a high likelihood of recurrence despite use of prophylactic medication and/or who experience high toxicity and therefore cannot tolerate prophylactic medications. For such patients, weekly or monthly treatments (usually on an outpatient basis) are prescribed, with careful monitoring of response and side effects. Following an effective course of ECT, the combination of continuation ECT and antidepressant drug therapy has been shown to have greater efficacy than use of medications alone (Gagné et al. 2000).

Despite the effectiveness of ECT, few deny that treatment may lead to memory difficulties. In a study by Frith et al. (1983), 70 severely depressed patients were randomly assigned to eight real or sham ECT treatments and were divided according to the degree of recovery from depression afterward. Compared with nondepressed control subjects, the depressed patients were impaired on a wide range of tests of memory and concentration before treatment, but after treatment, performance on most tests improved. Real ECT induced impairments in concentration, short-term memory, and learning but significantly facilitated access to remote memories. At 6-month follow-up, all differences between real and sham ECT groups had disappeared.

Family Therapy

The final component of therapy for the depressed elderly patient is work with the family. Not only may family dysfunction contribute to the depressive symptoms experienced by the older adult, but also family support is critical to a successful outcome in the treatment of depression in the elder. A clinician must attend to 1) those members of the family who will be available to the elder; 2) the frequency and quality of interactions between the older adult and family members, as well as among other family members; 3) the overall family atmosphere; 4) family values regarding psychiatric disorders; 5) family support and tolerance of symptoms (such as expressions of wishing not to live); and 6) stressors encountered by the family other than the depression experienced by the elder (Blazer 2002).

Most depressed elderly individuals do not resist interaction between the clinician and family members. With the patient's permission, the family should be instructed regarding the nature of the depressive disorder and the potential risks associated with depression in late life, especially suicide. Family members can assist the clinician in observing changes in the patient's behavior, such as an increase in discomfort (either physical or emotional), increased withdrawal and decreased verbalization, and preoccupation with medications or weapons. The family can assist by removing possible implements of suicide from places of easy access. The family can also take responsibility for administering medications to an older adult who is unreliable or whose potential for suicide is high.

When the symptoms of depression become so severe that hospitalization is required, family members are valuable in facilitating hospitalization. Without a proper alliance between clinician and family, a family may be resistant to hospitalization and undermine the clinician's attempts to treat the older adult appropriately. It is usually necessary for the clinician to take responsibility for saying that hospitalization is essential—that the situation has reached the point at which the family has no choice. The clinician informs the patient—in the presence of the family—of the necessity of hospitalization, and the family in turn can support the clinician's position. In such a situation, the patient rarely resists hospitalization for long.

References

Alexopoulos GS, Meyers BS, Young RC, et al: The course of geriatric depression with "reversible dementia": a controlled study. Am J Psychiatry 150:1693–1699, 1993

Alexopoulos GS, Meyers BS, Young RC, et al: Recovery in geriatric depression. Arch Gen Psychiatry 53:305–312, 1996

Ambelas A: Live events and mania. Br J Psychiatry 150:235–240, 1987

American Psychiatric Association: Practice guideline for the treatment of patients with bipolar disorder (revision). Am J Psychiatry 159(suppl):1–50, 2002

American Psychiatric Association: Diagnostic and Statistical Manual of Mental Disorders, 5th Edition. Arlington, VA, American Psychiatric Association, 2013

Arborelius L, Owens M, Plotsky P, et al: The role of corticotropin-releasing factor in depression and anxiety disorders. J Endocrinol 160:1–12, 1999

Avery D, Lubrano A: Depression treated with imipramine and ECT: the DeCarolis study reconsidered. Am J Psychiatry 136:559–562, 1979

Baldwin RC, Jolley DJ: The prognosis of depression in old age. Br J Psychiatry 149:574–583, 1986

Bharadwaj B, Kattimani S, Mukherjee A: Aripiprazole for acute mania in an elderly person. Ind Psychiatry J 20:142–144, 2011

Beck A: Cognitive model of depression. J Cogn Psychother 1:2–27, 1987

Beekman A, Deeg D, van Tilberg T, et al: Major and minor depression in later life: a study of prevalence and risk factors. J Affect Disord 36:65–75, 1995

Beekman AT, Deeg DJ, Geerlings SW, et al: Emergence and persistence of late life depression: a 3-year follow-up of the Longitudinal Aging Study Amsterdam. J Affect Disord 65:131–138, 2001

Beyer JL, Siegal A, Kennedy JS, et al: Olanzapine, divalproex, and placebo treatment non-head-to-head comparisons of older adult acute mania. Presented at the annual meeting of the International Psychogeriatric Association, Nice, France, September 2001

Blazer DG: Social support and mortality in an elderly community population. Am J Epidemiol 115:684–694, 1982

Blazer DG: Depression in Late Life, 3rd Edition. New York, Springer, 2002

Blazer DG: Depression in late life: review and commentary. J Gerontol A Biol Sci Med Sci 58:249–265, 2003

Blazer DG 2nd, Hybels CF: Origins of depression in later life. Psychol Med 35:1241–1252, 2005

Blazer D, Hughes DC, George LK: The epidemiology of depression in an elderly community population. Gerontologist 27:281–287, 1987

Blazer D, Burchett B, Service C, et al: The association of age and depression among the elderly: an epidemiologic exploration. J Gerontol 46:M210–M215, 1991

Blazer DG, Hybels CF, Pieper CF: The association of depression and mortality in elderly persons: a case for multiple independent pathways. J Gerontol A Biol Sci Med Sci 56A:M505–M509, 2001

Blazer DG, Burchett B, Fillenbaum G: APOE epsilon4 and low cholesterol as risks for depression in a biracial elderly community sample. Am J Geriatr Psychiatry 10:515–520, 2002a

Blazer DG, Moody-Ayers S, Craft-Morgan J, et al: Depression in diabetes and obesity: racial/ethnic/gender issues in older adults. J Psychosom Res 53:913–916, 2002b

Bowden CL, Lawson DM, Cunningham M, et al: The role of divalproex in the treatment of bipolar disorder. Psychiatr Ann 32:742–750, 2002

Bruce ML: Depression and disability in late life: directions for future research. Am J Geriatr Psychiatry 9:102–112, 2001

Bruce ML: Psychosocial risk factors for depressive disorders in late life. Biol Psychiatry 52:175–184, 2002

Bump GM, Mulsant BH, Pollock BG, et al: Paroxetine versus nortriptyline in the continuation and maintenance treatment of depression in the elderly. Depress Anxiety 13:38–44, 2001

Chen ST, Altshuler LL, Melnyk KA, et al: Efficacy of lithium vs. valproate in the treatment of mania in the elderly: a retrospective study. J Clin Psychiatry 60:181–185, 1999

Clayton PJ: Bereavement and depression. J Clin Psychiatry 51(suppl):34–40, 1990

Coffey CE, Hinkle PE, Weiner RD, et al: Electroconvulsive therapy of depression in patients with white matter hyperintensity. Biol Psychiatry 22:629–636, 1987

Coffey CE, Figiel GS, Djang WT: Subcortical hyperintensity on magnetic resonance imaging: a comparison of normal and depressed elderly subjects. Am J Psychiatry 147:187–189, 1990

Cohn CK, Shrivastava R, Mendels J, et al: Double-blind, multicenter comparison of sertraline and amitriptyline in elderly depressed patients. J Clin Psychiatry 51(suppl):28–33, 1990

Cole MG, Bellavance F, Mansour A: Prognosis of depression in elderly community and primary care populations: a systematic review and meta-analysis. Am J Psychiatry 156:1182–1189, 1999

Cole MG, Elie LM, McCusker J, et al: Feasibility and effectiveness of treatments of post-stroke depression in elderly inpatients: systematic review. J Geriatr Psychiatry Neurol 14:37–41, 2001

Cornoni-Huntley J, Blazer D, Lafferty M, et al (eds): Established Populations for Epidemiologic Studies of the Elderly: Resource Data Book, Vol 2. Bethesda, MD, National Institute on Aging, 1990

Cutler NR, Post RM: Life course of illness in untreated manic-depressive patients. Compr Psychiatry 23:101–115, 1982

Czéh B, Michaelis T, Watanabe T, et al: Stress-induced changes in cerebral metabolites, hippocampal volume, and cell proliferation are prevented by antidepressant treatment with tianeptine. Proc Natl Acad Sci USA 98:12796–12801, 2001

DeBattista C, Schatzberg AF: Current psychotropic dosing and monitoring guidelines. Primary Psychiatry 13:61–81, 2006 de Beurs E, Beekman A, Geerlings S, et al: On becoming depressed or anxious in late life: similar vulnerability factors but different effects of stressful life events. Br J Psychiatry 179:426–431, 2001

Depp CA, Jeste DV: Bipolar disorder in older adults: a critical review. Bipolar Disord 6:343–367, 2004

Devanand DP, Kim MK, Paykina N, et al: Adverse life events in elderly patients with major depression or dysthymia and in healthy-control subjects. Am J Geriatr Psychiatry 10:265–274, 2002

Dhingra U, Rabins PV: Mania in the elderly: a 5–7 year follow-up. J Am Geriatr Soc 39:581–583, 1991

Eastham JH, Jeste DV, Young RC: Assessment and treatment of bipolar disorder in the elderly. Drugs Aging 12:205–224, 1998

FDA Drug Safety Communication: Revised recommendations for Celexa (citalopram hydrobromide) related to a potential risk of abnormal heart rhythms with high doses. March 28, 2012. Available online at: http://www.fda.gov/Drugs/DrugSafety/ucm297391.htm. Accessed September 1, 2012.

Fiske A, Gatz M, Pedersen NL: Depressive symptoms and aging: the effects of illness and non-health-related events. J Gerontol B Psychol Sci Soc Sci 58:P320–P328, 2003

Folstein M, Folstein S, McHugh P: "Mini-mental state": a practical method for grading the cognitive state of patients for the clinician. J Psychiatr Res 12:189–198, 1975

Fried L: Frailty, in Principles of Geriatric Medicine and Gerontology, 3rd Edition. Edited by Hazzard W, Bierman E, Blass J, et al. New York, McGraw-Hill, 1994, pp 1149–1156

Frith CD, Stevens M, Johnstone EC, et al: Effects of ECT and depression on various aspects of memory. Br J Psychiatry 142:610–617, 1983

Frye MA, Altshuler LL, Bitran JA: Clozapine in rapid cycling bipolar disorder. J Clin Psychopharmacol 16:87–90, 1996

Gagné GG Jr, Furman MJ, Carpenter LL, et al: Efficacy of continuation ECT and antidepressant drugs compared to long-term antidepressants alone in depressed patients. Am J Psychiatry 157:1960–1965, 2000

Gatz M, Pedersen N, Plomin R, et al: Importance of shared genes and shared environments for symptoms of depression in older adults. J Abnorm Psychol 101:701–708, 1992

Glasser M, Rabins P: Mania in the elderly. Age Ageing 13:210–213, 1984

Glassman AH, Shapiro PA: Depression and the course of coronary artery disease. Am J Psychiatry 155:4–11, 1998

Gonzalez-Salvador MT, Arango C, Lyketsos CG, et al: The stress and psychological morbidity of the Alzheimer patient caregiver. Int J Geriatr Psychiatry 14:701–710, 1999

Gorwood P, Weiller E, Lemming O, et al: Escitalopram prevents relapse in older adults with major depressive disorder. Am J Geriatr Psychiatry 15:581–593, 2007

Gottfries CG: Neurochemical aspects on aging and diseases with cognitive impairment. J Neurosci Res 27:541–547, 1990

Guttmann CR, Jolesz F, Kikinis R, et al: White matter changes with normal aging. Neurology 50:972–978, 1998

Hays JC, Saunders WB, Flint EP, et al: Social support and depression as risk factors for loss of physical function in late life. Aging Ment Health 3:209–220, 1997

Heiligenstein JH, Ware JE Jr, Beusterien KM, et al: Acute effects of fluoxetine versus placebo on functional health and well-being in late-life depression. Int Psychogeriatr 7(suppl):125–137, 1995

Hickie I, Scott E, Naismith S, et al: Late-onset depression: genetic, vascular and clinical contributions. Psychol Med 31:1403–1412, 2001

Hirschfeld RMA: Guideline Watch: Practice Guideline for the Treatment of Patients With Bipolar Disorder, 2nd Edition. November 2005. Available at: http://psychiatryonline.org/content.aspx?bookid=28&sectionid=1682557. Accessed July 3, 2013

Hybels CF, Pieper CF, Blazer DG: Sex differences in the relationship between subthreshold depression and mortality in a community sample of older adults. Am J Geriatr Psychiatry 10:283–291, 2002

Hybels CF, Pieper CF, Blazer DG, et al: The course of depressive symptoms in older adults with comorbid major depression and dysthymia. Am J Geriatr Psychiatry 16:300–309, 2008

Jang Y, Haley WE, Small BJ: The role of mastery and social resources in the associations between disability and depression in later life. Gerontologist 42:807–813, 2002

Keller MB, Shapiro RW, Lavori PW, et al: Recovery in major depressive disorder: analyses with the life table and regression models. Arch Gen Psychiatry 39:905–910, 1982a

Keller MB, Shapiro RW, Lavori PW, et al: Relapse in major depressive disorder: analysis with the life table. Arch Gen Psychiatry 39:911–915, 1982b

Kennedy GJ, Kelman HR, Thomas C: The emergence of depressive symptoms in late life: the importance of declining health and increasing disability. J Community Health 15:93–104, 1990

Kessler RC, Chiu WT, Demler O, et al: Prevalence, severity, and comorbidity of 12-month DSM-IV disorders in the National Comorbidity Survey Replication [published erratum appears in Arch Gen Psychiatry 62:709, 2005]. Arch Gen Psychiatry 62:617–627, 2005

Koenig HG, Meador KG, Cohen HJ, et al: Depression in elderly hospitalized patients with medical illness. Arch Intern Med 148:1929–1936, 1988

Kondo DG, Speer MC, Krishnan KR, et al: Association of AGTR1 with 18-month treatment outcome in late-life depression. Am J Geriatr Psychiatry 15:564–572, 2007

Kraaij V, Arensman E, Spinhoven P: Negative life events and depression in elderly persons: a meta-analysis. J Gerontol B Psychol Sci Soc Sci 57:P87–P94, 2002

Krishnan KR, Goli V, Ellinwood EH, et al: Leukoencephalopathy in patients diagnosed as major depressive [published erratum appears in Biol Psychiatry 25:822, 1989]. Biol Psychiatry 23:519–522, 1988

Krishnan KR, Hays JC, Blazer DG: MRI-defined vascular depression. Am J Psychiatry 154:497–501, 1997

Krishnan KR, Doraiswamy PM, Clary CM: Clinical and treatment response characteristics of late-life depression associated with vascular disease: a pooled analysis of two multicenter trials with sertraline. Prog Neuropsychopharmacol Biol Psychiatry 25:347–361, 2001

Krishnan KR, Taylor WD, McQuoid DR, et al: Clinical characteristics of magnetic resonance imaging–defined subcortical ischemic depression. Biol Psychiatry 55:390–397, 2004

Kumar A, Mintz J, Bilker W, et al: Autonomous neurobiological pathways to late-life depressive disorders: clinical and pathophysiological implications. Neuropsychopharmacology 26:229–236, 2002

Lenze EJ, Munin MC, Skidmore ER, et al: Onset of depression in elderly persons after hip fracture: implications for prevention and early intervention of late-life depression. J Am Geriatr Soc 55:81–86, 2007

Li YS, Meyer JS, Thornby J: Longitudinal follow-up of depressive symptoms among normal versus cognitively impaired elderly. Int J Geriatr Psychiatry 16:718–727, 2001

Liverman C, Blazer D (eds): Testosterone and Aging: Clinical Research Directions. Washington, DC, National Academies Press, 2004

Lyketsos CG, Sheppard JM, Steele CD, et al: Randomized, placebo-controlled, double-blind, clinical trial of sertraline in the treatment of depression complicating Alzheimer's disease: initial results from the Depression in Alzheimer's Disease Study. Am J Psychiatry 157:1686–1689, 2000

Lyles KW: Osteoporosis and depression: shedding more light upon a complex relationship. J Am Geriatr Soc 49:827–828, 2001

Madhusoodanan S, Brenner R, Araujo L, et al: Efficacy of risperidone treatment for psychoses associated with schizophrenia, schizoaffective disorder, bipolar disorder, or senile dementia in 11 geriatric patients: a case series. J Clin Psychiatry 56:514–518, 1995

Madhusoodanan S, Brecher M, Brenner R, et al: Risperidone in the treatment of elderly patients with psychotic disorders. Am J Geriatr Psychiatry 7:132–138, 1999

Madhusoodanan S, Brenner R, Alcantra A: Clinical experience with quetiapine in elderly patients with psychotic disorders. J Geriatr Psychiatry Neurol 13:28–32, 2000

McDonald WM: Epidemiology, etiology, and treatment of geriatric mania. J Clin Psychiatry 61(suppl):3–11, 2000

Mischoulon D, Burger JK, Spillmann MK, et al: Anemia and macrocytosis in the prediction of serum folate and vitamin B_{12} status, and treatment outcome in major depression. J Psychosom Res 49:183–187, 2000

Mojtabai R, Olfson M: Major depression in community-dwelling middle-aged and older adults: prevalence and 2- and 4-year follow-up symptoms. Psychol Med 34:623–634, 2004

Morley J, Kraenzle D: Causes of weight loss in a community nursing home. J Am Geriatr Soc 42:583–585, 1994

Morse JQ, Lynch TR: A preliminary investigation of self-reported personality disorders in late life: prevalence, predictors of depressive severity, and clinical correlates. Aging Ment Health 8:307–315, 2004

Murphy E: Social origins of depression in old age. Br J Psychiatry 141:135–142, 1982

Murphy E: The prognosis of depression in old age. Br J Psychiatry 142:111–119, 1983

Musselman DL, Evans DL, Nemeroff CB: The relationship of depression to cardiovascular disease: epidemiology, biology, and treatment. Arch Gen Psychiatry 55:580–592, 1998

Nasreddine ZS, Phillips NA, Bédirian V, et al: The Montreal Cognitive Assessment: MoCA, a brief screening tool for cognitive assessment. J Am Geriatr Soc 53:695–699, 2005

Nyth AL, Gottfries CG: The clinical efficacy of citalopram in treatment of emotional disturbances in dementia disorders: a Nordic multicentre study. Br J Psychiatry 157:894–901, 1990

O'Conner M, Knapp R, Husain M, et al: The influence of age on the response of major depression to electroconvulsive therapy: a C.O.R.E. Report. Am J Geriatr Psychiatry 9:382–390, 2001

Olin J, Schneider L, Katz I, et al: Provisional diagnostic criteria for depression of Alzheimer disease. Am J Geriatr Psychiatry 10:125–128, 2002

Parmelee PA, Katz IR, Lawton MP: Depression among institutionalized aged: assessment and prevalence estimation. J Gerontol 44:M22–M29, 1989

Penninx BW, Leveille S, Ferrucci L, et al: Exploring the effect of depression on physical disability: longitudinal evidence from the Established Populations for Epidemiologic Studies of the Elderly. Am J Public Health 89:1346–1352, 1999

Pollock BG: Geriatric psychiatry: psychopharmacology: general principles, in Kaplan & Sadock's Comprehensive Textbook of Psychiatry, 7th Edition. Edited by Sadock BJ, Sadock VA. Philadelphia, PA, Lippincott Williams & Wilkins, 2000, pp 3086–3090

Post F: The Significance of Affective Symptoms at Old Age. London, Oxford University Press, 1962

Post F: The management and nature of depressive illnesses in late life: a follow-through study. Br J Psychiatry 121:393–404, 1972

Post F: The functional psychoses, in Geriatric Psychiatry. Edited by Isaacs A, Post F. New York, Wiley, 1978, pp 77–98

Prien RF, Caffey EM, Klett CJ: Relationship between serum lithium level and clinical response in acute mania treated with lithium. Br J Psychiatry 120:409–414, 1972

Prigerson H, Reynolds CF 3rd, Frank E, et al: Stressful life events, social rhythms, and depressive symptoms among the elderly: an examination of hypothesized causal linkages. Psychiatry Res 51:33–49, 1994

Prince MJ, Harwood RH, Thomas A, et al: A prospective population-based study of the effects of disablement and social milieu on the onset and maintenance of late-life depression: the Gospel Oak Project VII. Psychol Med 28:337–350, 1998

Rabkin JG, Charles E, Kass F: Hypertension and DSM-III depression in psychiatric outpatients. Am J Psychiatry 140:1072–1074, 1983

Radloff LS: The CES-D Scale: a self-report depression scale for research in the general population. Appl Psychol Meas 1:385–401, 1977

Raskin J, Xu JY, Kajdasz DK: Time to response for duloxetine 60 mg once daily versus placebo in elderly patients with major depressive disorder. Int Psychogeriatr 20:309–327, 2008

Regenold WT, Thapar RK, Marano C, et al: Increased prevalence of type 2 diabetes mellitus among psychiatric inpatients with bipolar I affective and schizoaffective disorders independent of psychotropic drug use. J Affect Disord 70:19–26, 2002

Reynolds CF 3rd, Frank E, Perel JM, et al: Combined pharmacotherapy and psychotherapy in the acute and continuation treatment of elderly patients with recurrent major depression: a preliminary report. Am J Psychiatry 149:1687–1692, 1992

Reynolds CF 3rd, Dew MA, Pollock BG, et al: Maintenance treatment of major depression in old age. N Engl J Med 354:1130–1138, 2006

Roberts RE, Kaplan GA, Shema SJ, et al: Does growing old increase the risk for depression? Am J Psychiatry 154:1384–1390, 1997

Robinson RG, Price TR: Post-stroke depressive disorders: a follow-up study of 103 patients. Stroke 13:635–641, 1982

Roose SP, Bone S, Haidorfer C, et al: Lithium treatment in older patients. Am J Psychiatry 136:843–844, 1979

Sajatovic M, Gyulai L, Calabrese JR, et al: Maintenance treatment outcomes in older patients with bipolar I disorder. Am J Geriatr Psychiatry 13:305–311, 2005a

Sajatovic M, Madhusoodanan S, Coconcea N: Managing bipolar disorder in the elderly: defining the role of the newer agents. Drugs Aging 22:39–54, 2005b

Sajatovic M, Ramsay E, Nanry K, et al: Lamotrigine therapy in elderly patients with epilepsy, bipolar disorder or dementia. Int J Geriatr Psychiatry 22:945–950, 2007

Sapolsky RM: Why stress is bad for your brain. Science 273:749–750, 1996

Sapolsky RM: Depression, antidepressants, and the shrinking hippocampus. Proc Natl Acad Sci USA 98:12320–12322, 2001

Seidman SN, Araujo AB, Roose SP, et al: Low testosterone levels in elderly men with dysthymic disorder. Am J Psychiatry 159:456–459, 2002

Sheline YI, Wang PW, Gado MH, et al: Hippocampal atrophy in recurrent major depression. Proc Natl Acad Sci USA 93:3908–3913, 1996

Sheline YI, Mintun MS, Moerlein SM, et al: Greater loss of 5-HT(2A) receptors in midlife than in late life. Am J Psychiatry 159:430–435, 2002

Sherwin B, Gelfand M: Sex steroids and affect in the surgical menopause: a double-blind, cross-over study. Psychoneuroendocrinology 10:325–335, 1985

Shulman KI: Mania in old age, in Affective Disorders in the Elderly. Edited by Murphy E. Edinburgh, Scotland, Churchill Livingstone, 1986, pp 203–216

Shulman K, Post F: Bipolar affective disorder in old age. Br J Psychiatry 136:26–32, 1980

Shulman KI, Tohen M, Satlin A, et al: Mania compared with unipolar depression in old age. Am J Psychiatry 149:341–345, 1992

Shulman RW, Singh A, Shulman KI: Treatment of elderly institutionalized bipolar patients with clozapine. Psychopharmacol Bull 33:113–118, 1997

Spiegel D: Cancer and depression. Br J Psychiatry 169(suppl):109–116, 1996

Staab JP, Evans DL: Efficacy of venlafaxine in geriatric depression. Depress Anxiety 12 (suppl 1):63–68, 2000

Steffens DC, Doraiswamy PM, McQuoid DR: Bupropion SR in the naturalistic treatment of elderly patients with major depression. Int J Geriatr Psychiatry 16:862–865, 2001

Steffens DC, Payne ME, Greenberg DL, et al: Hippocampal volume and incident dementia in geriatric depression. Am J Geriatr Psychiatry 10:62–71, 2002

Steffens DC, Fisher GG, Langa KM, et al: Prevalence of depression among older Americans: the Aging, Demographics and Memory Study. Int Psychogeriatr 21:878–888, 2009

Steffens DC, Nelson JC, Eudicone JM, et al: Efficacy and safety of adjunctive aripiprazole in major depressive disorder in older patients: a pooled subpopulation analysis. Int J Geriatr Psychiatry 26:564–572, 2011

Stoudemire A, Hill CD, Morris R, et al: Long-term outcome of treatment-resistant depression in older adults. Am J Psychiatry 150:1539–1540, 1993

Takeshita J, Masaki K, Ahmed I, et al: Are depressive symptoms a risk factor for mortality in elderly Japanese American men? The Honolulu-Asia Aging Study. Am J Psychiatry 159:1127–1132, 2002

Taylor WD, Steffens DC, MacFall JR, et al: White matter hyperintensity progression and late-life depression outcomes. Arch Gen Psychiatry 60:1090–1096, 2003

Taylor WD, Zücher S, McQuoid DR, et al: Allelic differences in the brain-derived neurotrophic factor Val66Met polymorphism in late-life depression. Am J Geriatr Psychiatry 15:850–857, 2007

Taylor WD, Steffens DC, Ashley-Koch A, et al: Angiotensin receptor gene polymorphisms and 2-year change in hyperintense lesion volume in men. Mol Psychiatry 15:816–822, 2010

Thomas C, Kelman HR, Kennedy GJ, et al: Depressive symptoms and mortality in elderly persons. J Gerontol 47:S80–S87, 1992

Weihs KL, Settle EC Jr, Batey SR, et al: Bupropion sustained release versus paroxetine for the treatment of depression in the elderly. J Clin Psychiatry 61:196–202, 2000

Weissman MM, Bruce ML, Leaf PJ, et al: Affective disorders, in Psychiatric Disorders in America: The Epidemiologic Catchment Area Study. Edited by Robins LN, Regier DA. New York, Free Press, 1991, pp 53–80

Wesner RB, Winokur G: The influence of age on the natural history of unipolar depression when treated with electroconvulsive therapy. Eur Arch Psychiatry Neurol Sci 238:149–154, 1989

Whooley MA, Browner WS: Association between depressive symptoms and mortality in older women. Study of Osteoporotic Fractures Research Group. Arch Intern Med 158:2129–2135, 1998

Williams SA, Kasl SV, Heiat A, et al: Depression and risk of heart failure among the elderly: a prospective community-based study. Psychosom Med 64:6–12, 2002

Wylie ME, Mulsant BH, Pollock BG, et al: Age of onset in geriatric bipolar disorder: effects on clinical presentation and treatment outcomes in an inpatient sample. Am J Geriatr Psychiatry 7:77–83, 1999

Yassa R, Nair V, Nastase C, et al: Prevalence of bipolar disorder in a psychogeriatric population. J Affect Disord 14:197–201, 1988

Yesavage JA, Brink TL, Rose TL, et al: Development and validation of a geriatric depression screening scale: a preliminary report. J Psychiatr Res 17:37–49, 1983

Young RC, Falk JR: Age, manic psychopathology, and treatment response. Int J Geriatr Psychiatry 4:73–78, 1989

Young RC, Klerman GL: Mania in late life: focus on age at onset. Am J Psychiatry 149:867–876, 1992

Young RC, Kalayam B, Tsuboyama G, et al: Mania: response to lithium across the age spectrum (abstract). Soc Neurosci 18:669, 1992

Young RC, Gyulai L, Mulsant BH, et al: Pharmacotherapy of bipolar disorder in old age: review and recommendations. Am J Geriatr Psychiatry 12:342–357, 2004

Zesiewicz TA, Gold M, Chari G, et al: Current issues in depression in Parkinson's disease. Am J Geriatr Psychiatry 7:110–118, 1999

Zhang X, Gainetdinov RR, Beaulieu JM, et al: Loss-of-function mutation in tryptophan hydroxylase-2 identified in unipolar major depression. Neuron 45:11–16, 2005

Suggested Readings

Alexopoulos GS, Meyers BS, Young RC, et al: The course of geriatric depression with "reversible dementia": a controlled study. Am J Psychiatry 150:1693–1699, 1993

Blazer DG: Psychiatry and the oldest old. Am J Psychiatry 157:1915–1924, 2000

Blazer DG: Depression in Late Life, 3rd Edition. New York, Springer, 2002

Blazer DG: Depression in late life: review and commentary. J Gerontol A Biol Sci Med Sci 58:249–265, 2003

Blazer DG 2nd, Hybels CF: Origins of depression in later life. Psychol Med 35:1241–1252, 2005

Koenig HG, Meador KG, Cohen HJ, et al: Depression in elderly hospitalized patients with medical illness. Arch Intern Med 148:1929–1936, 1988

Krishnan KR, Goli V, Ellinwood EH, et al: Leukoencephalopathy in patients diagnosed as major depressive [published erratum appears in Biol Psychiatry 25:822, 1989]. Biol Psychiatry 23:519–522, 1988

Reynolds CF 3rd, Dew MA, Pollock BG, et al: Maintenance treatment of major depression in old age. N Engl J Med 354:1130–1138, 2006

Steffens DC, Payne ME, Greenberg DL, et al: Hippocampal volume and incident dementia in geriatric depression. Am J Geriatr Psychiatry 10:62–71, 2002

Taylor WS, Steffens DC, MacFall JR, et al: White matter hyperintensity progression and late-life depression outcomes. Arch Gen Psychiatry 60:1090–1096, 2003

6

Schizophrenia and Paranoid Disorders

Ipsit V. Vahia, M.D.

Nicole M. Lanouette, M.D.

Dilip V. Jeste, M.D.

Delusions, hallucinations, and other psychotic symptoms in late life may be more common than previously thought. A Swedish investigation (Ostling et al. 2007) found that the prevalence of any psychotic symptom in a population-based sample of 95-year-old individuals who did not have dementia was 7.1%, with 6.7% experiencing hallucinations, 10.4% having delusions, and 0.6% experiencing paranoid ideation. In this chapter, we review the epidemiology, presentation, diagnosis, and treatment of chronic late-life psychotic disorders not secondary to a mood disorder or a general medical condition other than dementia. Thus, we discuss early-onset schizophrenia, late-onset schizophrenia, and very-late-onset schizophrenia-like psychosis (VLOSLP) (i.e., onset after age 60); delusional disorder; psychosis of Alzheimer's disease (AD); and psychosis associated with other dementias.

Psychotic Disorders in Late Life

Schizophrenia

Early-Onset Schizophrenia

The prevalence of schizophrenia among adults ages 45–64 is approximately 0.6%, and prevalence estimates for schizophrenia among elderly individuals range from 0.1% to 0.5%. Typically, individuals with schizophrenia develop the disease in the second or third decade of life (American Psychiatric Association 2000). Although mortality rates in general, and suicide and homicide rates in particular, are higher among individuals with schizophrenia than in the general population, many of these patients with early-onset schizophrenia are now living into older adulthood. Thus, most older adults with schizophrenia typically have had an early onset of the disease and have a chronic course of illness spanning several decades.

Longitudinal follow-up of schizophrenia patients indicates considerable heterogeneity of outcome. A minority of patients experience remission of both positive and negative symptoms. Auslander and Jeste (2004) reported that in approximately 10% of patients, the criteria for remission may be met, and although the course of illness over time is unchanged in the majority of patients, there is generally an improvement in positive symptoms.

Cognition in older schizophrenia patients.   Among community-dwelling older outpatients with schizophrenia, cognitive functioning seems to remain relatively stable other than the changes expected from normal aging (Harvey et al. 1999; Heaton et al. 2001). In general, cognitive functioning is better in persons with later ages at onset (Rajji et al. 2009).

Depression in older schizophrenia patients.   Studies have shown depressive symptoms to be distinct from negative symptoms. Depression is also a major predictor of suicidality in older patients with schizophrenia. Recent studies of depression in this population highlight the role of subsyndromal depression in increasing morbidity (Zisook et al. 2007).

Functional capacity. The level of functional impairment varies considerably among older adults with schizophrenia (Palmer et al. 2003). In general, worse neuropsychological test performance, lower educational level, and negative symptoms, but not positive symptoms, are associated with poorer functional capacity in older outpatients with schizophrenia.

Late-Onset Schizophrenia

A literature review found that approximately 23% of patients with schizophrenia reportedly had onset of the disorder after age 40, with 3% being older than 60 (Harris and Jeste 1988). One investigation of first-contact patients reported that 29% of the patients had onset after age 44, with 12% reporting onset after age 64 (Jeste et al. 1997). The consensus statement by the International Late-Onset Schizophrenia Group (Howard et al. 2000) suggested that schizophrenia with an onset after age 40 should be called "late-onset schizophrenia" and considered a subtype of schizophrenia rather than a related disorder.

Risk factors and clinical presentation are similar between individuals with early- and late-onset schizophrenia. The self-reported proportion of individuals with positive family history of schizophrenia (10%–15%), genetic risk, and levels of childhood maladjustment is similar in earlier- and late-onset patients (Sachdev et al. 1999). A long-term neuropsychological follow-up of a group of late-onset schizophrenia patients found no evidence of cognitive decline, suggesting a neurodevelopmental rather than a neurodegenerative process (Palmer et al. 2003).

Women predominate among individuals with onset of schizophrenia in middle to late life. It has been speculated that estrogen may serve as an endogenous antipsychotic, masking schizophrenic symptoms in vulnerable women until after menopause, but treatments targeting estrogen have not been found effective (Seeman 1996).

In a study conducted at our center, we used a comprehensive battery of measurements of psychopathology, cognition, and functioning to compare 110 subjects with late-onset schizophrenia with 744 early-onset schizophrenia patients. In our study, we noted that persons with late-onset schizophrenia were more likely to be women and to have less severe positive symptoms and lower scores on measures of general psychopathology. We also noted that patients with late-onset schizophrenia did better on cognitive tasks measuring abstraction, cognitive flexibility, and verbal memory. Patients with late-onset schizophrenia had better physical and emotional functioning and were receiving lower average dosages of antipsychotic medications (Vahia et al. 2010). A meta-analysis also noted that cognitive deficits in late-onset schizophrenia are specific rather than just a function of age (Rajji et al. 2009).

Very-Late-Onset Schizophrenia-Like Psychosis

The consensus statement by the International Late-Onset Schizophrenia Group proposed the diagnostic term *very-late-onset schizophrenia-like psychosis* for patients in whom onset of psychosis is after age 60. Table 6–1 compares risk factors for and clinical features of early-onset schizophrenia, late-onset schizophrenia, and VLOSLP. VLOSLP may be difficult to diagnose clinically because its clinical picture can be confused with other conditions such as delirium or psychosis due to underlying medical illness. Nevertheless, new-onset primary psychotic symptoms have been described in adults as old as 100 (Cervantes et al. 2006).

Factors distinguishing VLOSLP patients from "true" schizophrenia patients include a lower genetic load, less evidence of early childhood maladjustment, a relative lack of thought disorder and negative symptoms (including blunted affect), greater risk of tardive dyskinesia (TD), and evidence of a neurodegenerative rather than a neurodevelopmental process (Moore et al. 2006; Palmer et al. 2003).

Clinical vigilance must be exercised when the clinician is treating apparent primary-onset psychotic symptoms in older patients, and "organic" causes should be meticulously ruled out.

Delusional Disorder

The essential feature of a delusional disorder is a nonbizarre delusion (e.g., persecutory, somatic, erotomanic, grandiose, or jealous) without prominent auditory or visual hallucinations. Symptoms must be present for at least 1 month. When delusional disorder arises in late life, basic personality features, intellectual performance, and occupational function are preserved, but social functioning is compromised. To diagnose delusional disorder, the clinician must rule out other organic causes (Evans et al. 1996).

The lifetime prevalence of delusional disorder, according to DSM-5 (American Psychiatric Association 2013), is about 0.2% and is slightly higher among women than among men. Delusional disorder typically first appears in

Table 6–1. Comparison of early-onset schizophrenia, late-onset schizophrenia, and very-late-onset schizophrenia-like psychosis (VLOSLP)

	Early-onset schizophrenia	Late-onset schizophrenia	VLOSLP
Age at onset	Before 40	Middle age (~40–60)	Late life (>60)
Female preponderance	−	+	++
Negative symptoms	++	+	−
Minor physical anomalies	+	+	−
Neuropsychological impairment			
Learning	++	+	?++
Retention	−	−	?++
Progressive cognitive deterioration	−	−	++
Brain structure abnormalities (e.g., strokes, tumors)	−	−	++
Family history of schizophrenia	+	+	−
Early childhood maladjustment	+	+	−
Daily antipsychotic dose	++	+	+
Risk of tardive dyskinesia	+	+	++

Note.   + = mildly present; ++ = strongly present; ?++ = probably strongly present, but limited data exist; − = absent.
Source.   Adapted from Palmer et al. 2001.

middle to late adulthood, with an average age at onset of 40–49 for men and 60–69 for women (Copeland et al. 1998).

Risk factors for delusional disorder include a family history of schizophrenia and avoidant, paranoid, or schizoid personality disorder (Kendler and Davis 1981). Evans et al. (1996) compared middle-aged and older patients with schizophrenia and delusional disorder and found no differences in neuropsychological impairment but more severe psychopathology associated with delusional disorder.

Psychosis of Alzheimer's Disease

Ropacki and Jeste (2005) estimated the median prevalence of psychosis in AD to be about 41% (range, 12.2%–74.1%) in their review of 55 studies. Psychosis is associated with more rapid cognitive decline. Some studies have reported a significant association between psychosis and age, age at onset of AD, and illness duration. Paulsen et al. (2000) found a cumulative incidence of psychotic symptoms of 20% at 1 year, 36% at 2 years, 50% at 3 years, and 51% at 4 years in a large sample of patients with probable AD. Active suicidal ideation and history of psychosis are rare. Because psychotic symptoms in dementia patients tend to remit in the late stages of the disease, very-long-term maintenance therapy with antipsychotics is typically unnecessary.

AD patients with and without psychosis differ in several important ways. Neuropsychologically, AD patients with psychosis show greater impairment in executive functioning, more rapid cognitive decline, and a greater prevalence of extrapyramidal symptoms (EPS) than do AD patients without psychosis. Neuropathologically, dementia patients with psychosis show increased neurodegenerative changes in the cortex, increased norepinephrine in subcortical regions, and reduced serotonin levels in both cortical and subcortical areas.

Jeste and Finkel (2000) recommended specific diagnostic criteria for psychosis of AD: presence of visual or auditory hallucinations or delusions, a primary diagnosis of AD, and duration (at least 1 month) and time-of-onset (symptoms of AD preceding those of psychosis) criteria. Alternative causes of psychosis must be excluded, and sufficient functional impairment should be present for this diagnosis to be made.

Psychosis in Other Dementias

Psychosis is also common in other dementias. Visual hallucinations and secondary delusions are common in Lewy body disease, and vascular dementia also may be accompanied by delusions or hallucinations (Schneider et al. 2006). Naimark et al. (1996) found psychotic symptoms in approximately one-third of a sample of patients with Parkinson's disease, with hallucinations being more common than delusions. Psychosis in frontotemporal dementias is poorly characterized but may be as common as that in AD.

Diagnostic Approach to Patients With New Onset of Suspiciousness and Paranoia[1]

A careful psychiatric evaluation and history are key components of the initial approach to the suspicious or paranoid patient. Interviews of family members may be necessary for establishing a diagnosis, particularly if delusions and agitation are present. Part of the task of the clinician is to determine whether the suspicious behavior is warranted. Older adults are occasionally abused or neglected; therefore, confronting family members about a patient's accusations of harm or neglect is often part of the assessment. If, after such a confrontation, the clinician is not convinced that the accusations are totally explained by the delusion, a social services agency or department should be requested to investigate further.

Challenging the delusional patient usually is not recommended. It is important to seek an understanding of the patient's thought processes, so providing an atmosphere of acceptance (although not necessarily agreement) will allow the patient to express his or her beliefs and feelings. Reassurance should be provided in a manner conveying that although the clinician may not fully understand the whole situation, the goal is for the patient to feel better and more secure.

A laboratory workup is usually needed in new cases of paranoia to rule out an organic delusional syndrome. Blood chemistry, a complete blood count, and a thyroid profile should be obtained. If respiratory symptoms are present, a chest X ray may be needed. A computed tomography or magnetic resonance imaging brain scan may be indicated, especially if cognitive impairment or focal neurological findings are present. Because suspiciousness is often associated with sensory impairment, particularly visual and auditory deficits, audiometric and visual testing may identify potential areas for further intervention.

---

[1]We wish to thank Lisa Gwyther, M.S.W., and Harold Goforth, M.D., for providing this section on the diagnostic approach to patients with new onset of suspiciousness and paranoia.

Treatment

Although conventional agents substantially improve the positive symptoms of schizophrenia (e.g., hallucinations and delusions), several treatment liabilities, such as movement disorders, sedation, orthostatic hypotension, elevated prolactin concentrations, and most notably TD, have been recognized over the years. Atypical antipsychotics have been linked to increased risk of metabolic dysfunction, including diabetes, dyslipidemia, and obesity, leading to a worsened cardiovascular risk profile. In elderly patients with dementia, atypical antipsychotics have been associated with increased risk of cerebrovascular adverse events and mortality compared with placebo, leading pharmaceutical regulatory agencies to issue warnings about their use. However, lack of evidence-based alternatives restricts clinicians to off-label treatments, which must be used with caution and close monitoring. Psychosocial treatments for older adults with psychosis show promise as adjunctive treatments.

Schizophrenia and Delusional Disorder

Pharmacological Treatment

Pharmacotherapy for schizophrenia and delusional disorder in older adults is restricted by a paucity of randomized placebo-controlled, double-blind clinical trials in this population. Maintenance pharmacotherapy is usually required for older patients with schizophrenia because of risk of relapse. Older patients are at higher risk for adverse antipsychotic effects as a result of age-related pharmacokinetic and pharmacodynamic factors, coexisting medical illnesses, and concomitant medications. Therefore, the recommended doses of antipsychotics in older individuals are 25%–50% lower than the usual doses in younger adults (American Psychiatric Association 2004).

Few efficacy comparisons between conventional and atypical antipsychotics have been done in patients with schizophrenia older than 65 (Jeste et al. 1999). The National Institute of Mental Health's Clinical Antipsychotic Trials of Intervention Effectiveness (CATIE) study, which included adults ages 18–65 years, found no significant differences in effectiveness between the conventional antipsychotic perphenazine and the atypical antipsychotics risperidone, olanzapine, quetiapine, and ziprasidone, but it is unknown how these findings would translate to patients older than 65 (Lieberman et al. 2005).

Use of conventional or typical antipsychotics in this population is problematic given the higher incidence of TD in older patients. Aging appears to be the most important risk factor for the development of TD (American Psychiatric Association 2000; Yassa and Nair 1992). Atypical antipsychotics have a less favorable side-effect profile in terms of metabolic function. Common metabolic side effects include excessive weight gain and obesity, glucose intolerance, new-onset type 2 diabetes mellitus, diabetic ketoacidosis, and dyslipidemia (Jin et al. 2004). Although no guidelines are available for management of these side effects specifically in older patients with schizophrenia, monitoring recommendations of the American Diabetes Association et al. (2004) are potentially applicable. Because elderly patients tend to be at higher risk for cardiovascular disease than are younger patients, closer monitoring would be necessary for older adults.

The only large-scale randomized, double-blind, controlled trial comparing two atypical antipsychotics in adults older than 60 is Jeste et al.'s (2003) multisite international study of risperidone and olanzapine. In that trial, 175 patients with schizophrenia or schizoaffective disorder age 60 years and older were randomly assigned to receive risperidone (1–3 mg/day; median, 2 mg/day) or olanzapine (5–20 mg/day; median, 10 mg/day). Both groups had significant improvement in symptoms and reduction in EPS rating scale scores. Clinically relevant weight gain was significantly less frequent in patients taking risperidone.

Given the dearth of randomized controlled data, Alexopoulos et al. (2004) conducted a consensus survey of 48 American experts on antipsychotic treatment in older adults. The experts' first-line recommendation for late-life schizophrenia was risperidone (1.25–3.5 mg/day). The second-line recommendations included quetiapine (100–300 mg/day), olanzapine (7.5–15 mg/day), and aripiprazole (15–30 mg/day). Support for the use of clozapine, ziprasidone, and high-potency conventional antipsychotics was limited. In a more recent trial (Scott et al. 2010), atypical antipsychotics at geriatric doses were effective in treating VLOSLP as well.

Given the data on the increased risk of strokes and mortality in elderly patients with dementia treated with atypical antipsychotics (Gill et al. 2005) and the consequent U.S. Food and Drug Administration (FDA) black box warnings (discussed in the subsection "Psychosis of Alzheimer's Disease and

Other Dementias" later in this chapter), clinicians should exercise caution when using these drugs in older patients with schizophrenia.

Few data are available specifically on the pharmacological treatment of delusional disorder in late life. Alexopoulos et al.'s (2004) survey of 48 experts in geriatric care concluded that antipsychotics are the only recommended treatment, and their first-line recommendation for older adults with delusional disorder was risperidone (0.75–2.5 mg/day), followed by olanzapine (5–10 mg/day) and quetiapine (50–200 mg/day).

Psychosocial Treatments

Recent years have seen the development and testing of psychosocial interventions for older adults with chronic psychotic disorders. In a randomized controlled trial, Granholm et al. (2005) noted that cognitive-behavioral social skills training (CBSST), which combines cognitive and behavioral coping techniques, training in social functioning and problem solving, and compensatory aids for neurocognitive impairments, led to significantly increased frequency of social functioning activities, greater cognitive insight (more objectivity in reappraising psychotic symptoms), and greater skill mastery. An increase in cognitive insight was significantly correlated with greater reduction in positive symptoms. At 12-month follow-up (Granholm et al. 2007), the CBSST group had maintained their greater skill acquisition and performance of everyday living skills.

Patterson et al. (2006) conducted a randomized controlled trial of a behavioral group intervention called Functional Adaptation Skills Training (FAST), a manualized behavioral intervention designed to improve everyday living skills such as medication management, social skills, communication skills, organization and planning, transportation, and financial management. The researchers noted that the FAST group showed significant improvement in daily living skills and social skills but not medication management.

In an examination of employment outcomes among middle-aged and older adults with schizophrenia, Twamley et al. (2005) reported that the highest rates of volunteer or paid work (81%) and competitive or paid work (69%) occurred for the patients who were placed in a job chosen with a vocational counselor and who then received individualized on-site support.

Psychosis of Alzheimer's Disease and Other Dementias

Since their introduction in the 1990s, the atypical antipsychotics have for the most part replaced conventional antipsychotics in treating psychosis, aggression, and agitation in patients with dementia because of greater tolerability, lower risk for acute EPS, and comparatively lower risk of TD (Kindermann et al. 2002). Most antipsychotic prescriptions in older adults are for behavioral disturbances associated with dementia, despite their lacking this FDA-approved indication (Ballard et al. 2006). Only a few randomized controlled trials have compared typical and atypical classes of antipsychotics for dementia, and results have been inconclusive (De Deyn et al. 1999).

In the CATIE-AD trial (Schneider et al. 2006), which was the largest (*N*=421) non-industry-sponsored trial of atypical antipsychotics for psychosis or agitation/aggression in people with dementia, olanzapine, quetiapine, and risperidone were no better than placebo for the primary outcome (time to discontinuation for any reason). Time to discontinuation due to lack of efficacy favored olanzapine and risperidone, whereas time to discontinuation due to adverse events favored placebo.

In addition to the lack of evidence described earlier, use of atypical antipsychotics in elderly dementia patients has been associated with cerebrovascular adverse events and death, leading to black box warnings by the FDA. Retrospective database reviews did not find any difference in incidence of cerebrovascular adverse events for typical versus atypical antipsychotic use (Gill et al. 2005, 2007), although none of these studies were originally designed to examine cerebrovascular adverse event risk. The data on risk of mortality associated with typical versus atypical antipsychotics have been mixed (Jeste et al. 2008).

Unfortunately, data are also insufficient to support systematic use of any of the alternatives to antipsychotics, and few well-designed randomized controlled trials of behavioral and psychosocial interventions have been done in patients with dementia. There are, however, promising possibilities (e.g., behavioral management techniques, caregiver education) (Ayalon et al. 2006; Cohen-Mansfield 2001; Livingston et al. 2005).

Patients with Lewy body dementia and parkinsonian dementia are especially sensitive to side effects such as EPS and anticholinergic effects, so very low doses and slow titration schedules should be used to avoid worsening of motor symptoms (Chou et al. 2007; Masand 2000). Low-dose clozapine has shown efficacy in reducing symptoms of psychosis, and clozapine does not worsen and can even improve the parkinsonian tremor.

References

Alexopoulos GS, Streim JE, Carpenter D, et al; Expert Consensus Panel for Using Antipsychotic Drugs in Older Patients: Using antipsychotic agents in older patients. J Clin Psychiatry 65:5–99, 2004

American Diabetes Association, American Psychiatric Association, American Association of Clinical Endocrinologists, et al: Consensus development conference on antipsychotic drugs and obesity and diabetes. Diabetes Care 27:596–601, 2004

American Psychiatric Association: Diagnostic and Statistical Manual of Mental Disorders, 4th Edition, Text Revision. Washington, DC, American Psychiatric Association, 2000

American Psychiatric Association: Practice guideline for the treatment of patients with schizophrenia, 2nd Edition. Arlington, VA, American Psychiatric Association, April 2004. Available at: http://psychiatryonline.org/content.aspx?bookid=28&sectionid=1665359. Accessed July 3, 2013.

Auslander LA, Jeste DV: Sustained remission of schizophrenia among community-dwelling older outpatients. Am J Psychiatry 161:1490–1493, 2004

Ayalon L, Gum AM, Feliciano L, et al: Effectiveness of nonpharmacological interventions for the management of neuropsychiatric symptoms in patients with dementia: a systematic review. Arch Intern Med 166:2182–2188, 2006

Ballard CG, Waite J, Birks J: Atypical antipsychotics for aggression and psychosis in Alzheimer's disease. Cochrane Database of Systematic Reviews 2006, Issue 1, Art. No. CD003476. DOI: 10.1002/14651858. CD003476.pub2.

Cervantes AN, Rabins PV, Slavney PR: Onset of schizophrenia at age 100. Psychosomatics 47:356–359, 2006

Chou KL, Borek LL, Friedman JH: The management of psychosis in movement disorder patients. Expert Opin Pharmacother 8:935–943, 2007

Cohen-Mansfield J: Nonpharmacologic interventions for inappropriate behaviors in dementia: a review and critique. Am J Geriatr Psychiatry 9:361–381, 2001

Copeland JRM, Dewey ME, Scott A, et al: Schizophrenia and delusional disorder in older age: community prevalence, incidence, comorbidity and outcome. Schizophr Bull 19:153–161, 1998

De Deyn P, Rabheru K, Rasmussen A, et al: A randomized trial of risperidone, placebo, and haloperidol for behavioral symptoms of dementia. Neurology 53:946–955, 1999

Evans JD, Paulsen JS, Harris MJ, et al: A clinical and neuropsychological comparison of delusional disorder and schizophrenia. J Neuropsychiatry Clin Neurosci 8:281–286, 1996

Gill SS, Rochon PA, Herrmann N, et al: Atypical antipsychotic drugs and risk of ischaemic stroke: population based retrospective cohort study. BMJ 330(7489):445, 2005

Gill SS, Bronskill SE, Normand SL, et al: Antipsychotic drug use and mortality in older adults with dementia. Ann Intern Med 146(11):775–786, 2007

Granholm E, McQuaid JR, McClure FS, et al: A randomized, controlled trial of cognitive behavioral social skills training for middle-aged and older outpatients with chronic schizophrenia. Am J Psychiatry 162:520–529, 2005

Granholm E, McQuaid JR, McClure FS, et al: Randomized controlled trial of cognitive behavioral social skills training for older people with schizophrenia: 12-month follow-up. J Clin Psychiatry 68:730–737, 2007

Harris MJ, Jeste DV: Late-onset schizophrenia: an overview. Schizophr Bull 14:39–55, 1988

Harvey PD, Silverman JM, Mohs RC, et al: Cognitive decline in late-life schizophrenia: a longitudinal study of geriatric chronically hospitalized patients. Biol Psychiatry 45:32–40, 1999

Heaton RK, Gladsjo JA, Palmer BW, et al: Stability and course of neuropsychological deficits in schizophrenia. Arch Gen Psychiatry 58:24–32, 2001

Howard R, Rabins PV, Seeman MV, et al: Late-onset schizophrenia and very-late-onset schizophrenia-like psychosis: an international consensus. Am J Psychiatry 157:172–178, 2000

Jeste DV, Finkel SI: Psychosis of Alzheimer's disease and related dementias: diagnostic criteria for a distinct syndrome. Am J Geriatr Psychiatry 8:29–34, 2000

Jeste DV, Symonds LL, Harris MJ, et al: Non-dementia non-praecox dementia praecox? Late-onset schizophrenia. Am J Geriatr Psychiatry 5:302–317, 1997

Jeste DV, Rockwell E, Harris MJ, et al: Conventional versus newer antipsychotics in elderly patients. Am J Geriatr Psychiatry 7:70–76, 1999

Jeste DV, Barak Y, Madhusoodanan S, et al: International multisite double-blind trial of the atypical antipsychotics risperidone and olanzapine in 175 elderly patients with chronic schizophrenia. Am J Geriatr Psychiatry 11:638–647, 2003

Jeste DV, Blazer D, Casey DE, et al: ACNP White Paper: update on the use of antipsychotic drugs in elderly persons with dementia. Neuropsychopharmacology 33:957–970, 2008

Jin H, Meyer JM, Jeste DV: Atypical antipsychotics and glucose dysregulation: a systematic review. Schizophr Res 71:195–212, 2004

Kendler S, Davis KL: The genetics and biochemistry of paranoid schizophrenia and other paranoid psychoses. Schizophr Bull 7:689–709, 1981

Kindermann SS, Dolder CR, Bailey A, et al: Pharmacologic treatment of psychosis and agitation in elderly patients with dementia: four decades of experience. Drugs Aging 19:257–276, 2002

Lieberman JA, Stroup TS, McEvoy JP, et al: Effectiveness of antipsychotic drugs in patients with chronic schizophrenia. N Engl J Med 353:1209–1223, 2005

Livingston G, Johnston K, Katona C, et al: Systematic review of psychological approaches to the management of neuropsychiatric symptoms of dementia. Am J Psychiatry 162:1996–2021, 2005

Masand PS: Atypical antipsychotics for elderly patients with neurodegenerative disorders and medical conditions. Psychiatr Ann 30:203–208, 2000

Moore R, Blackwood N, Corcoran R, et al: Misunderstanding the intentions of others: an exploratory study of the cognitive etiology of persecutory delusions in very late-onset schizophrenia-like psychosis. Am J Geriatr Psychiatry 14:410–418, 2006

Naimark D, Jackson E, Rockwell E, et al: Psychotic symptoms in Parkinson's disease patients with dementia. J Am Geriatr Soc 44:296–299, 1996

Ostling S, Börjesson-Hanson A, Skoog I: Psychotic symptoms and paranoid ideation in a population-based sample of 95-year-olds. Am J Geriatr Psychiatry 15:999–1004, 2007

Palmer BW, McClure FS, Jeste DV: Schizophrenia in late life: findings challenge traditional concepts. Harv Rev Psychiatry 9(2):51–58, 2001

Palmer BW, Bondi MW, Twamley EW, et al: Are late-onset schizophrenia-spectrum disorders a neurodegenerative condition? Annual rates of change on two dementia measures. J Neuropsychiatry Clin Neurosci 15:45–52, 2003

Patterson TL, Mausbach BT, McKibbin C, et al: Functional adaptation skills training (FAST): a randomized trial of a psychosocial intervention for middle-aged and older patients with chronic psychotic disorders. Schizophr Res 86:291–299, 2006

Paulsen JS, Salmon DP, Thal LJ, et al: Incidence of and risk factors for hallucinations and delusions in patients with probable AD. Neurology 54:1965–1971, 2000

Rajji TK, Ismail Z, Mulsant BH: Age at onset and cognition in schizophrenia: a meta-analysis. Br J Psychiatry 195:286–293, 2009

Ropacki SA, Jeste DV: Epidemiology of and risk factors for psychosis of Alzheimer's disease: a review of 55 studies published from 1990 to 2003. Am J Psychiatry 162:2022–2030, 2005

Sachdev P, Brodaty H, Rose N, et al: Schizophrenia with onset after age 50 years, 2: neurological, neuropsychological and MRI investigation. Br J Psychiatry 175:416–421, 1999

Schneider LS, Tariot PN, Dagerman KS, et al: Effectiveness of atypical antipsychotic drugs in patients with Alzheimer's disease. N Engl J Med 355:1525–1538, 2006

Scott J, Greenwald BS, Kramer E, et al: Atypical (second generation) antipsychotic treatment response in very late-onset schizophrenia-like psychosis. Int Psychogeriatr 1:1–7, 2010

Seeman MV: The role of estrogen in schizophrenia. J Psychiatr Neurosci 21:123–127, 1996

Twamley EW, Padin DS, Bayne KS, et al: Work rehabilitation for middle-aged and older people with schizophrenia: a comparison of three approaches. J Nerv Ment Dis 193:596–601, 2005

Vahia IV, Palmer BW, Depp C, et al: Is late-onset schizophrenia a subtype of schizophrenia? Acta Psychiatr Scand 122:414–426, 2010

Yassa R, Nair NPV: A 10-year follow-up study of tardive dyskinesia. Acta Psychiatr Scand 86:262–266, 1992

Zisook S, Montross L, Kasckow J, et al: Subsyndromal depressive symptoms in middle-aged and older persons with schizophrenia. Am J Geriatr Psychiatry 15:1005–1014, 2007

7

Anxiety Disorders

Eric J. Lenze, M.D.
Julie Loebach Wetherell, Ph.D.
Carmen Andreescu, M.D.

Anxiety disorders are common in older adults and cause considerable distress and functional impairment. However, they are typically not assessed or managed properly. In this chapter, we briefly discuss the epidemiology and neurobiology, neuropsychiatry, and neuropsychology of anxiety disorders in late life. We then review treatment outcome studies and discuss guidelines for assessment and management.

Epidemiology

Prevalence

Epidemiological studies have produced wide variation in prevalence estimates of anxiety disorders in elderly persons (Bryant et al. 2008), ranging from 1.2%

to 15% in community samples and from 1% to 28% in medical settings. Likewise, the prevalence of clinically relevant anxiety symptoms ranges from 15% to 52% in community samples and from 15% to 56% in medical settings. Some have questioned whether diagnostic criteria, and the methods used to observe them, are adequate in detecting mental disorders in older adults (Jeste et al. 2005). For example, older adults commonly have fear of falling (Gagnon et al. 2005; Nagaratnam et al. 2005), which may not be discerned by standard epidemiological assessments or methodology.

The one anxiety disorder that seems to commonly present in late life is generalized anxiety disorder (GAD): approximately one-half of older adults with GAD have onset later in life (Chou 2009; Lenze et al. 2005a; Le Roux et al. 2005). Otherwise, anxiety disorders, particularly social phobia and panic disorder, are usually considered to have onset in childhood or early adulthood. On the contrary, several anxiogenic stressors are associated with aging, such as chronic illness and disability, caregiver status, and bereavement, and many elderly anxiety disorder patients in clinical samples have late onset of anxiety disorders (Lenze et al. 2005a; Le Roux et al. 2005; Sheikh et al. 2004b). Also, many common conditions in older adults could exacerbate anxiety. Dementia can cause anxiety that often manifests as agitation (Mintzer and Brawman-Mintzer 1996), hoarding syndrome (Saxena et al. 2002), or other atypical symptoms (Starkstein et al. 2007). Many common medical conditions are anxiogenic, such as heart disease (Todaro et al. 2007), lung disease (Yohannes et al. 2006), and neurological diseases (such as Parkinson's disease). Comorbid anxiety is extremely common in late-life depression (Beekman et al. 2000; Lenze et al. 2000).

Course

The few longitudinal studies that have been carried out in older adults with anxiety suggest that it is persistent in this age group (Schuurmans et al. 2005). Of the anxious older adults in epidemiological and treatment-seeking samples, 60%–70% retrospectively reported an onset in or before early adulthood (Blazer et al. 1991; Lenze et al. 2005a; Le Roux et al. 2005; Sheikh et al. 1991).

Anxiety increases disability (Brenes et al. 2005) and potentially elevates mortality risk (Brenes et al. 2007a). Significant quality of life impairment has been noted in older adults with GAD, similar to that seen in those with late-life depression (Porensky et al. 2009; Wetherell et al. 2004).

Comorbidity With Depression

Depressed elderly patients with comorbid anxiety have greater somatic symptoms, greater likelihood of suicidal ideation (Jeste et al. 2006; Lenze et al. 2000), and a higher risk of suicide (Allgulander and Lavori 1993). Longitudinally, anxiety symptoms appear to be more stable over time than depressive symptoms and more likely to lead to depressive symptoms than vice versa (Wetherell et al. 2001). Conversely, anxiety and depression may appear simultaneously (Lenze et al. 2005a); in such cases, anxiety symptoms often persist after remission of depression and increase risk for depressive relapse (Dombrovski et al. 2007; Flint and Rifat 1997). Comorbid anxiety predicts greater decline in memory during long-term follow-up of late-life depression (DeLuca et al. 2005). In summary, anxious depression is a severe, treatment-relevant subtype of late-life depression.

Neurobiology, Neuropsychiatry, and Neuropsychology

Neurobiology of Anxiety

Understanding the neuropsychiatry of anxiety in older adults requires an understanding of the neuroanatomy of anxiety. Midlife studies have found amygdala hyperactivation in panic disorders and specific phobias; insula hyperactivation in GAD, phobias, and posttraumatic stress disorder (PTSD); and right prefrontal hyperactivation and altered coupling of the amygdala–prefrontal circuit in anxious arousal (Bishop 2007). The amygdala–prefrontal circuit enables both representations of salient emotions and implementation of top-down control mechanisms to influence interpretive processes. Disruption of this circuitry, including deficient recruitment of prefrontal control mechanisms and amygdala hyperresponsivity to threat, leads to a sustained threat-related processing bias in anxious individuals.

Anxiety-regulation strategies typically involve higher-level cognitive restructuring through the medial prefrontal cortex (mPFC). Top-down conscious reinterpretation reappraises potentially threatening stimuli as less threatening

(Arce et al. 2008; Bishop 2007) through the activation of the cingulate cortex and the mPFC.

Within the large area of the mPFC involved in the top-down reappraisal of threatening stimuli, recent research has delineated the subgenual anterior cingulate cortex (sACC; the affective division of ACC) as a key region in assessing the salience of emotional information and the regulation of emotional response (Bissiere et al. 2008). Inappropriate recruitment of the sACC during emotional events is one of the functional neuroanatomical bases of clinical anxiety (Simmons et al. 2008).

Neuropsychiatric Conditions in Older Adults That Are Associated With Anxiety

In patients with neurodegenerative disease that results in pathological anxiety, the pathophysiology is likely to be network dysregulation, including centrally the dysregulation of the sACC-amygdala axis (Bissiere et al. 2008). Given this disconnectivity hypothesis, neuropsychiatric conditions that affect subcortical white matter, or the functioning of cortical and subcortical components of this network, are likely to be anxiogenic. Of course, the anxiety that frequently arises in stroke and other medical conditions also may reflect their status as anxiogenic life stressors (e.g., leading to sudden or chronic loss of control).

Parkinson's disease may be a particularly anxiogenic neurodegenerative illness because of its association not only with subcortical disease but also with autonomic dysfunction (potentially leading to panic attacks or similar autonomic symptoms) and uncontrollability over basic movements and activities (Lauterbach et al. 2003; Marsh 2000; Richard et al. 1996). Huntington's disease is another subcortical neurodegenerative disease with a high prevalence of anxiety symptoms (Paulsen et al. 2001). Stroke can cause anxiety symptoms (De Wit et al. 2008), GAD (Aström 1996; Castillo et al. 1995), or obsessive-compulsive disorder (Swoboda and Jenike 1995). As with depression, some evidence indicates that left hemisphere lesions may be more likely to cause anxiety (Barker-Collo 2007), although the pathophysiology underlying this link is unclear.

Dementing illness can cause anxiety symptoms (Ballard et al. 2000; Lyketsos et al. 2002) or GAD (Starkstein et al. 2007). Anxiety symptoms or disorders in elderly adults are associated with accelerated cognitive decline (DeLuca et al. 2005; Palmer et al. 2007; Sinoff and Werner 2003). Several potential mechanisms exist for anxiety-induced neurodegeneration. Pathological anxiety in late life is associated with activation of the hypothalamic-pituitary-adrenal axis, leading to higher cortisol levels, which may adversely affect hippocampal and prefrontal function (Lenze et al. 2011; Mantella et al. 2008). Anxiety may induce cerebrovascular disease via insulin resistance, endothelial reactivity, and impaired autonomic function (Narita et al. 2008). Chronic mood disorders lead, via oxidative stress, to decreased telomerase activity and telomere shrinking, resulting in accelerated cellular aging (Simon et al. 2006). Finally, altering serotonin function in an aging model modifies not only stress responsivity but also age-related neurodegeneration (Sibille et al. 2007).

Neuropsychological Impairments in Late-Life Anxiety

Anxiety and cognitive impairment have a consistent and bidirectional relation in older adults (Beaudreau and O'Hara 2008). Recent investigations have found a variety of memory and executive impairments in geriatric GAD, including poorer short-term memory and executive dysfunction (Butters et al. 2011; Caudle et al. 2007; Mantella et al. 2007; Mohlman and Gorman 2005). Some evidence indicates that cognitive impairment predicts poorer long-term psychotherapy outcome with cognitive-behavioral therapy (CBT) for geriatric GAD (Caudle et al. 2007).

Treatment Outcome Studies

Both psychotherapy and pharmacotherapy appear to be effective treatment options in this age group (Wetherell et al. 2005b). A meta-analysis and one direct randomized comparison of pharmacotherapy and psychotherapy found medications more effective than CBT in the acute phase of treatment (Pinquart and Duberstein 2007; Schuurmans et al. 2006). Nevertheless, patient and provider preferences most likely will be the deciding factor in whether to initiate pharmacotherapy or psychotherapy.

Psychotherapy

CBT is currently the dominant formal psychotherapy for anxiety disorders; it might be particularly effective for anxiety disorders in older adults who are able to learn new skills in CBT and use them effectively (Wetherell et al. 2005a). As such, consideration of cognition, motivation, and ability to practice skills should be part of an evaluation for psychotherapy. CBT for late-life anxiety typically involves psychoeducation, relaxation, cognitive therapy, problem-solving skills training, exposure exercises (i.e., exposure and habituation to anxiogenic situations), and sleep hygiene when necessary for the common problem of insomnia (Brenes et al. 2009), similar to treatment in younger adults (Stanley et al. 2004). In elderly persons, the most effective ingredient of CBT may be relaxation (Thorp et al. 2009). CBT has been shown to be effective in the primary care setting (Stanley et al. 2009), although the lack of highly skilled CBT practitioners with experience in late-life anxiety may be a barrier to widespread implementation.

Booster sessions to prevent loss of efficacy during maintenance treatment are particularly important for older adults because aging is associated with poorer performance on attention and memory tasks for which internally generated and maintained strategies are required (Prull et al. 2006). Booster sessions are also responsive to life events, which appear to play a role in long-term outcomes from late-life GAD (Wetherell and Stein 2009). With respect to long-term management, follow-up studies of older patients with GAD treated with CBT have reported maintenance of gains for up to 1 year following discontinuation of treatment (Barrowclough et al. 2001; Stanley et al. 2003).

Adaptations of CBT for older adults include a slower pace with increased repetition, less abstract cognitive restructuring techniques and correspondingly more focus on behavior change, more focus on health-related problems, and a family session, reflecting the importance of engaging family in geriatric mental health treatment. In addition to in-session discussion and a written summary of material, we audiotape sessions for participants to consolidate learning. Another possible adaptation is the integration of religion into CBT (Paukert et al. 2009).

Another promising treatment is bibliotherapy (Brenes et al. 2007b). One study of late-life anxiety and depression prevention used a stepped-care approach, in which bibliotherapy, the first intervention, was effective at preventing anxiety and depressive episodes (van't Veer-Tazelaar et al. 2009). Many self-help workbooks exist for anxiety disorders, although none to our knowledge are focused on older adults.

Pharmacotherapy

The evidence base for pharmacotherapy in older adults is limited and consists mainly of small clinical trials. Benzodiazepines are still commonly used for geriatric anxiety (Benitez et al. 2008), despite the association of these medications with falls (Landi et al. 2005) and cognitive impairment and decline (Paterniti et al. 2002). Generally, their long-term use for late-life anxiety is discouraged.

Two small randomized controlled trials (RCTs; Lenze et al. 2005b; Schuurmans et al. 2006) and a full-scale RCT (Lenze et al. 2009) showed the efficacy of selective serotonin reuptake inhibitors (SSRIs) in the acute treatment of anxiety disorders, predominantly GAD, in older adults. In the latter study, which involved 177 older adults with GAD, escitalopram was superior to placebo in cumulative response (69% vs. 51%). The effect size for most outcome measures in that study was in the small to moderate range.

With respect to serotonin-norepinephrine reuptake inhibitors (SNRIs), retrospective examinations of venlafaxine extended release and duloxetine studies found them to be efficacious in adults age 60 and older (Davidson et al. 2008; Katz et al. 2002). Additionally, a large-scale study with pregabalin found it to be efficacious in geriatric GAD (Montgomery et al. 2008). Pregabalin has not been approved by the U.S. Food and Drug Administration to treat anxiety disorders.

In addition to the studies of mainly GAD, some other medication studies should be noted. One supports the use of citalopram in PTSD (English et al. 2006), another supports superiority of mirtazapine over an SSRI (Chung et al. 2004), and a third finds evidence that the α-adrenergic antagonist prazosin is efficacious for sleep-related concerns in PTSD (Raskind et al. 2007). Additionally, in late-life panic disorder, one study found evidence for the superiority of escitalopram over citalopram in time to response (Rampello et al. 2006), and a small open-label study found evidence of benefit from sertraline (Sheikh et al. 2004a). Finally, nortriptyline was efficacious in a merged dataset of several RCTs in poststroke depression, in which patients with comorbid GAD were analyzed (Kimura et al. 2003).

The only published augmentation study in late-life anxiety disorders is a small study with risperidone (Morinigo et al. 2005). The use of atypical antipsychotics in elderly patients is problematic given concerns about higher mortality with antipsychotics compared with placebo in older patients with dementia. It remains unclear whether these risks apply to elderly persons without dementia.

The long-term or maintenance treatment of late-life anxiety with medication has not been studied, and no augmentation strategies can be recommended with confidence, although a pilot study has suggested benefits of sequencing SSRIs with CBT (Wetherell et al. 2011). No data exist on the efficacy and safety of complementary and alternative medications for anxiety in older adults.

Treatment Guidelines for Assessing and Managing Anxiety in Older Adults

Goals of Assessment

Clinicians should measure severity and provide objective criteria for assessing response, as well as assess comorbidity, prior treatment, cognitive status, and need for a medical workup. Anxiety assessment is challenging in older adults, who may find terms such as *anxiety* or *worry* not to be relevant (instead preferring words like *concern*). A helpful introduction to the topic is to inquire about stress, such as by asking, "Older adults often deal with stress; how do you feel in times of stress?" Geriatric anxiety disorders are defined, in presence and severity, by 1) level of distress (how much the anxiety symptoms bother the patient, and what strategies are being used to control or avoid anxiety); 2) amount of time consumed by anxiety symptoms, including associated somatic and psychic symptoms; and 3) avoidance. Avoidance is one of the most disabling components of anxiety disorders and often is not recognized by patients. For example, older adults may downplay changes in behavior patterns as being a result of poor health. Paradoxically, avoidance also may take the form of intrusive overinvolvement with family members as an attempt to decrease perceived loss of control.

Inquiring about somatic symptoms is helpful. For example, patients may not endorse "panic attacks" but may admit to brief periods with multiple physical symptoms (particularly autonomic symptoms such as palpitations). Likewise, patients with GAD may downplay the effects of worrying on their lives but more readily complain about distress from sleep disturbance or difficulty concentrating.

Most older adults who present with an anxiety disorder describe long-term, often lifelong, anxiety symptoms or proneness. Thus, a report that "I was never an anxious person, until just recently" should elicit consideration of 1) depression, 2) cognitive impairment (dementia, delirium), 3) anxiety-inducing medications (or recent discontinuation of sedatives), and 4) common and rare medical conditions that could masquerade as an anxiety disorder. Medical conditions might include thyroid disease, vitamin B_{12} deficiency, hypoxia, ischemia, metabolic changes (e.g., hypercalcemia or hypoglycemia), and arrhythmia.

Cautious Use of Benzodiazepines

No knee-jerk benzodiazepine prescription should be given. Benzodiazepines, like any sedatives, have a poor risk-benefit ratio in elderly persons. Even benzodiazepines with shorter half-lives and less complicated elimination (such as lorazepam) are associated with an increased risk of falling in elderly persons. Furthermore, in this age group, benzodiazepines appear to cause cognitive impairment, particularly in recall (Pomara et al. 1989, 1998a, 1998b). This cognitive problem is more likely with higher dosages of benzodiazepines and in elderly persons who are already predisposed to cognitive impairment. Therefore, long-term use of benzodiazepines appears unfavorable in this age group, and patients should be warned about the risks associated with these medications.

Psychoeducation

Psychoeducation about anxiety and treatment, including potential health benefits, should be provided. Of paramount importance, psychoeducation will improve treatment adherence and thereby improve quality of life, health, and cognition.

Choice of Treatment and Follow-Up

First-line treatment should be based on the patient's preference, the provider's preference and competence, and treatment availability. First-line options include use of one or more of the following: SSRI, SNRI, relaxation training, and CBT.

Frequent follow-up, particularly within the first month of treatment or a dosage change, is necessary to encourage adherence and monitor treatment response. Antidepressants can initially have a stimulating or mildly anxiogenic effect. Older adults with anxiety disorders often report that they are sensitive or intolerant to antidepressant medications; this report appears to stem from their anticipatory concern about side effects, their vigilance toward interoceptive stimuli, and their tendency to catastrophize about any sensations they detect. The management of this fear is part of the process of engaging the patient in treatment. The clinician should describe how such antidepressant medications have established efficacy and good tolerability in his or her experience with other patients. He or she should state that side effects are possible but no particular side effect is inevitable, and that most patients will have either no side effects or brief, self-limited side effects that subside in a few weeks. Family involvement can help with adherence. We recommend weekly visits with the clinician, or biweekly visits with interim telephone contacts (as well as availability of the clinician by phone as needed), for the first month of treatment and the month subsequent to a dosage increase, because this is when patients are most likely to develop concerns about side effects.

Dosing

Dosing of medications should start low, go slow, but go—as aggressively as required to treat symptoms to remission. Older and frailer or medically ill individuals need close monitoring (e.g., of gait, vital signs, or any incident medical issues that arise) along with lower starting dosages. However, the main acute goal is a treatment course of sufficient intensity and duration to alleviate symptoms. Thus, inadequate treatment is at least as significant a problem as medication intolerance.

Augmentation Treatment

A clinician should consider augmentation treatment and refer the patient to experts if necessary. Monotherapy is usually inadequate, and persistence is required. If a single adequate trial of medication monotherapy does not help sufficiently, additional trials and/or augmentation therapy should be tried. After the clinician has exhausted options, he or she should refer the patient to someone with expertise in geriatrics or other empirically supported forms of treatment for anxiety (e.g., a psychotherapist skilled at treating anxiety disorders).

Maintenance Treatment

The clinician should provide maintenance treatment or evaluate the need for such if treatment is discontinued. Maintenance pharmacotherapy tends to be simpler, and less frequent oversight is necessary, although continued monitoring of side effects, changes in coprescribed medications, and patient concerns is important.

Tapering Off Medication

A patient who chooses to taper off a medication may need to resume it at some future point. A taper should be very gradual to avoid rebound anxiety symptoms. In our experience, relapse following discontinuation of medication typically occurs within the first 3 months, whereas relapse following discontinuation of psychotherapy is often conditional on stressful life events coupled with the failure to continue practicing anxiety management skills.

Conclusion

The high prevalence of anxiety disorders in older adults, as well as the close and reciprocal relationship of these disorders with cognitive impairment and with disability, highlights their importance for public health. Effective treatments include antidepressants and psychotherapy. By following simple management strategies as outlined in this chapter, clinicians can effectively manage anxiety disorders in older patients.

References

Allgulander C, Lavori PW: Causes of death among 936 elderly patients with "pure" anxiety neurosis in Stockholm County, Sweden, and in patients with depressive neurosis or both diagnoses. Compr Psychiatry 34:299–302, 1993

Arce E, Simmons AN, Lovero KL, et al: Escitalopram effects on insula and amygdala BOLD activation during emotional processing. Psychopharmacology (Berl) 196:661–672, 2008

Aström M: Generalized anxiety disorder in stroke patients: a 3-year longitudinal study. Stroke 27:270–275, 1996

Ballard C, Neill D, O'Brien J, et al: Anxiety, depression and psychosis in vascular dementia: prevalence and associations. J Affect Disord 59:97–106, 2000

Barker-Collo SL: Depression and anxiety 3 months post stroke: prevalence and correlates. Arch Clin Neuropsychol 22:519–531, 2007

Barrowclough C, King P, Colville J, et al: A randomized trial of the effectiveness of cognitive-behavioral therapy and supportive counseling for anxiety symptoms in older adults. J Consult Clin Psychol 69:756–762, 2001

Beaudreau SA, O'Hara R: Late-life anxiety and cognitive impairment: a review. Am J Geriatr Psychiatry 16:790–803, 2008

Beekman AT, de Beurs E, van Balkom AJ, et al: Anxiety and depression in later life: co-occurrence and communality of risk factors. Am J Psychiatry 157:89–95, 2000

Benitez CI, Smith K, Vasile RG, et al: Use of benzodiazepines and selective serotonin reuptake inhibitors in middle-aged and older adults with anxiety disorders: a longitudinal and prospective study. Am J Geriatr Psychiatry 16:5–13, 2008

Bishop SJ: Neurocognitive mechanisms of anxiety: an integrative account. Trends Cogn Sci 11:307–316, 2007

Bissiere S, Plachta N, Hoyer D, et al: The rostral anterior cingulate cortex modulates the efficiency of amygdala-dependent fear learning. Biol Psychiatry 63:821–831, 2008

Blazer D, George KL, Hughes D: The epidemiology of anxiety disorders: an age comparison, in Anxiety in the Elderly: Treatment and Research. Edited by Salzman C, Lebowitz BD. New York, Springer, 1991, pp 17–30

Brenes GA, Guralnik JM, Williamson JD, et al: The influence of anxiety on the progression of disability. J Am Geriatr Soc 53:34–39, 2005

Brenes GA, Kritchevsky SB, Mehta KM, et al: Scared to death: results from the Health, Aging, and Body Composition study. Am J Geriatr Psychiatry 15:262–265, 2007a

Brenes GA, McCall WV, Williamson JD, et al: Feasibility and acceptability of bibliotherapy and telephone sessions for the treatment of late-life anxiety disorders. Clin Gerontol 33:62–68, 2007b

Brenes GA, Miller ME, Stanley MA, et al: Insomnia in older adults with generalized anxiety disorder. Am J Geriatr Psychiatry 17:465–472, 2009

Bryant C, Jackson H, Ames D: The prevalence of anxiety in older adults: methodological issues and a review of the literature. J Affect Disord 109:233–250, 2008

Butters MA, Bhalla RK, Andreescu C, et al: Changes in neuropsychological functioning following treatment for late-life generalised anxiety disorder. Br J Psychiatry 199:211–218, 2011

Castillo CS, Schultz SK, Robinson RG: Clinical correlates of early onset and late-onset poststroke generalized anxiety. Am J Psychiatry 152:1174–1179, 1995

Caudle DD, Senior AC, Wetherell JL, et al: Cognitive errors, symptom severity, and response to cognitive behavior therapy in older adults with generalized anxiety disorder. Am J Geriatr Psychiatry 15:680–689, 2007

Chou KL: Age at onset of generalized anxiety disorder in older adults. Am J Geriatr Psychiatry 17:455–464, 2009

Chung MY, Min KH, Jun YJ, et al: Efficacy and tolerability of mirtazapine and sertraline in Korean veterans with posttraumatic stress disorder: a randomized open label trial. Hum Psychopharmacol 19:489–494, 2004

Davidson J, Allgulander C, Pollack MH, et al: Efficacy and tolerability of duloxetine in elderly patients with generalized anxiety disorder: a pooled analysis of four randomized, double-blind, placebo-controlled studies. Hum Psychopharmacol 23:519–526, 2008

DeLuca AK, Lenze EJ, Mulsant BH, et al: Comorbid anxiety disorder in late life depression: association with memory decline over four years. Int J Geriatr Psychiatry 20:848–854, 2005

De Wit L, Putman K, Baert I, et al: Anxiety and depression in the first six months after stroke: a longitudinal multicentre study. Disabil Rehabil 30:1858–1866, 2008

Dombrovski AY, Mulsant BH, Houck PR, et al: Residual symptoms and recurrence during maintenance treatment of late-life depression. J Affect Disord 103:77–82, 2007

English BA, Jewell M, Jewell G, et al: Treatment of chronic posttraumatic stress disorder in combat veterans with citalopram: an open trial. J Clin Psychopharmacol 26:84–88, 2006

Flint AJ, Rifat SL: Two-year outcome of elderly patients with anxious depression. Psychiatry Res 66:23–31, 1997

Gagnon N, Flint AJ, Naglie G, et al: Affective correlates of fear of falling in elderly persons. Am J Geriatr Psychiatry 13:7–14, 2005

Jeste DV, Blazer DG, First M: Aging-related diagnostic variations: need for diagnostic criteria appropriate for elderly psychiatric patients. Biol Psychiatry 58:265–271, 2005

Jeste ND, Hays JC, Steffens DC: Clinical correlates of anxious depression among elderly patients with depression. J Affect Disord 90:37–41, 2006

Katz IR, Reynolds CF 3rd, Alexopoulos GS, et al: Venlafaxine ER as a treatment for generalized anxiety disorder in older adults: pooled analysis of five randomized placebo-controlled clinical trials. J Am Geriatr Soc 50:18–25, 2002

Kimura M, Tateno A, Robinson RG: Treatment of poststroke generalized anxiety disorder comorbid with poststroke depression: merged analysis of nortriptyline trials. Am J Geriatr Psychiatry 11:320–327, 2003

Landi F, Onder G, Cesari M, et al: Psychotropic medications and risk for falls among community-dwelling frail older people: an observational study. J Gerontol A Biol Sci Med Sci 60:622–626, 2005

Lauterbach EC, Freeman A, Vogel RL: Correlates of generalized anxiety and panic attacks in dystonia and Parkinson disease. Cogn Behav Neurol 16:225–233, 2003

Lenze EJ, Mulsant BH, Shear MK, et al: Comorbid anxiety disorders in depressed elderly patients. Am J Psychiatry 157:722–728, 2000

Lenze EJ, Mulsant BH, Mohlman J, et al: Generalized anxiety disorder in late life: lifetime course and comorbidity with major depressive disorder. Am J Geriatr Psychiatry 13:77–80, 2005a

Lenze EJ, Mulsant BH, Shear MK, et al: Efficacy and tolerability of citalopram in the treatment of late-life anxiety disorders: results from an 8-week randomized, placebo-controlled trial. Am J Psychiatry 162:146–150, 2005b

Lenze EJ, Rollman BL, Shear MK, et al: Escitalopram for older adults with generalized anxiety disorder: a placebo-controlled trial. JAMA 301:295–303, 2009

Lenze EJ, Mantella RC, Shi P, et al: Elevated cortisol in older adults with generalized anxiety disorder is reduced by treatment: a placebo-controlled evaluation of escitalopram. Am J Geriatr Psychiatry 19:482–490, 2011

Le Roux H, Gatz M, Wetherell JL: Age at onset of generalized anxiety disorder in older adults. Am J Geriatr Psychiatry 13:23–30, 2005

Lyketsos CG, Lopez O, Jones B, et al: Prevalence of neuropsychiatric symptoms in dementia and mild cognitive impairment: results from the Cardiovascular Health Study. JAMA 288:1475–1483, 2002

Mantella RC, Butters MA, Dew MA, et al: Cognitive impairment in late-life generalized anxiety disorder. Am J Geriatr Psychiatry 15:673–679, 2007

Mantella RC, Butters MA, Amico JA, et al: Salivary cortisol is associated with diagnosis and severity of late-life generalized anxiety disorder. Psychoneuroendocrinology 33:773–781, 2008

Marsh L: Neuropsychiatric aspects of Parkinson's disease. Psychosomatics 41:15–23, 2000

Mintzer JE, Brawman-Mintzer O: Agitation as a possible expression of generalized anxiety disorder in demented elderly patients: toward a treatment approach. J Clin Psychiatry 57(suppl):55–63; discussion 73–75, 1996

Mohlman J, Gorman JM: The role of executive functioning in CBT: a pilot study with anxious older adults. Behav Res Ther 43:447–465, 2005

Montgomery S, Chatamra K, Pauer L, et al: Efficacy and safety of pregabalin in elderly people with generalised anxiety disorder. Br J Psychiatry 193:389–394, 2008

Morinigo A, Blanco M, Labrador J, et al: Risperidone for resistant anxiety in elderly persons. Am J Geriatr Psychiatry 13:81–82, 2005

Nagaratnam N, Ip J, Bou-Haidar P: The vestibular dysfunction and anxiety disorder interface: a descriptive study with special reference to the elderly. Arch Gerontol Geriatr 40:253–264, 2005

Narita K, Murata T, Hamada T, et al: Associations between trait anxiety, insulin resistance, and atherosclerosis in the elderly: a pilot cross-sectional study. Psychoneuroendocrinology 33:305–312, 2008

Palmer K, Berger AK, Monastero R, et al: Predictors of progression from mild cognitive impairment to Alzheimer disease. Neurology 68:1596–1602, 2007

Paterniti S, Dufouil C, Alperovitch A: Long-term benzodiazepine use and cognitive decline in the elderly: the Epidemiology of Vascular Aging Study. J Clin Psychopharmacol 22:285–293, 2002

Paukert AL, Phillips L, Cully JA, et al: Integration of religion into cognitive-behavioral therapy for geriatric anxiety and depression. J Psychiatr Pract 15:103–112, 2009

Paulsen JS, Ready RE, Hamilton JM, et al: Neuropsychiatric aspects of Huntington's disease. J Neurol Neurosurg Psychiatry 71:310–314, 2001

Pinquart M, Duberstein PR: Treatment of anxiety disorders in older adults: a meta-analytic comparison of behavioral and pharmacological interventions. Am J Geriatr Psychiatry 15:639–651, 2007

Pomara N, Deptula D, Medel M, et al: Effects of diazepam on recall memory: relationship to aging, dose, and duration of treatment. Psychopharmacol Bull 25:144–148, 1989

Pomara N, Tun H, DaSilva D, et al: The acute and chronic performance effects of alprazolam and lorazepam in the elderly: relationship to duration of treatment and self-rated sedation. Psychopharmacol Bull 34:139–153, 1998a

Pomara N, Tun H, DaSilva D, et al: Benzodiazepine use and crash risk in older patients. JAMA 279:113–114; author reply 115, 1998b

Porensky EK, Dew MA, Karp JF, et al: The burden of late-life generalized anxiety disorder: effects on disability, health-related quality of life, and healthcare utilization. Am J Geriatr Psychiatry 17:473–482, 2009

Prull MW, Dawes LL, Martin AM 3rd, et al: Recollection and familiarity in recognition memory: adult age differences and neuropsychological test correlates. Psychol Aging 21:107–118, 2006

Rampello L, Alvano A, Raffaele R, et al: New possibilities of treatment for panic attacks in elderly patients: escitalopram versus citalopram. J Clin Psychopharmacol 26:67–70, 2006

Raskind MA, Peskind ER, Hoff DJ, et al: A parallel group placebo controlled study of prazosin for trauma nightmares and sleep disturbance in combat veterans with post-traumatic stress disorder. Biol Psychiatry 61:928–934, 2007

Richard IH, Schiffer RB, Kurlan R: Anxiety and Parkinson's disease. J Neuropsychiatry Clin Neurosci 8:383–392, 1996

Saxena S, Maidment KM, Vapnik T, et al: Obsessive-compulsive hoarding: symptom severity and response to multimodal treatment. J Clin Psychiatry 63:21–27, 2002

Schuurmans J, Comijs HC, Beekman AT, et al: The outcome of anxiety disorders in older people at 6-year follow-up: results from the Longitudinal Aging Study Amsterdam. Acta Psychiatr Scand 111:420–428, 2005

Schuurmans J, Comijs H, Emmelkamp PM, et al: A randomized, controlled trial of the effectiveness of cognitive-behavioral therapy and sertraline versus a waitlist control group for anxiety disorders in older adults. Am J Geriatr Psychiatry 14:255–263, 2006

Sheikh JI, King RJ, Taylor CB: Comparative phenomenology of early onset versus late-onset panic attacks: a pilot survey. Am J Psychiatry 148:1231–1233, 1991

Sheikh JI, Lauderdale SA, Cassidy EL: Efficacy of sertraline for panic disorder in older adults: a preliminary open-label trial (letter). Am J Geriatr Psychiatry 12:230, 2004a

Sheikh JI, Swales PJ, Carlson EB, et al: Aging and panic disorder: phenomenology, comorbidity, and risk factors. Am J Geriatr Psychiatry 12:102–109, 2004b

Sibille E, Su J, Leman S, et al: Lack of serotonin1B receptor expression leads to age-related motor dysfunction, early onset of brain molecular aging and reduced longevity. Mol Psychiatry 12:1042–1056, 975, 2007

Simmons A, Matthews SC, Feinstein JS, et al: Anxiety vulnerability is associated with altered anterior cingulate response to an affective appraisal task. Neuroreport 19:1033–1037, 2008

Simon NM, Smoller JW, McNamara KL, et al: Telomere shortening and mood disorders: preliminary support for a chronic stress model of accelerated aging. Biol Psychiatry 60:432–435, 2006

Sinoff G, Werner P: Anxiety disorder and accompanying subjective memory loss in the elderly as a predictor of future cognitive decline. Int J Geriatr Psychiatry 18:951–959, 2003

Stanley MA, Beck JG, Novy DM, et al: Cognitive-behavioral treatment of late-life generalized anxiety disorder. J Consult Clin Psychol 71:309–319, 2003

Stanley MA, Diefenbach GJ, Hopko DR: Cognitive behavioral treatment for older adults with generalized anxiety disorder: a therapist manual for primary care settings. Behav Modif 28:73–117, 2004

Stanley MA, Wilson NL, Novy DM, et al: Cognitive behavior therapy for generalized anxiety disorder among older adults in primary care: a randomized clinical trial. JAMA 301:1460–1467, 2009

Starkstein SE, Jorge R, Petracca G, et al: The construct of generalized anxiety disorder in Alzheimer disease. Am J Geriatr Psychiatry 15:42–49, 2007

Swoboda KJ, Jenike MA: Frontal abnormalities in a patient with obsessive-compulsive disorder: the role of structural lesions in obsessive-compulsive behavior. Neurology 45:2130–2134, 1995

Thorp SR, Ayers CR, Nuevo R, et al: Meta-analysis comparing different behavioral treatments for late-life anxiety. Am J Geriatr Psychiatry 17:105–115, 2009

Todaro JF, Shen BJ, Raffa SD, et al: Prevalence of anxiety disorders in men and women with established coronary heart disease. J Cardiopulm Rehabil Prev 27:86–91, 2007

van't Veer-Tazelaar PJ, van Marwijk HW, van Oppen P, et al: Stepped-care prevention of anxiety and depression in late life: a randomized controlled trial. Arch Gen Psychiatry 66:297–304, 2009

Wetherell JL, Stein MB: Geriatric psychiatry: anxiety disorders, in Kaplan & Sadock's Comprehensive Textbook of Psychiatry, 9th Edition. Edited by Kaplan BJ, Sadock VA, Ruiz P. Philadelphia, PA, Wolters Kluwer Health/Lippincott Williams & Wilkins, 2009, pp 4040–4046

Wetherell JL, Gatz M, Pedersen NL: A longitudinal analysis of anxiety and depressive symptoms. Psychol Aging 16:187–195, 2001

Wetherell JL, Thorp SR, Patterson TL, et al: Quality of life in geriatric generalized anxiety disorder: a preliminary investigation. J Psychiatr Res 38:305–312, 2004

Wetherell JL, Hopko DR, Diefenbach GJ, et al: Cognitive-behavioral therapy for late-life generalized anxiety disorder: who gets better? Behav Ther 36:147–156, 2005a

Wetherell JL, Lenze EJ, Stanley MA: Evidence-based treatment of geriatric anxiety disorders. Psychiatr Clin North Am 28:871–896, ix, 2005b

Wetherell JL, Stoddard JA, White KS, et al: Augmenting antidepressant medication with modular CBT for geriatric generalized anxiety disorder: a pilot study. Int J Geriatr Psychiatry 26:869–875, 2011

Yohannes AM, Baldwin RC, Connolly MJ: Depression and anxiety in elderly patients with chronic obstructive pulmonary disease. Age Ageing 35:457–459, 2006

Suggested Readings

Beaudreau SA, O'Hara R: Late-life anxiety and cognitive impairment: a review. Am J Geriatr Psychiatry 16:790–803, 2008

Bryant C, Jackson H, Ames D: The prevalence of anxiety in older adults: methodological issues and a review of the literature. J Affect Disord 109:233–250, 2008

Lenze EJ, Wetherell JL: Bringing the bedside to the bench, and then to the community: a prospectus for intervention research in late-life anxiety disorders. Int J Geriatr Psychiatry 24:1–14, 2009

Lenze EJ, Rollman BL, Shear MK, et al: Escitalopram for older adults with generalized anxiety disorder: a placebo-controlled trial. JAMA 301:296–303, 2009

Stanley MA, Wilson NL, Novy DM, et al: Cognitive behavior therapy for generalized anxiety disorder among older adults in primary care: a randomized clinical trial. JAMA 301:1460–1467, 2009

van't Veer-Tazelaar PJ, van Marwijk HW, van Oppen P, et al: Stepped-care prevention of anxiety and depression in late life: a randomized controlled trial. Arch Gen Psychiatry 66:297–304, 2009

Wetherell JL, Lenze EJ, Stanley MA: Evidence-based treatment of geriatric anxiety disorders. Psychiatr Clin North Am 28:871–896, ix, 2005

8

Sleep and Circadian Rhythm Disorders

Andrew D. Krystal, M.D., M.S.

Jack D. Edinger, Ph.D.

William K. Wohlgemuth, Ph.D.

Sleep disorders are an important aspect of geriatric psychiatry. In the United States, more than half of noninstitutionalized individuals age 65 years and older report chronic sleep difficulties (Foley et al. 1995; "National Institutes of Health Consensus Development Conference Statement" 1991; Prinz et al. 1990). These problems affect quality of life, increase the risk of accidents and falls, and may lead to long-term-care placement (Pollak and Perlick 1991; Pollak et al. 1990; Sanford 1975). Working effectively with elderly individuals requires expertise in the diagnosis and treatment of sleep disorders.

DSM-5 (American Psychiatric Association 2013) includes eight general sleep disorders categories: insomnia disorder, hypersomolence disorder, narcolepsy, breathing-related sleep disorders, circadian rhythm sleep-wake disorders, parasomnias, restless legs syndrome, and substance/medication-induced sleep disorder. Patients with these conditions generally complain about some aspect of their sleep and/or waking function. For some patients, the sleep-focused concerns pertain to the quality, timing, amounts, or discontinuity in their sleep. For other patients, primary complaints may focus more on daytime sleepiness or impairment. For a subset of patients, complaints may focus on unusual behaviors occurring in sleep.

In this chapter we consider those sleep-wake disorders most commonly encountered in geriatric psychiatry. Among these are those insomnia disorders involving a difficulty initiating or maintaining sleep with associated daytime impairment or distress, as well as those that present as disorders of excessive daytime somnolence characterized by persistent daytime sleepiness that causes significant distress or impairment in function (American Psychiatric Association 2000; American Sleep Disorders Association 1997). The most important disorders of excessive sleepiness are sleep apnea, restless legs syndrome/periodic limb movement disorder (PLMD), and narcolepsy. Circadian rhythm disorders manifest as a misalignment between an individual's sleep-wake cycle and the pattern that is desired or required (American Psychiatric Association 2000; American Sleep Disorders Association 1997). The circadian rhythm is important for function because it is a cycle not only of sleep and wakefulness but also of many physiological processes and phenomena, including body temperature, alertness, cognitive performance, and hormone release (Czeisler et al. 1990; Folkard and Totterdell 1994; Minors et al. 1994).

Influence of Aging on Sleep and Circadian Functions

Extensive research has shown that marked changes in the duration, continuity, and depth of nocturnal sleep accompany normal aging (Hirshkowitz et al. 1992). Nocturnal sleep time steadily decreases across the life span, and nocturnal wake time increases because of an increase in arousals (Figure 8–1). Accompanying these changes are marked reductions in stage 3 and 4 sleep ("deeper" stages of non–rapid eye movement sleep). Although the clinical sig-

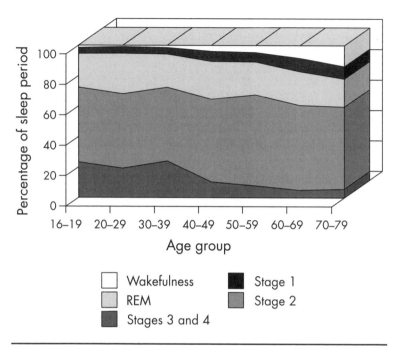

Figure 8–1.   Sleep-stage distributions across age groups.
Note.   REM = rapid eye movement.

nificance of these changes is unknown, they may relate to the reported reduction in subjective sleep quality and lowering of the arousal threshold with age (Riedel and Lichstein 1998; Zepelin et al. 1984).

The amplitudes of both the sleep-wake cycle and the 24-hour body temperature rhythm appear to decrease with aging as well (Bliwise 2000; Czeisler et al. 1999). Older adults also tend to awaken at an earlier phase and show a greater propensity to awaken during the later portions of their sleep episodes (Dijk et al. 1997; Duffy et al. 1998). Furthermore, psychosocial changes that accompany aging may alter important zeitgebers ("time markers") for the circadian system and promote the onset of sleep difficulties.

Disorders Associated With Sleep and Circadian Rhythm Disturbances

Several medical and psychiatric conditions are associated with sleep difficulties, and these conditions occur more frequently with increasing age. The emerging view is that sleep disorders occurring with medical and psychiatric disorders have been undertreated and that the sleep problems are best thought of as comorbid and not secondary conditions (National Institutes of Health 2005).

Primary Sleep Disorders

Sleep Apnea

In sleep apnea, breathing ceases for periods of 10 seconds or more (Aldrich 2000) either because no effort is made to breathe (central sleep apnea) or because the oropharynx collapses (obstructive sleep apnea). The frequency of obstructive sleep apnea increases with age (Ancoli-Israel 1989; Ancoli-Israel et al. 1991; Dickel and Mosko 1990; Roehrs et al. 1983). Apnea generally causes sleepiness, although mild to moderate apnea can be associated with insomnia. Referral to a sleep disorders specialist is required for diagnosis and treatment. The treatment of choice for obstructive sleep apnea is continuous positive airway pressure (CPAP). This treatment involves blowing air through the nose at night to increase pressure within the upper airway, thereby preventing the collapse that leads to apnea. Individuals with anatomical anomalies predisposing them to apnea are treated with upper airway surgery. Central sleep apnea is relatively rare (4%–10% of apnea cases; White 2000) and has many causes, including alveolar hypoventilation, congestive heart failure, neurological disorders, and nasal and upper airway obstruction. Therapy should be targeted to the underlying process, and when no such problem can be identified, CPAP is usually attempted (White 2000).

PLMD and Restless Legs Syndrome

In PLMD, repetitive muscular contractions occur during sleep; these contractions most commonly involve the legs and often cause sleep disturbances. The frequency of these events is characterized in terms of the number of movements associated with arousal per hour of sleep (the movement-arousal index). Thresholds for abnormality ranging from 5 to 15 movements per hour have been suggested (Ancoli-Israel et al. 1991; Dickel and Mosko 1990). Some authors have suggested that a higher threshold for abnormality should be applied to elderly patients (Ancoli-Israel 1989), in whom PLMD is more prevalent (Roehrs et al. 1983). Several studies indicate that clinically significant PLMD is seen in 30%–45% of adults age 60 years and older, compared with 5%–6% of all adults (Ancoli-Israel et al. 1991).

Individuals with PLMD may complain of leg kicks, cold feet, excessive daytime sleepiness, and insomnia (Ancoli-Israel 1989; Ancoli-Israel et al. 1991; Roehrs et al. 1983). The insomnia may be characterized by difficulty in falling asleep or staying asleep (Ancoli-Israel 1989). Unfortunately, PLMD is difficult to predict reliably on the basis of a patient's history (Ancoli-Israel 1989; Dickel and Mosko 1990). Furthermore, a high level of confidence in the diagnosis is needed before beginning treatment because treatment typically involves long-term use of medications that can have significant side effects. Therefore, when a history is suggestive of PLMD, standard practice is to make a referral for a polysomnogram for definitive diagnosis (Ancoli-Israel 1989). Polysomnography is also indicated when an individual has significant insomnia or hypersomnia that does not respond to usual treatment. Such a patient may have significant undetected PLMD.

Restless legs syndrome (RLS) is often associated with PLMD and is described as an uncomfortable feeling in the lower extremities that creates an irresistible urge to move. RLS occurs in 6% of the adult population and is present in up to 28% of patients older than 65 years (Clark 2001). Polysomnography is not needed for a diagnosis of RLS.

RLS and PLMD have been associated with anemia (O'Keeffe et al. 1994). Ferritin levels less than 45 µg/L are associated with an increased risk of RLS, and such patients often benefit from administration of supplemental iron (O'Keeffe et al. 1994). Also associated with PLMD and RLS are diabetes mellitus, pregnancy, iron deficiency anemia, and use of certain medications, including antidepressants (Bliwise et al. 1985). The same medications are effective for both RLS and PLMD. The primary treatment for these conditions is dopaminergic agonists (Bliwise et al. 2005; Montplaisir et al. 1999). Second-line treatment options include anticonvulsants (gabapentin) and benzodiazepines (clonazepam). Opiates are typically reserved for patients whose symptoms do not respond to these other drugs.

Neuropsychiatric Disorders

Bereavement

Psychological factors that most commonly affect sleep in elderly persons are reactions to loss. Although bereavement is normal, it is often associated with substantial sleep disturbance (American Psychiatric Association 2000). Antidepressant medication may be helpful. A short course of sedative-hypnotic therapy may provide substantial symptomatic relief. If all symptoms of bereavement have resolved except insomnia, cognitive-behavioral therapy for insomnia should be considered. Grief counseling also should be considered.

Major Depression

Depression is frequently associated with sleep disruption in individuals age 60 years and older. The most frequent sleep complaints in affected individuals are 1) experiencing a decrease in total sleep time and 2) waking earlier than desired.

Major depression is the condition for which the evidence is strongest for a complex bidirectional relation with sleep disturbance (Krystal 2006). Although insomnia has long been viewed as a secondary symptom of underlying depression, the results of a series of studies are inconsistent with this point of view (National Institutes of Health Consensus Conference 1984). The findings include evidence that those with insomnia have an increased future risk of major depression, that insomnia is an independent risk factor for suicide in depressed individuals, that antidepressant treatment frequently does not result in resolution of insomnia, and that this residual insomnia is associated with an increased risk of depression relapse (Breslau et al. 1996; Fawcett et al. 1990; Livingston et al. 1994; Reynolds et al. 1997).

The strongest evidence of the importance of depression in sleep disturbance is a study indicating that adding an insomnia medication (eszopiclone) to fluoxetine not only improved sleep but also led to greater and more rapid improvement in non-sleep-related depression symptoms (Fava et al. 2006; Krystal et al. 2007). However, the available research literature provides little guidance on the optimal management of insomnia occurring in individuals with depression.

Alzheimer's Disease

Individuals with Alzheimer's disease have been found to experience an increased number of arousals and awakenings, to take more daytime naps, and to have a diminished amount of rapid eye movement (REM) sleep and slow-wave sleep (Prinz et al. 1982). Individuals with dementia often experience evening or nocturnal agitation and confusion. This phenomenon, called *sundowning*, is among the leading reasons that individuals with dementia become institutionalized (Pollak and Perlick 1991; Pollak et al. 1990; Sanford 1975). Several features appear to increase the risk of sundowning, including greater dementia severity, pain, fecal impaction, malnutrition, polypharmacy, infections, REM sleep behavior disorder, PLMD, and environmental sleep disruptions (Bliwise 2000).

Treatment of sundowning should begin with an assessment for such conditions. If no causative condition can be found, or if attempts to eliminate the cause are unsuccessful, treatment such as light therapy, melatonin, structured activity programs, and eliminating naps should be considered. In terms of medications, benzodiazepines are ineffective (Bliwise 2000). Antipsychotic medications have the most evidence supporting efficacy (Bliwise 2000); however, most studies involved older agents. The newer antipsychotics may have fewer side effects (Bliwise 2000), but they have been linked to an increased risk of mortality in this population (Kales et al. 2007).

Parkinson's Disease

Sleep complaints are noted in 60%–90% of individuals with Parkinson's disease (Trenkwalder 1998). Most Parkinson's disease patients experience difficulty in initiating and maintaining sleep, daytime fatigue, RLS, and an inability to turn over in bed. Another sleep problem seen in patients with Parkinson's disease is REM sleep behavior disorder, in which the patient acts out dreams because the paralysis that usually occurs during REM sleep is absent (Clarenbach 2000). No study findings indicate how to manage sleep difficulties in patients with Parkinson's disease.

Medical Conditions

Pain

Pain is a central feature of many conditions that occur with increased frequency in elderly individuals, including arthritis, neuropathies, angina, reflux esophagitis, and peptic ulcer disease (Aldrich 2000), and pain frequently disrupts sleep (Pilowsky et al. 1985). Attempts to ameliorate the condition causing the pain should be the first step. When these attempts fail, treatment for the pain should be instituted. Often, combined behavioral and pharmacological treatment is needed. Some evidence indicates that as with depression, pain may have a bidirectional relationship with sleep disturbance in that the treatment of insomnia improves pain (Edinger et al. 2005; Walsh et al. 1996).

Chronic Obstructive Pulmonary Disease

Individuals with chronic obstructive pulmonary disease (COPD) have been found to have both subjective and objective evidence of disturbed sleep (Douglas 2000). Polysomnography is not routinely indicated for individuals with COPD who have sleep difficulties (Connaughton et al. 1988). Nocturnal oxygen may be needed in some patients (Connaughton et al. 1988). Oral theophyllines, which are frequently used in COPD treatment, are adenosine receptor antagonists and may have a sleep-disruptive effect (Douglas 2000). Also, patients with COPD should be instructed to avoid alcohol, which can exacerbate hypoxemia and promote other complications. In severe COPD, the benzodiazepines triazolam and flunitrazepam, but not the non-benzodiazepine zolpidem, adversely affected oxygenation (Murciano et al. 1993). However, in patients with mild to moderate COPD, both zolpidem and triazolam improved awakenings compared with placebo, and neither had an adverse effect on respiration compared with placebo (Steens et al. 1993). The melatonin receptor agonist ramelteon also has been found to improve sleep without adversely affecting respiration in patients with mild to moderate COPD (Kryger et al. 2008).

Cerebrovascular Disease

The sleep pathology associated with cerebrovascular disease depends on which areas of the brain are affected by the condition. Hypersomnia has been associated with lesions of the midbrain and paramedian region of the thalamus (Bassetti and Chervin 2000). Insomnia directly related to damage of specific areas of the brain is uncommon (Bassetti and Chervin 2000).

Nocturia

Nocturia (excessive urination at night) is the most common explanation given by elderly individuals for difficulty in maintaining sleep (Middelkoop et al. 1996). The most common causes of nocturia are conditions that increase in frequency with age: benign prostatic hypertrophy in men and decreased urethral resistance due to decreased estrogen levels in women (Bliwise 2000). Sleep apnea can also lead to nocturia (Bliwise 2000). Thus, when evaluating elderly individuals with complaints regarding sleep maintenance, the clinician should assess for nocturia and the associated conditions that increase the risk for nocturia.

Menopause

Evidence shows that many menopausal women experience sleep disruption in association with vasomotor symptoms (night sweats and hot flashes) that are caused by decreased levels of circulating estrogen and progesterone (Bliwise 2000; Krystal et al. 1998). Elderly women with insomnia should be evaluated for underlying causes of sleep disturbance (e.g., medical and psychiatric conditions, primary sleep disorders), and clinicians should determine whether an association exists between changes in menstrual periods, vasomotor symptoms, and insomnia symptoms. If an association between insomnia and menopausal changes appears to exist, a trial of hormone replacement therapy could be considered. If hormone replacement therapy ameliorates vasomotor symptoms but insomnia complaints persist, behavior therapy should be considered. If hormone replacement therapy is contraindicated or if use of this treatment is not preferred, other treatments such as pharmacological management of insomnia or cognitive-behavioral sleep therapy should be considered. Two studies (Dorsey et al. 2004; Soares et al. 2006) documented the efficacy of zolpidem, 10 mg, and eszopiclone, 3 mg, for improving sleep difficulties that occur in association with hot flashes.

Loss of Hearing, Vision, and Mobility

Many elderly individuals experience decrements in hearing, vision, and mobility (e.g., walking, driving). Changes in these vital functions can have a profound effect on sleep, which stems from a loss of activities in which the affected individual can engage. To pass the time, the person takes unplanned naps or tries to sleep more than he or she is physiologically able to. The result is fragmentation of sleep and loss of circadian rhythmicity. Although this problem should be easily solved by increasing activity and developing new activity options, in practice, making these changes is difficult.

Treatment of Insomnia

Cognitive-Behavioral Treatment

Myriad lifestyle changes that accompany aging increase risks of insomnia among older adults (Morgan 2000). Currently, a variety of behavioral interventions are available for treating insomnia in these patients, including relaxation therapies, cognitive therapies, and treatments that target disruptive sleep habits. Among the more effective of these interventions is stimulus control therapy, developed by Bootzin (1972). This treatment is particularly useful for older adults who have fallen out of a normal sleep-wake routine and for those who compromise their nighttime sleep by excessive daytime napping. Stimulus control therapy addresses such problems by curtailing daytime napping and by enforcing a consistent sleep-wake schedule. In addition, this treatment enhances sleep-inducing qualities of the bedroom by eliminating sleep-incompatible behaviors in bed. The patient with insomnia is instructed to go to bed only when sleepy; establish a standard wake-up time; get out of bed whenever he or she is awake for more than 15–20 minutes; avoid reading, watching television, eating, worrying, and engaging in other sleep-incompatible behaviors in bed and in the bedroom; and refrain from daytime napping.

Because older adults appear to have a reduced homeostatic sleep drive (Dijk et al. 1997) as well as a propensity to spend excessive time in bed (Carskadon et al. 1982), measures are often needed to reduce the amount of time older patients with insomnia allot for nocturnal sleep. Such a reduction is the aim of sleep restriction therapy (Spielman et al. 1987; Wohlgemuth and Edinger 2000). Typically, this treatment begins with the patient maintaining a sleep log. After 2–3 weeks, the average total sleep time (TST)—that is, the time actually spent asleep as estimated by the patient—is calculated. Subsequently, an initial time-in-bed (TIB) prescription may be set either at the average TST or at a value equal to the average TST plus an amount of time that is deemed to represent normal nocturnal wakefulness (e.g., 30 minutes). The TIB prescription is increased by 15- to 20-minute increments after weeks in which the person with insomnia sleeps more than 85%–90% of the TIB, on average, and continues to report daytime sleepiness. Conversely, TIB is usually reduced by similar increments after weeks in which the individual sleeps less than 80% of the time spent in bed, on average. Research suggests that stimulus-control and sleep-restriction therapies are more effective than most other nonpharmacological interventions (Morin et al. 1999, 2006; Murtagh and Greenwood 1995). Clinical trials also have generally suggested that therapies combining stimulus control, sleep restriction, and cognitive strategies to alter dysfunctional sleep-related beliefs hold particular promise for treatment of the sleep maintenance difficulties so common in older age groups (Edinger et al. 2001, 2007; Morin et al. 1999).

Pharmacological Treatment

Studies of treatment for up to 2 weeks have established the risk-benefit profile for seven agents available in the United States for the treatment of insomnia. These are the benzodiazepines flurazepam, triazolam, and temazepam; the nonbenzodiazepines eszopiclone, zaleplon, and zolpidem; and the melatonin agonist ramelteon (Krystal 2009). Some of the benzodiazepines have half-lives that are so long that they are unsuitable insomnia agents because of inevitable daytime impairment. Only triazolam and temazepam have half-lives in a range that makes them reasonable to use in the treatment of insomnia. Of the medications most frequently used to treat insomnia, the nonbenzodiazepine hypnotic zaleplon and the melatonin receptor agonist ramelteon have the shortest half-lives (approximately 1 hour), making them well suited for treating problems in falling asleep. Because of its short half-life, zaleplon also may be useful in the middle of the night for individuals who sometimes wake up at that time (Stone et al. 2002). Zolpidem, with a half-life of approximately 2.5 hours, is another agent approved for the treatment of difficulties in falling asleep. Although the agent with the shortest half-life that effectively treats the sleep difficulty should always be used in order to minimize risks, individuals with difficulty staying asleep generally need longer-acting agents. Of the agents available in the United States, eszopiclone is the only one shown to improve the ability to fall and stay asleep in older adults with insomnia (McCall et al. 2006). The tricyclic antidepressant doxepin, 3 mg, has been found to have significant benefit for sleep maintenance and early-morning awakening in older adults, and a very favorable side-effect profile (Krystal et al. 2010). Although other antidepressants are widely used to treat insomnia in the United States (most notably, trazodone, mirtazapine, and amitriptyline), there has yet to be a study of any of these agents in older adults with insomnia (Walsh 2004).

The primary adverse effects of the benzodiazepines and nonbenzodiazepines are motor and cognitive impairments. Many older adults may be particularly vulnerable to adverse outcomes because of these effects. In terms of motor impairment, these agents might be expected to increase the risk for falls in older adults. Although evidence indicates an association of falls with benzodiazepines, nonbenzodiazepines, and medications with anticholinergic and antiadrenergic effects (including antihistamines and antidepressants), studies also suggest that untreated insomnia increases the risk for falls (Allain et al. 2005; Avidan et al. 2005; Brassington et al. 2000; Koski et al. 1998; Nebes et al. 2007; Neutel et al. 2002; Suzuki et al. 1992). Further research will be needed to provide guidance, when managing insomnia in clinical practice, as to how to take into account the risks of falls caused by being awake at night versus the risks of falls caused by medications.

Conclusion

Although sleep disorders are not an inevitable consequence of aging, elderly persons are more prone to primary sleep disorders and medical and psychiatric conditions that cause sleep difficulties. Therefore, evaluation of a sleep complaint in an elderly individual should include a thorough workup to determine whether primary sleep pathology and associated psychiatric and medical disorders are present. Effective behavioral and medication treatments exist for treating sleep and circadian rhythm disorders in elderly patients, but these treatments have significant limitations. More research is needed to develop and assess nonmedication therapies that are effective in treating insomnia and normalizing the circadian rhythm. Particularly promising areas include cognitive-behavioral sleep therapy and exercise programs.

References

Aldrich MS: Cardinal manifestations of sleep disorders, in Principles and Practice of Sleep Medicine, 3rd Edition. Edited by Kryger MH, Roth T, Dement WC. Philadelphia, PA, WB Saunders, 2000, pp 526–534

Allain H, Bentué-Ferrer D, Polard E, et al: Postural instability and consequent falls and hip fractures associated with use of hypnotics in the elderly: a comparative review. Drugs Aging 22:749–765, 2005

American Psychiatric Association: Diagnostic and Statistical Manual of Mental Disorders, 4th Edition, Text Revision. Washington, DC, American Psychiatric Association, 2000

American Psychiatric Association: Diagnostic and Statistical Manual of Mental Disorders, 5th Edition. Arlington, VA, American Psychiatric Association, 2013

American Sleep Disorders Association: The International Classification of Sleep Disorders: Diagnostic and Coding Manual, Revised Edition. Rochester, MN, American Sleep Disorders Association, 1997

Ancoli-Israel S: Epidemiology of sleep disorders. Clin Geriatr Med 5:347–362, 1989

Ancoli-Israel S, Kripke DF, Klauber MR, et al: Periodic limb movements in sleep in community-dwelling elderly. Sleep 14:496–500, 1991

Avidan AY, Fries BE, James ML, et al: Insomnia and hypnotic use, recorded in the minimum data set, as predictors of falls and hip fractures in Michigan nursing homes. J Am Geriatr Soc 53:955–962, 2005

Bassetti C, Chervin R: Cerebrovascular diseases, in Principles and Practice of Sleep Medicine, 3rd Edition. Edited by Kryger MH, Roth T, Dement WC. Philadelphia, PA, WB Saunders, 2000, pp 1072–1086

Bliwise DL: Normal aging, in Principles and Practice of Sleep Medicine, 3rd Edition. Edited by Kryger MH, Roth T, Dement WC. Philadelphia, PA, WB Saunders, 2000, pp 26–42

Bliwise DL, Petta D, Seidel W, et al: Periodic leg movements during sleep in the elderly. Arch Gerontol Geriatr 4:273–281, 1985

Bliwise DL, Freeman A, Ingram CD, et al: Randomized, double-blind, placebo-controlled, short-term trial of ropinirole in restless legs syndrome. Sleep Med 6:141–147, 2005

Bootzin RR: A stimulus control treatment for insomnia. Proceedings of the American Psychological Association 7:395–396, 1972

Brassington GS, King AC, Bliwise DL: Sleep problems as a risk factor for falls in a sample of community-dwelling adults aged 64–99 years. J Am Geriatr Soc 48:1234–1240, 2000

Breslau N, Roth T, Rosenthal L, et al: Sleep disturbance and psychiatric disorders: a longitudinal epidemiological study of young adults. Biol Psychiatry 39:411–418, 1996

Carskadon MA, Brown ED, Dement WC: Sleep fragmentation in the elderly: relationship to daytime sleep tendency. Neurobiol Aging 3:321–327, 1982

Clarenbach P: Parkinson's disease and sleep. J Neurol 247(suppl):IV20–IV23, 2000

Clark MM: Restless legs syndrome. J Am Board Fam Pract 14:368–374, 2001

Connaughton JJ, Catterall JR, Elton RA, et al: Do sleep studies contribute to the management of patients with severe chronic obstructive pulmonary disease? Am Rev Respir Dis 138:341–344, 1988

Czeisler CA, Johnson MP, Duffy JF, et al: Exposure to bright light and darkness to treat physiologic maladaptation to night work. N Engl J Med 322:1253–1259, 1990

Czeisler CA, Duffy JF, Shanahan TL, et al: Stability, precision, and near-24-hour period of the human circadian pacemaker. Science 284:2177–2181, 1999

Dickel MJ, Mosko SS: Morbidity cut-offs for sleep apnea and periodic leg movements in predicting subjective complaints in seniors. Sleep 13:155–166, 1990

Dijk DJ, Duffy JF, Riel E, et al: Altered interaction of circadian and homeostatic aspects of sleep propensity results in awakening at an earlier circadian phase in older people. Sleep Res 26:710, 1997

Dorsey CM, Lee KA, Scharf MB: Effect of zolpidem on sleep in women with perimenopausal and postmenopausal insomnia: a 4-week, randomized, multicenter, double-blind, placebo-controlled study. Clin Ther 26:1578–1586, 2004

Douglas NJ: Chronic obstructive pulmonary disease, in Principles and Practice of Sleep Medicine, 3rd Edition. Edited by Kryger MH, Roth T, Dement WC. Philadelphia, PA, WB Saunders, 2000, pp 965–975

Duffy JF, Dijk DJ, Klerman EB, et al: Later endogenous circadian temperature nadir relative to an earlier wake time in older people. Am J Physiol 275:R1478–R1487, 1998

Edinger JD, Wohlgemuth WK, Radtke RA, et al: Cognitive behavioral therapy for treatment of chronic primary insomnia: a randomized controlled trial. JAMA 285:1856–1864, 2001

Edinger JD, Wohlgemuth WK, Krystal AD, et al: Behavioral insomnia therapy for fibromyalgia patients: a randomized clinical trial. Arch Intern Med 165:2527–2535, 2005

Edinger JD, Wohlgemuth WK, Radtke RA, et al: Dose response effects of cognitive-behavioral insomnia therapy: a randomized clinical trial. Sleep 30:203–212, 2007

Fava M, McCall WV, Krystal A, et al: Eszopiclone co-administered with fluoxetine in patients with insomnia co-existing with major depressive disorder. Biol Psychiatry 59:1052–1060, 2006

Fawcett J, Scheftner WA, Fogg L, et al: Time-related predictors of suicide in major affective disorder. Am J Psychiatry 147:1189–1194, 1990

Foley DJ, Monjan AA, Brown SL, et al: Sleep complaints among elderly persons: an epidemiologic study of three communities. Sleep 18:425–432, 1995

Folkard S, Totterdell P: "Time since sleep" and "body clock" components of alertness and cognition. Acta Psychiatr Belg 94:73–74, 1994

Hirshkowitz M, Moore CA, Hamilton CR, et al: Polysomnography of adults and elderly: sleep architecture, respiration, and leg movement. J Clin Neurophysiol 9:56–62, 1992

Kales HC, Valenstein M, Kim HM, et al: Mortality risk in patients with dementia treated with antipsychotics versus other psychiatric medications. Am J Psychiatry 164:1568–1576, 2007

Koski K, Luukinen H, Laippala P, et al: Risk factors for major injurious falls among the home-dwelling elderly by functional abilities: a prospective population-based study. Gerontology 44:232–238, 1998

Kryger M, Wang-Weigand S, Zhang J, et al: Effect of ramelteon, a selective MT(1)/MT (2)-receptor agonist, on respiration during sleep in mild to moderate COPD. Sleep Breath 12:243–250, 2008

Krystal AD: Sleep and psychiatry: future directions. Psychiatr Clin North Am 29:1115–1130, 2006

Krystal AD: A compendium of placebo-controlled trials of the risks/benefits of pharmacological treatments for insomnia: the empirical basis for U.S. clinical practice. Sleep Med Rev 13:265–274, 2009

Krystal AD, Edinger J, Wohlgemuth W, et al: Sleep in peri-menopausal and postmenopausal women. Sleep Med Rev 2:243–253, 1998

Krystal AD, Fava M, Rubens R, et al: Evaluation of eszopiclone discontinuation after co-therapy with fluoxetine for insomnia with co-existing depression. J Clin Sleep Med 3:48–55, 2007

Krystal AD, Durrence HH, Scharf M, et al: Efficacy and safety of doxepin 1 mg and 3 mg in a 12-week sleep laboratory and outpatient trial of elderly subjects with chronic primary insomnia. Sleep 33:1553–1561, 2010

Livingston G, Blizard B, Mann A: Does sleep disturbance predict depression in elderly people? A study in inner London. Br J Gen Pract 44:445–448, 1994

McCall WV, Erman M, Krystal AD, et al: A polysomnography study of eszopiclone in elderly patients with insomnia. Curr Med Res Opin 22:1633–1642, 2006

Middelkoop HA, Smilde-van den Doel DA, Neven AK, et al: Subjective sleep characteristics of 1,485 males and females aged 50–93: effects of sex and age and factors related to self-evaluated quality of sleep. J Gerontol A Biol Sci Med Sci 51:M108–M115, 1996

Minors DS, Waterhouse JM, Akerstedt T: The effect of the timing, quality, and quantity of sleep upon the depression (masking) of body temperature on an irregular sleep/wake schedule. J Sleep Res 3:45–51, 1994

Montplaisir J, Nicolas A, Denesle R, et al: Restless legs syndrome improved by pramipexole: a double-blind randomized trial. Neurology 52:938–943, 1999

Morgan K: Sleep and aging, in Treatment of Late-Life Insomnia. Edited by Lichstein KL, Morin CM. Thousand Oaks, CA, Sage, 2000, pp 3–36

Morin CM, Colecchi C, Stone J, et al: Behavioral and pharmacological therapies for late-life insomnia: a randomized controlled trial. JAMA 281:991–1035, 1999

Morin CM, Bootzin R, Buysse DJ, et al: Psychological and behavioral treatment for insomnia. Sleep 29:1398–1414, 2006

Murciano D, Armengaud MH, Cramer PH, et al: Acute effects of zolpidem, triazolam and flunitrazepam on arterial blood gases and control of breathing in severe COPD. Eur Respir J 6:625–629, 1993

Murtagh DR, Greenwood KM: Identifying effective psychological treatments for insomnia: a meta-analysis. J Consult Clin Psychol 63:79–89, 1995

National Institutes of Health: National Institutes of Health State of the Science Conference statement on manifestations and management of chronic insomnia in adults, June 13–15, 2005. Sleep 28:1049–1057, 2005

National Institutes of Health Consensus Conference: Drugs and insomnia: the use of medications to promote sleep. JAMA 251:2410–2414, 1984

National Institutes of Health Consensus Development Conference Statement: the treatment of sleep disorders in older people, March 26–28, 1990. Sleep 14:169–177, 1991

Nebes RD, Pollock BG, Halligan EM, et al: Serum anticholinergic activity and motor performance in elderly persons. J Gerontol A Biol Sci Med Sci 62:83–85, 2007

Neutel CI, Perry S, Maxwell C: Medication use and risk of falls. Pharmacoepidemiol Drug Saf 11:97–104, 2002

O'Keeffe ST, Gavin K, Lavan JN: Iron status and restless legs syndrome in the elderly. Age Ageing 23:200–203, 1994

Pilowsky I, Crettenden I, Townley M: Sleep disturbance in pain clinic patients. Pain 23:27–33, 1985

Pollak CP, Perlick D: Sleep problems and institutionalization of the elderly. J Geriatr Psychiatry Neurol 4:204–210, 1991

Pollak CP, Perlick D, Linsner JP, et al: Sleep problems in the community elderly as predictors of death and nursing home placement. J Community Health 15:123–135, 1990

Prinz PN, Peskind ER, Vitaliano PP, et al: Changes in the sleep and waking EEGs of nondemented and demented elderly subjects. J Am Geriatr Soc 30:86–93, 1982

Prinz PN, Vitiello MV, Raskind MA, et al: Geriatrics: sleep disorders and aging. N Engl J Med 323:520–526, 1990

Reynolds CF 3rd, Frank E, Houck PR, et al: Which elderly patients with remitted depression remain well with continued interpersonal psychotherapy after discontinuation of antidepressant medication? Am J Psychiatry 154:958–962, 1997

Riedel BW, Lichstein KL: Objective sleep measures and subjective sleep satisfaction: how do older adults with insomnia define a good night's sleep? Psychol Aging 13:159–163, 1998

Roehrs T, Zorick F, Sicklesteel J, et al: Age-related sleep-wake disorders at a sleep disorder center. J Am Geriatr Soc 31:364–370, 1983

Sanford JRA: Tolerance of debility in elderly dependants by supporters at home: its significance for hospital practice. Br Med J 3:471–473, 1975

Soares CN, Joffe H, Rubens R, et al: Eszopiclone in patients with insomnia during perimenopause and early postmenopause: a randomized controlled trial. Obstet Gynecol 108:1402–1410, 2006

Spielman AJ, Saskin P, Thorpy MJ: Treatment of chronic insomnia by restriction of time in bed. Sleep 10:45–55, 1987

Steens RD, Pouliot Z, Millar TW, et al: Effects of zolpidem and triazolam on sleep and respiration in mild to moderate chronic obstructive pulmonary disease. Sleep 16:318–326, 1993

Stone BM, Turner C, Mills SL, et al: Noise-induced sleep maintenance insomnia: hypnotic and residual effects of zaleplon. Br J Clin Pharmacol 53:196–202, 2002

Suzuki M, Okamura T, Shimazu Y, et al: A study of falls experienced by institutionalized elderly. Nippon Koshu Eisei Zasshi 39:927–940, 1992

Trenkwalder C: Sleep dysfunction in Parkinson's disease. Clin Neurosci 5:107–114, 1998

Walsh JK: Drugs used to treat insomnia in 2002: regulatory-based rather than evidence-based medicine. Sleep 27:14441–14442, 2004

Walsh JK, Muehlbach MJ, Lauter SA, et al: Effects of triazolam on sleep, daytime sleepiness, and morning stiffness in patients with rheumatoid arthritis. J Rheumatol 23:245–252, 1996

White DP: Central sleep apnea, in Principles and Practice of Sleep Medicine, 3rd Edition. Edited by Kryger MH, Roth T, Dement WC. Philadelphia, PA, WB Saunders, 2000, pp 827–839

Wohlgemuth WK, Edinger JD: Sleep restriction therapy, in Treatment of Late-Life Insomnia. Edited by Lichstein KL, Morin CM. Thousand Oaks, CA, Sage, 2000, pp 147–184

Zepelin H, McDonald CS, Zammit GK: Effects of age on auditory awakening thresholds. J Gerontol 39:294–300, 1984

Suggested Readings

Ancoli-Israel S, Richardson GS, Mangano RM, et al: Long-term use of sedative hypnotics in older patients with insomnia. Sleep Med 6:107–113, 2005

Bliwise DL: Sleep in normal aging and dementia. Sleep 16:40–81, 1993

National Institutes of Health Consensus Development Conference Statement: the treatment of sleep disorders in older people, March 26–28, 1990. Sleep 14:169–177, 1991

Pollak CP, Perlick D: Sleep problems and institutionalization of the elderly. J Geriatr Psychiatry Neurol 4:204–210, 1991

Pollak CP, Perlick D, Linsner JP, et al: Sleep problems in the community elderly as predictors of death and nursing home placement. J Community Health 15:123–135, 1990

9

Alcohol and Drug Problems

David W. Oslin, M.D.

Shahrzad Mavandadi, Ph.D.

Alcohol and drug misuse are associated with a wide array of negative physical and mental health outcomes that are exacerbated with advancing age, such as functional and cognitive decline, compromised immune function, and depression. However, relatively little work has examined the correlates and consequences of substance use among older adults. Accordingly, substance misuse in later life has been called an "invisible epidemic" (Widlitz and Marin 2002). Epidemiological work determined that beginning when people are in their mid- to late 20s, overall rates of alcohol and illicit drug use begin to decline, and most older adults report no substance use. Nevertheless, changes in demographic and cohort trends suggest that substance misuse in later life is a pressing public health matter and that older adults represent a group in growing need of specialized substance treatment programs and services (Gfroerer et al. 2003). Most notable among demographic changes is the aging of the "baby boom" generation, a cohort that poses unique challenges; in addition to reporting higher rates of illicit drug and alcohol use and addiction than earlier aging cohorts, the baby boom cohort is significantly larger than previous cohorts (Koenig et al. 1994).

The potential public health effect of these demographic trends is highlighted by examining changes in rates of substance use and misuse in the last several decades. For example, it has been estimated that from the early 1990s until 2002, the prevalence of alcohol abuse or dependence tripled to 3.1% among adults age 65 and older (Grant et al. 2004). Heavy and binge drinking among adults older than 65 also has increased, with reports citing rates near 7.6% (Office of Applied Studies 2007). Substance use among the baby boomers has been reported to be notably higher; 22% of adults ages 50–54 were heavy or binge drinkers in 2006, and rates of illicit drug use among those in this age group increased from 3.4% to 6.0% from 2002 to 2006 (Office of Applied Studies 2007).

Guidelines and Classification: A Spectrum of Use

Proper screening, diagnosis, and treatment of individuals with drug and/or alcohol problems require an understanding of both drinking guidelines and the full range of substance use behavior seen among older adults. Because physiological factors render older adults more sensitive not only to alcohol and illicit drugs but also to over-the-counter (OTC) and prescription medications, guidelines and recommendations for use of these substances by older adults differ from those applied to younger adults. For example, lean body mass and total water volume decrease relative to total fat volume in later life. As a result, total body volume decreases, thereby increasing the serum concentration, absorption, and distribution of alcohol and drugs in the body (Moore et al. 2007).

Because of these age-related factors, guidelines for alcohol use specify lower consumption for older relative to younger adults. Recommendations set forth by the Center for Substance Abuse Treatment's Treatment Improvement Protocol on older adults state that adults age 65 and older should consume no more than one standard drink per day (Table 9–1) (Blow 1998; National Institute on Alcohol Abuse and Alcoholism 1995). Moreover, older adults should not consume more than two standard drinks on any one occasion (binge drinking). These drinking-limit recommendations are in accord with data concerning the relationship between heavy consumption and alcohol-related problems (Chermack et al. 1996) as well as evidence for the beneficial health effects of low-risk drinking among older adults (Klatsky and Armstrong 1993; Poikolainen 1991).

There are no accepted safe limits for tobacco, marijuana, or other illicit drugs.

In addition to the quantity of consumption, diagnostic categories that include clinical effect are considered. Table 9–2 describes six categories that are based on patterns of alcohol use and reflect both the clinical experience and the research findings of addiction specialists (Blow 1998).

Epidemiology of Late-Life Substance Use

Alcohol

The most recent National Survey on Drug Use and Health reported that 51.6% of adults ages 60–64 had consumed alcohol in the past month, with 37.8% currently reporting nonbinge or nonheavy use, 10.5% reporting bingeing behavior, and 3.3% reporting heavy use (Substance Abuse and Mental Health Services Administration 2011). With respect to alcohol abuse or dependence, it is estimated, based on epidemiological census–based work, that diagnostic criteria for alcohol abuse are met in 2.4% of older men and 0.4% of older women, and criteria for alcohol dependence are met in an additional 0.4% and 0.1% of older men and older women, respectively (Grant et al. 2004).

Because substance misuse is more likely to be present in health care settings, rates of alcohol problems and dependence are higher among clinical than among community-based samples. For example, Kirchner et al. (2007) reported that of the 24,863 individuals screened in primary care settings, 21.5% drank within the recommended levels (1–7 drinks per week), 4.1% were at-risk drinkers (8–14 drinks per week), and 4.5% were heavy drinkers (>14 drinks per week) or binge drinkers. Rates of abuse and dependence appear to be particularly high among patients in mental health clinics and nursing homes. In their study of 140 patients enrolled in a geriatric mental health outpatient clinic, Holroyd and Duryee (1997) found that DSM-IV (American Psy-

Table 9–1.   Alcohol conversion chart

"ONE STANDARD DRINK"

Beverage type	Quantity
Beer	12 oz.
Wine	5 oz.
Fortified wine	3 oz.
Hard liquor (80-proof distilled spirits)	1½ oz. (i.e., "a shot")
Malt liquor	8 oz.
Liqueur or aperitif	4 oz.

ADDITIONAL CONVERSIONS

Beverage type/quantity	No. of standard drinks
Beer	
1 6-pack of 16-oz. cans/bottles	8
1 quart	3
Wine (e.g., red, white, Chianti)	
1 bottle (750 mL)	5
1 magnum	12
½ gallon	16
Fortified wine (e.g., sherry, port; low-end wines [e.g., Thunderbird, "bum wine"])	
1 bottle (750 mL)	8
Hard liquor (e.g., bourbon, rum, gin, tequila, vodka)	
"Fifth" (750 mL)	17
"Pint" (250 mL)	5

Source.   Data from National Institute on Alcohol Abuse and Alcoholism 2005.

chiatric Association 1994) criteria for alcohol dependence were met in 8.6% of patients. Oslin et al. (1997b) found that 29% of male nursing home residents had a lifetime diagnosis of alcohol abuse or dependence, with criteria for abuse or dependence being met in 10% of residents within 1 year of admission to the home.

Table 9–2. Diagnostic categories of alcohol/drug use based on patterns of use

Use category	Description	Comments
Abstinence	<1–2 drinks in previous year	This pattern is reported by 50%–70% of older adults. They may or may not have a history of prior use.
Low-risk, social, or moderate use	≤1 drink/day, no alcohol-related problems	
Low-risk medication/drug use	Adheres to physician's prescriptions	
At-risk or excessive substance use	>1 drink/day, minimal or no substance-related health, social, or emotional problems	Individuals with this pattern are at risk for developing health problems (e.g., falls, liver disease, alcohol-medication interactions).
Abuse[a] or problem use	Excessive use, with social/medical psychological consequences	
Dependence[a]/addiction	Clinically significant distress/impairment coupled with preoccupation with alcohol or drugs, loss of control, continued substance use despite adverse consequences, and/or physiological symptoms such as tolerance and withdrawal	DSM-IV criteria for dependence are based on younger subjects and may not accurately capture older subjects. These individuals are susceptible to self-reporting bias (e.g., poor recall, poor insight).

[a]DSM-IV criteria for alcohol abuse and dependence have, in DSM-5 (American Psychiatric Association 2013), been combined into a single alcohol use disorder, which is divided into mild, moderate, and severe subtypes. Moreover, the DSM-5 diagnosis for mild alcohol use disorder requires endorsement of at least two symptoms (as opposed to one in DSM-IV).

Source. American Psychiatric Association 2000; Blow 1998; Kirchner et al. 2007; Moore et al. 2000.

Prescription and Over-the-Counter Medications

The use of pharmaceutical drugs is prevalent in older adulthood, and the risk of misusing prescription and OTC medications, which include substances such as sedative-hypnotics, narcotic and nonnarcotic analgesics, diet aids, and decongestants, also increases with age. According to a review of the scant literature on this topic, up to 11% of older women misuse prescription drugs, and it is projected that 2.7 million adults will be using prescription drugs for nonmedical purposes by the year 2020 (Simoni-Wastila and Yang 2006).

Illicit Drugs

Unlike alcohol and prescription/OTC medication use, illicit drug use among older adults is rare. According to the most recent National Survey on Drug Use and Health, the percentage of adults ages 55–59 using illicit drugs in the month preceding the survey increased from 1.9% in 2002 to 4.1% in 2010 (Substance Abuse and Mental Health Services Administration 2011). Although this increase in drug use may not seem significant, it is important to keep in mind that the baby boomers represent the only age group that showed notable increases in illicit substance use during the designated time period.

Correlates and Consequences of Substance Use Problems

Correlates of and Risk Factors for Substance Abuse

Several studies have sought to identify factors that are related to increased vulnerability to substance misuse and the maintenance of problematic substance use patterns in later life. Factors such as gender, medical comorbidity, history of past use, and social and family environment are all correlated with problematic substance use. Longitudinal work, for instance, suggests that older men tend to drink greater quantities of alcohol than do women and are more likely to have alcohol-related problems (Moore et al. 2005). Furthermore, increases in free time coupled with a reduction in role obligations may have a large effect on problem drinking in older women (Wilsnack and Wilsnack 1995). Indeed, age-related losses in social, physical, and occupational/role domains, such as widowhood, the death of family and friends, reduced physical function, and retirement, help contribute to the adoption or maintenance of abusive drinking patterns in later life among men and women (Blow 1998). Finally, longitudinal work has found that additional social context and life history factors, such as friends' approval of drinking and a history of heavy drinking or alcohol problems, also are related to a higher likelihood of late-life drinking problems (Moos et al. 2004).

With respect to prescription and OTC drugs, factors such as decline in physical health and physiological changes that accompany the aging process increase exposure and reactivity to medications and, thus, the potential for misuse of these substances in later life. Women are less likely than men to use and abuse alcohol but are more likely than men to use and misuse psychoactive medications (Simoni-Wastila and Yang 2006), particularly if the women are divorced or widowed, have lower socioeconomic status (e.g., education and income), or have received a mood disorder diagnosis such as depression or anxiety (Closser and Blow 1993). Comorbid psychiatric diagnoses, in general, increase the risk for prescription drug abuse and dependence, regardless of gender (Simoni-Wastila and Yang 2006).

Consequences of Substance Use

Although the literature presented thus far has alluded to the adverse effects of problematic substance use and dependence, some evidence suggests that low-risk or moderate alcohol consumption may have a positive effect on physical health and mental well-being. For example, low-risk or moderate alcohol consumption is associated with a reduced risk of cardiovascular disease in both men and women and a reduced risk of cardiovascular disease–related disability (Rimm et al. 1991; Stampfer et al. 1988). With respect to functional decline, findings from cross-sectional work suggest that among older men, low to moderate alcohol consumption is associated with lower odds of reporting physical limitations when compared with abstinence or heavy use (Cawthon et al. 2007). Finally, light to moderate alcohol use has beneficial effects on subjective well-being for both men and women (Lang et al. 2007) and improves self-esteem, reduces stress, and provides relaxation, particularly in social situations (Dufour et al. 1992).

Although the literature cited previously does suggest that low to moderate use of alcohol can lead to various health benefits among older adults, it is important to recognize that no evidence supports the notion that recommending that nondrinkers initiate drinking will translate into reduced health risks. Moreover, no evidence suggests that an individual with a medical condition, such as cardiovascular disease, will benefit from continued drinking or the initiation of drinking. In fact, abstinence should still be recommended for individuals who are taking certain medications, those who have been diagnosed with certain acute or chronic conditions (e.g., diabetes, cardiovascular disease), and those who present with a history of alcohol or drug abuse, because substance use is detrimental in these cases. Indeed, low to moderate consumption of alcohol also has been shown to impair one's ability to drive and may increase the risk of accidents and fatal injuries caused by falls, motor vehicle crashes, and suicide (Sorock et al. 2006). Moderate alcohol use has been linked to depression, memory problems, liver disease, cardiovascular disease, cognitive changes, and sleep problems (Gambert and Katsoyannis 1995; Liberto et al. 1992), whereas alcohol dependence is associated with an increased probability of morbidity and mortality from disease-specific disorders such as acute pancreatitis, alcohol-induced cirrhosis, or alcohol-related cardiomyopathy. When assessing and treating older adults, clinicians not only should take the previously mentioned factors into account but also should consider the potential interaction between alcohol and both prescribed and OTC medications, especially psychoactive medications such as benzodiazepines, barbiturates, and antidepressants. Finally, mental health providers should be well versed in the effect of moderate alcohol consumption on other mental health disorders. In a study of more than 2,000 elderly patients, Oslin et al. (2000) reported that reducing moderate alcohol use (defined as 1–7 drinks per week) while treating a depressive disorder enhanced treatment outcomes. Results further indicated that the greater the alcohol consumption, the larger the negative effect on the treatment of depression. Although data are sparse, there is speculation that moderate alcohol use also may have a negative effect on the prognosis and course of dementing illnesses such as Alzheimer's disease. Moreover, alcohol use may elicit the onset of, or exacerbate preexisting, personality changes or behavioral disturbances in patients with dementia.

Screening and Diagnosis of Substance Use Problems

Potential Barriers to Screening and Diagnosis

As outlined previously, alcohol and drug problems are common in later life. However, substance misuse remains largely underrecognized and undertreated among older adults. It has been suggested that adults older than 60 years be screened for alcohol and prescription drug use as part of their routine mental and physical health care (Blow 1998). Routine screening would enable the identification not only of those older adults who have problematic substance use but also of those who are at risk for misusing drugs and alcohol (Table 9–3). Furthermore, proper screening helps determine whether additional assessment is needed. Nonetheless, various factors may interfere with screening and diagnostic processes.

At the patient level, confusion as to what constitutes a substance use problem and who might benefit from an intervention affects patients' behavior with regard to seeking assessment. Like providers, older adults may perceive physical symptoms (e.g., fatigue, sleep problems, anxiety, confusion) as normative or attribute them to other medical illnesses. Older adults and their families also may not think that their substance use is problematic because of either denial or lack of knowledge about recommendations and guidelines for acceptable drinking and prescription and OTC drug use levels. In addition to these factors, age- and substance-related declines in memory may contribute to underreporting of past and current alcohol or drug use. Despite these potential issues, research suggests that retrospective self-report is as reliable as a prospective diet record in identifying patterns of alcohol use (Werch 1989).

Standardized Screening Instruments

Brief, low-cost, convenient, standardized assessments that can be used to screen not only for frequency and quantity of alcohol use but also for drinking consequences and alcohol or medication interactions are essential in the success of efforts targeted toward prevention and early intervention for older adults at risk. To complement questions assessing the quantity and frequency of use, the Short Michigan Alcoholism Screening Test—Geriatric Version (Figure 9–1) (University of Michigan 1991), the Alcohol Use Disorders Iden-

Table 9–3. Common signs and symptoms of potential substance misuse and abuse in older adults

Anxiety	Incontinence
Blackouts, dizziness	Increased tolerance to alcohol/medications
Depression, mood swings	Legal difficulties
Disorientation	Memory loss
Falls, bruises, and burns	New difficulties in decision making
Family problems	Poor hygiene
Financial problems	Poor nutrition
Headaches	Sleep problems
Idiopathic seizures	Social isolation

Source. Adapted from Barry KL, Blow FC, Oslin DW: "Substance Abuse in Older Adults: Review and Recommendations for Education and Practice in Medical Settings," in *Strategic Plan for Interdisciplinary Faculty Development: Arming the Nation's Health Professional Workforce for a New Approach to Substance Use Disorders.* Edited by Haack MR, Adger H. Providence, RI, Association for Medical Education and Research in Substance Abuse (AMERSA), September 2002, pp 105–131.

tification Test (AUDIT; Bradley et al. 1998), and the CAGE questionnaire (Mayfield et al. 1974) often are used to screen for at-risk substance use or misuse among older adults.

The AUDIT and its abbreviated version, the Alcohol Use Disorders Identification Test—Consumption (AUDIT-C; Figure 9–2), are simple screening measures that capture the frequency of drinking and bingeing in the past year (Bush et al. 1998; Dawson et al. 2005). The AUDIT-C is scored on a scale of 0 to 12, with a score of 0 indicating no alcohol use during the preceding year. For older adults, a score of 3 or more reflects a positive screen and suggests the need for further evaluation. Generally, the higher the AUDIT-C score, the more likely it is that the individual's drinking is affecting his or her health and safety (Bush et al. 1998; Dawson et al. 2005).

The CAGE questionnaire (Mayfield et al. 1974) is the most widely used alcohol screening test in clinical practice. A modified version of the original CAGE questionnaire asks only about recent problems, and the threshold is often reduced to one positive response as an indicator of problems in older adults. This modified version of the CAGE has demonstrated high specificity for detecting alcohol abuse but relatively low sensitivity for alcohol dependence or problem drinking (Buchsbaum et al. 1992).

In the past year:	Yes	No
1. When talking with others, do you ever underestimate how much you actually drink?	(1)	(0)
2. After a few drinks, have you sometimes not eaten or been able to skip a meal because you didn't feel hungry?	(1)	(0)
3. Does having a few drinks help decrease your shakiness or tremors?	(1)	(0)
4. Does alcohol sometimes make it hard for you to remember parts of the day or night?	(1)	(0)
5. Do you usually take a drink to relax or calm your nerves?	(1)	(0)

In the past year:	Yes	No
6. Do you drink to take your mind off your problems?	(1)	(0)
7. Have you ever increased your drinking after experiencing a loss in your life?	(1)	(0)
8. Has a doctor or nurse ever said they were worried or concerned about your drinking?	(1)	(0)
9. Have you ever made rules to manage your drinking?	(1)	(0)
10. When you feel lonely, does having a drink help?	(1)	(0)

TOTAL SMAST-G SCORE (0–10) ———

Figure 9–1. Short Michigan Alcohol Screening Test—Geriatric Version (SMAST-G).

A total of three or more positive responses is indicative of an alcohol abuse problem.
Source. Reprinted from the University of Michigan Alcohol Research Center. Copyright 1991, The Regents of the University of Michigan. Used with permission.

Following administration of a screening instrument, clinicians can ask follow-up questions about consequences, health risks, and social and family issues related to substance use. In accordance with DSM-IV-TR criteria (American Psychiatric Association 2000), to assess dependence, the clinician should ask questions about alcohol-related problems, a history of failed attempts to stop or to cut back, and withdrawal symptoms (e.g., anxiety, tremors, sleep disturbance). Of note, DSM-5 diagnostic categories have been modified such that alcohol abuse and dependence have been combined into a

1. How often did you have a drink containing alcohol in the past year?

_____	Never	(0 points)
_____	Monthly or less	(1 point)
_____	Two to four times a month	(2 points)
_____	Two to three times per week	(3 points)
_____	Four or more times a week	(4 points)

If you answered "never," score questions 2 and 3 as zero.

2. How many drinks did you have on a typical day when you were drinking in the past year?

_____	1 or 2	(0 points)
_____	3 or 4	(1 point)
_____	5 or 6	(2 points)
_____	7 to 9	(3 points)
_____	10 or more	(4 points)

3. How often did you have six or more drinks on one occasion in the past year?

_____	Never	(0 points)
_____	Less than monthly	(1 point)
_____	Monthly	(2 points)
_____	Weekly	(3 points)
_____	Daily or almost daily	(4 points)

Possible range = 0–12. For older adults, a score of 3 or more is considered positive.

Figure 9–2. Alcohol Use Disorders Identification Test–Consumption (AUDIT-C).

Source. Adapted from Bush K, Kivlahan DR, McDonell MB, et al.: "The AUDIT Alcohol Consumption Questions (AUDIT-C): An Effective Brief Screening Test for Problem Drinking." _Archives of Internal Medicine_ 158:1789–1795, 1998. Copyright 1998, American Medical Association. All rights reserved. Used with permission.

single category—alcohol use disorder (American Psychiatric Association 2013). Thus, assessments should be modified accordingly, and clinicians should ask about symptoms in order to determine the extent to which individuals' symptoms meet criteria for mild, moderate, or severe disorder (American Psychiatric Association 2013).

Use of Biological Markers for Screening

Biological markers of alcohol and drug use have proved to be less accepted in clinical practice but can be useful. Several laboratory values indicate recent use or abuse, including levels of blood alcohol or acetate, which is a metabolite of alcohol (Salaspuro 1994). Long-term markers of alcohol use include γ-glutamyltransferase, mean corpuscular volume, high-density lipoprotein level, and carbohydrate-deficient transferrin (Oslin et al. 1998b). Also, urine drug screens are useful both as screening tools and for confirmation of self-report when assessing prescription or OTC medication and illicit drug abuse. Most drugs of abuse will remain detectable in urine for 4 or more days, with some still detectable after several weeks.

Treatments for Substance Use Problems

Although numerous treatment options are available for substance use in later life, little formal research has been conducted to compare the relative efficacy of these various approaches among older adults. Nevertheless, results from naturalistic studies are promising: older adults who engage in treatment not only have outcomes that are comparable to or significantly better than those of their younger counterparts (Lemke and Moos 2003b; Oslin et al. 2002; Satre et al. 2003, 2004), but also are more likely to complete treatment than are younger patients (Schuckit and Pastor 1978; Wiens et al. 1982).

Brief Interventions and Therapies

Low-intensity brief interventions or brief therapies are cost-effective and practical techniques that can be used in the initial treatment of at-risk and problem drinkers in a variety of clinical settings (Barry 1999). Brief interventions are time-limited and nonconfrontational in their approach. Given that these interventions are based on concepts and techniques from the behavioral self-control literature, one of the hallmarks of brief interventions is to encourage individuals to change behavior through motivational interviewing (Miller and Rollnick 1991). Randomized clinical trials of brief interventions for alcohol problems among older populations reveal that older adults can be engaged in brief intervention protocols and find the protocols acceptable. Results also point to a greater reduction in alcohol consumption among at-risk drinkers receiving interventions than among control groups. For example, in one randomized clinical study, older primary care patients randomly assigned to a brief intervention arm received two 10- to 15-minute physician counseling visits and two follow-up telephone calls from clinic staff that involved advice, education, and the creation of contracts (Fleming et al. 1999). Results from this study demonstrated that rates of alcohol use at 12-month follow-up were significantly lower for patients randomly assigned to the brief intervention arm than for those in the control group.

Psychosocial Treatments

Please refer to Chapter 10, "Individual and Group Psychotherapy," for discussion of one form of psychological therapy, cognitive-behavioral therapy, for the treatment of substance abuse and dependence in older adulthood.

Twelve-Step Programs

A large proportion of community-based and residential treatment programs incorporate the traditional 12-Step peer support model of recovery and rehabilitation. Participants share their experiences with one another and follow the 12 steps, which include admitting to one's addiction, recognizing the influence of a greater power as a source of strength, and acknowledging and atoning for past mistakes (Alcoholics Anonymous Services 2004).

Although self-help groups have been associated with positive outcomes for many individuals, findings regarding rates of group engagement and outcomes among older adults remain mixed. In their matched comparison of older versus younger and middle-aged adults who participated in age-integrated residential treatment, Lemke and Moos (2003a) found that older patients engaged in 12-Step programs as frequently as their younger and middle-aged counterparts when assessed at follow-up. Similarly, an investigation of patients who had completed an outpatient treatment program for chemical dependency yielded no age-group differences in Alcoholics Anonymous (AA) affiliation 5 years posttreatment (Satre et al. 2004). However, despite the fact that rates of attendance appeared to be comparable across age groups, the depth of involvement differed; older adults were less likely than middle-aged adults to self-identify as being a 12-Step group member and were less likely than younger and middle-aged adults to report calling a fellow group member for help. Comparable results were observed in examining 1-month postdischarge outcomes among alcohol-dependent patients admitted to a 12-Step residential rehabilitation program (Oslin et al. 2005). Although rates of postdischarge abstinence and AA attendance did not differ across middle-aged and older adults, older adults were significantly less likely to contact a sponsor. Furthermore, older adults were less likely than middle-aged adults to engage in formal aftercare (31.2% vs. 56.4%).

Taken together, these findings highlight the importance of more careful examination of factors that may be related to 12-Step program attendance, degree of engagement, and outcomes among older adults. These factors include but are not limited to perceived stigma, level of comfort regarding disclosure of personal information in group settings, degree to which age-relevant issues are addressed during group meetings, and logistical barriers such as lack of transportation and health problems that may preclude older adults from attending group sessions and engaging with sponsors (Oslin et al. 2005; Satre et al. 2004).

Pharmacotherapy

Until recently, the long-term treatment of alcohol dependence in older adults did not involve the use of pharmacological agents. Although disulfiram was originally the only medication approved for the treatment of alcohol dependence, it was seldom used in older patients because of the potential for adverse effects. More recently, naltrexone has been shown to be effective among older adults. For example, results from a double-blind, placebo-controlled, randomized trial indicated that among older veterans ages 50–70, half as many naltrexone-treated subjects relapsed to significant drinking when compared with those who received placebo (Oslin et al. 1997a). Acamprosate is another promising agent in the treatment of alcohol dependence. Although the exact action of acamprosate is still unclear, it is believed to reduce glutamate response (Pelc et al. 1997). Unfortunately, no studies of the efficacy or safety of acamprosate among older patients have been conducted to date.

Detoxification and Withdrawal

When patients stop consuming substances or drastically cut down their consumption after heavy use, withdrawal symptoms are likely to occur. During hospitalizations, patients may be particularly vulnerable to alcohol or benzodiazepine withdrawal if the clinical team is unaware of problems with these substances. In light of the potential for life-threatening complications, clinicians caring for patients who abuse substances, particularly in settings in which withdrawal management or treatment is available, need to have a fundamental understanding of withdrawal symptoms and be able to provide detoxification management. The classic set of symptoms associated with alcohol withdrawal includes autonomic hyperactivity (increased pulse rate, increased blood pressure, and increased temperature), restlessness, disturbed sleep, anxiety, nausea, and tremor. Severe withdrawal is marked by auditory, visual, or tactile hallucinations; delirium; seizures; and/or coma. It is important to recognize that among older patients, the duration of withdrawal symptoms is longer, and withdrawal has the potential to complicate other medical and psychiatric illnesses. Nonetheless, no evidence suggests that older patients are more prone to alcohol withdrawal or require longer treatment for withdrawal symptoms (Brower et al. 1994).

Moderators and Correlates of Treatment Response and Adherence

Some evidence indicates that certain factors may have an effect on the degree of treatment response and adherence among older adults receiving treatment. For example, age-specific treatment, or age matching, has been shown to improve treatment completion and to result in higher rates of attendance at group meetings when compared with mixed-age treatments. In one study of male veterans with alcohol problems who were randomly assigned after detoxification to either age-specific or standard mixed-age treatment, outcomes showed that elder-specific program patients were 2.9 times more likely at 6 months and 2.1 times more likely at 1 year to report abstinence compared with mixed-age group patients (Kashner et al. 1992).

The type of treatment setting also may affect rates of adherence. In a study comparing engagement outcomes among older primary care patients referred to specialty mental health providers and those referred to an integrated care model using a brief intervention, 60.4% of at-risk drinkers attended at least one visit in the integrated care model (Bartels et al. 2004). In contrast, only 33% of the patients attended at least one visit to a specialty provider. It is important to note that these differences emerged despite efforts to address barriers to specialty care, such as copayments and insurance claims, and to ensure appointments within 2 weeks of patients being identified with at-risk drinking.

Medical and Psychiatric Comorbidity

The co-occurrence of problematic substance use and other medical and psychiatric conditions deserves special attention because such comorbidity may affect the course, treatment, and prognosis of both conditions. For example, in a review of 3,986 Veterans Affairs hospital patients between ages 60 and 69 presenting for alcohol abuse treatment, the most common comorbid psychiatric disorder was an affective disorder (present in 21% of the patients) (Blow et al. 1992). Of these patients, 43% had major depression. Similarly, in a study of community-dwelling elderly, of the 4.5% of older adults who had a history of alcohol abuse, almost half had a comorbid diagnosis of depression or dysthymia (Blazer et al. 1987).

Comorbid symptoms of depression and alcohol misuse not only are common in late life but also may have a reciprocal effect on one another. Individuals with comorbid depression and alcoholism have a more complicated clinical course, marked by an increased risk of suicide and more social dysfunction, than individuals with alcoholism alone (Conwell 1994; Cook et al. 1991; Waern 2003). In the same vein, alcohol use prior to late life has been shown to influence treatment of late-life depression; for example, a history of alcohol abuse is associated with a more severe and chronic course of depression (Cook et al. 1991).

Co-occurrence of alcohol use and dementing illnesses such as Alzheimer's disease is also a complex issue. Although Wernicke-Korsakoff syndrome is well defined and often caused by alcohol dependence, alcohol-related dementia may be difficult to differentiate from Alzheimer's disease because of a lack of well-specified diagnostic criteria. As a result, clinical diagnostic criteria for alcohol-related dementia have been proposed and validated in at least one trial examining a method for distinguishing alcohol-related dementia, including Wernicke-Korsakoff syndrome, from other types of dementia (Oslin and Cary 2003; Oslin et al. 1998a). Despite these diagnostic issues, it is generally agreed that alcohol abuse contributes to cognitive deficits in later life.

Sleep disorders and disturbances also frequently co-occur with excessive alcohol use. It is well established that alcohol causes changes in sleep patterns, such as decreased sleep latency, decreased stage 4 sleep, and precipitation or aggravation of sleep apnea (Wagman et al. 1977). Age-related changes in sleep patterns also occur with advancing age and include increased rapid eye movement (REM) episodes, a decrease in REM length and stage 3 and 4 sleep, and increased awakenings. Age-associated changes in sleep can be exacerbated by factors such as alcohol use and depression. For instance, in their study of younger subjects, Moeller et al. (1993) found that alcohol and depression had additive effects on sleep disturbances when occurring together. Furthermore, Wagman et al. (1977) reported that abstinent alcoholic individuals had poor sleep as a result of insomnia, frequent awakenings, and REM sleep fragmentation. Nevertheless, after alcohol was consumed, sleep periodicity normalized and REM sleep was temporarily suppressed, suggesting that these patients may have been using alcohol to self-medicate for sleep disturbances.

Future Directions

In light of changes in demographic and cohort trends, recent years have seen an increase in the number of older adults who misuse or abuse alcohol and drugs. Moreover, there is a growing awareness that older adults often engage in at-risk or problem substance use. Nevertheless, individuals in need of treatment or at risk for future problems often go unidentified and untreated. Thus, research and clinical efforts aimed at improving screening efforts and identifying system, provider, and patient factors that may interfere with screening and referral processes for older adults at risk are warranted.

References

Alcoholics Anonymous Services: Twelve Steps and Twelve Traditions. New York, Alcoholics Anonymous, 2004

American Psychiatric Association: Diagnostic and Statistical Manual of Mental Disorders, 4th Edition. Washington, DC, American Psychiatric Association, 1994

American Psychiatric Association: Diagnostic and Statistical Manual of Mental Disorders, 4th Edition, Text Revision. Washington, DC, American Psychiatric Association, 2000

American Psychiatric Association: Diagnostic and Statistical Manual of Mental Disorders, 5th Edition. Arlington, VA, American Psychiatric Association, 2013

Barry KL (consensus panel chair): Brief Interventions and Brief Therapies for Substance Abuse. Treatment Improvement Protocol (TIP) Series 34 (DHHS SAMHSA Publ No SMA-99-3353). Rockville, MD, Center for Substance Abuse Treatment, 1999

Bartels S, Coakley E, Zubritsky C, et al: Improving access to geriatric mental health services: a randomized trial comparing treatment engagement with integrated versus enhanced referral care for depression, anxiety, and at-risk alcohol use. Am J Psychiatry 16:1455–1462, 2004

Blazer DG, Hughes DC, George LK: The epidemiology of depression in an elderly community population. Gerontologist 27:281–287, 1987

Blow FC (consensus panel chair): Substance Abuse Among Older Adults. Treatment Improvement Protocol (TIP) Series 26. Center for Substance Abuse Treatment. Rockville, MD, U.S. Department of Health and Human Services, 1998

Blow F, Cook CL, Booth B, et al: Age-related psychiatric comorbidities and level of functioning in alcoholic veterans seeking outpatient treatment. Hosp Community Psychiatry 43:990–995, 1992

Bradley KA, Bush K, McDonell MB, et al: Screening for problem drinking: comparison of CAGE and AUDIT. J Gen Intern Med 13:379–388, 1998

Brower KJ, Mudd S, Blow FC, et al: Severity and treatment of alcohol withdrawal in elderly versus younger patients. Alcohol Clin Exp Res 18:196–201, 1994

Buchsbaum DG, Buchanan R, Welsh J, et al: Screening for drinking disorders in the elderly using the CAGE questionnaire. J Am Geriatr Soc 40:662–665, 1992

Bush K, Kivlahan DR, McDonell MB, et al: The AUDIT alcohol consumption questions (AUDIT-C): an effective brief screening test for problem drinking. Ambulatory Care Quality Improvement Project (ACQUIP). Alcohol Use Disorders Identification Test. Arch Intern Med 158:1789–1795, 1998

Cawthon PM, Fink HA, Barrett-Connor E, et al: Alcohol use, physical performance, and functional limitations in older men. J Am Geriatr Soc 55:212–220, 2007

Chermack ST, Blow FC, Hill EM, et al: The relationship between alcohol symptoms and consumption among older drinkers. Alcohol Clin Exp Res 20:1153–1158, 1996

Closser MH, Blow FC: Special populations: women, ethnic minorities, and the elderly. Psychiatr Clin North Am 16:199–209, 1993

Conwell Y: Suicide in elderly patients, in Diagnosis and Treatment of Depression in Late Life. Edited by Schneider LS, Reynolds CF, Lebowitz BD, et al. Washington, DC, American Psychiatric Press, 1994, pp 397–418

Cook B, Winokur G, Garvey M, et al: Depression and previous alcoholism in the elderly. Br J Psychiatry 158:72–75, 1991

Dawson DA, Grant BF, Stinson FS, et al: Effectiveness of the derived Alcohol Use Disorders Identification Test (AUDIT-C) in screening for alcohol use disorders and risk drinking in the U.S. general population. Alcohol Clin Exp Res 29:844–854, 2005

Dufour MC, Archer L, Gordis E: Alcohol and the elderly. Clin Geriatr Med 8:127–141, 1992

Fleming MF, Manwell LB, Barry KL, et al: Brief physician advice for alcohol problems in older adults: a randomized community-based trial. J Fam Pract 48:378–384, 1999

Gambert S, Katsoyannis K: Alcohol-related medical disorders of older heavy drinkers, in Alcohol and Aging. Edited by Beresford T, Gomberg E. New York, Oxford University Press, 1995, pp 70–81

Gfroerer J, Penne M, Pemberton M, et al: Substance abuse treatment need among older adults in 2020: the impact of the aging baby-boom cohort. Drug Alcohol Depend 69:127–135, 2003

Grant BF, Dawson DA, Stinson FS, et al: The 12-month prevalence and trends in DSM-IV alcohol abuse and dependence: United States, 1991–1992 and 2001–2002. Drug Alcohol Depend 74:223–234, 2004

Holroyd S, Duryee J: Substance use disorders in a geriatric psychiatry outpatient clinic: prevalence and epidemiologic characteristics. J Nerv Ment Dis 185:627–632, 1997

Kashner TM, Rodell DI, Ogden SR, et al: Outcomes and costs of two VA inpatient treatment programs for older alcoholic patients. Hosp Community Psychiatry 43:985–989, 1992

Kirchner JE, Zubritsky C, Cody M, et al: Alcohol consumption among older adults in primary care. J Gen Intern Med 22:92–97, 2007

Klatsky AL, Armstrong A: Alcohol use, other traits and risk of unnatural death: a prospective study. Alcohol Clin Exp Res 17:1156–1162, 1993

Koenig HG, George LK, Schneider R: Mental health care for older adults in the year 2020: a dangerous and avoided topic. Gerontologist 34:674–679, 1994

Lang I, Wallace RB, Huppert FA, et al: Moderate alcohol consumption in older adults is associated with better cognition and well-being than abstinence. Age Ageing 36:256–261, 2007

Lemke S, Moos RH: Outcomes at 1 and 5 years for older patients with alcohol disorders. J Subst Abuse Treat 24:43–50, 2003a

Lemke S, Moos RH: Treatment and outcomes of older patients with alcohol use disorders in community residential programs. J Stud Alcohol 64:219–226, 2003b

Liberto JG, Oslin DW, Ruskin PE: Alcoholism in older persons: a review of the literature. Hosp Community Psychiatry 43:975–984, 1992

Mayfield D, McLeod G, Hall P: The CAGE questionnaire: validation of a new alcoholism instrument. Am J Psychiatry 131:1121–1123, 1974

Miller W, Rollnick S: Motivational Interviewing: Preparing People to Change Addictive Behavior. New York, Guilford, 1991

Moeller FG, Gillin JC, Irwin M, et al: A comparison of sleep EEGs in patients with primary major depression and major depression secondary to alcoholism. J Affect Disord 27:39–42, 1993

Moore AA, Hays RD, Reuben DB, et al: Using a criterion standard to validate the Alcohol-Related Problems Survey (ARPS): a screening measure to identify harmful and hazardous drinking in older persons. Aging (Milano) 12:221–227, 2000

Moore AA, Gould R, Reuben DB, et al: Longitudinal patterns and predictors of alcohol consumption in the United States. Am J Public Health 95:458–465, 2005

Moore AA, Whiteman EJ, Ward KT: Risks of combined alcohol/medication use in older adults. Am J Geriatr Pharmacother 5:64–74, 2007

Moos RH, Schutte K, Brennan P, et al: Ten-year patterns of alcohol consumption and drinking problems among older women and men. Addiction 99:829–838, 2004

National Institute on Alcohol Abuse and Alcoholism: Diagnostic criteria for alcohol abuse. Alcohol Alert No 30 (October) PH 359, 1995. Bethesda, MD, U.S. Department of Health and Human Services, Public Health Service, National Institutes of Health, 1995, pp 1–6

National Institute on Alcohol Abuse and Alcoholism: Helping Patients Who Drink Too Much: A Clinician's Guide, Updated 2005 Edition (NIH Publ No. 07-3769). National Institutes of Health, U.S. Dept of Health and Human Services, 2005. Available at: http://pubs.niaaa.nih.gov/publications/Practitioner/CliniciansGuide2005/clinicians_guide.htm. Accessed July 11, 2013.

Office of Applied Studies: Results from the 2006 National Survey on Drug Use and Health: National Findings (DHHS Publ No SMA 07-4293, NSDUH Series H-32). Rockville, MD, Substance Abuse and Mental Health Services Administration, 2007

Oslin DW, Cary MS: Alcohol-related dementia: validation of diagnostic criteria. Am J Geriatr Psychiatry 11:441–447, 2003

Oslin D, Liberto JG, O'Brien J, et al: Naltrexone as an adjunctive treatment for older patients with alcohol dependence. Am J Geriatr Psychiatry 5:324–332, 1997a

Oslin D, Streim JE, Parmelee P, et al: Alcohol abuse: a source of reversible functional disability among residents of a VA nursing home. Int J Geriatr Psychiatry 12:825–832, 1997b

Oslin D, Atkinson RM, Smith DM, et al: Alcohol related dementia: proposed clinical criteria. Int J Geriatr Psychiatry 13:203–212, 1998a

Oslin DW, Pettinati HM, Luck G, et al: Clinical correlations with carbohydrate-deficient transferrin levels in women with alcoholism. Alcohol Clin Exp Res 22:1981–1985, 1998b

Oslin DW, Katz IR, Edell WS, et al: Effects of alcohol consumption on the treatment of depression among elderly patients. Am J Geriatr Psychiatry 8:215–220, 2000

Oslin DW, Pettinati HM, Volpicelli JR: Alcoholism treatment adherence: older age predicts better adherence and drinking outcomes. Am J Geriatr Psychiatry 10:740–747, 2002

Oslin DW, Slaymaker VJ, Blow FC, et al: Treatment outcomes for alcohol dependence among middle-aged and older adults. Addict Behav 30:1431–1436, 2005

Pelc I, Verbanck P, Le Bon O, et al: Efficacy and safety of acamprosate in the treatment of detoxified alcohol-dependent patients: a 90 day placebo-controlled dose-finding study. Br J Psychiatry 171:73–77, 1997

Poikolainen K: Epidemiologic assessment of population risks and benefits of alcohol use. Alcohol Alcohol Suppl 1:27–34, 1991

Rimm EB, Giovannucci EL, Willett WC, et al: Prospective study of alcohol consumption and risk of coronary disease in men. Lancet 338:464–468, 1991

Salaspuro M: Biological state markers of alcohol abuse. Alcohol Health Res World 18:131–135, 1994

Satre DD, Mertens JR, Arean PA, et al: Contrasting outcomes of older versus middle-aged and younger adult chemical dependency patients in a managed care program. J Stud Alcohol 64:520–530, 2003

Satre DD, Mertens JR, Arean PA, et al: Five-year alcohol and drug treatment outcomes of older adults versus middle-aged and younger adults in a managed care program. Addiction 99:1286–1297, 2004

Schuckit M, Pastor P: The elderly as a unique population. Alcohol Clin Exp Res 2:31–38, 1978

Simoni-Wastila L, Yang HK: Psychoactive drug abuse in older adults. Am J Geriatr Pharmacother 4:380–394, 2006

Sorock GS, Chen LH, Gonzalgo SR, et al: Alcohol-drinking history and fatal injury in older adults. Alcohol 40:193–199, 2006

Stampfer MJ, Colditz GA, Willett WC, et al: A prospective study of moderate alcohol consumption and the risk of coronary disease and stroke in women. N Engl J Med 319:267–273, 1988

Substance Abuse and Mental Health Services Administration: Results from the 2010 National Survey on Drug Use and Health: Summary of National Findings (NSDUH Series H-41, HHS Publ No [SMA] 11-4658). Rockville, MD, Substance Abuse and Mental Health Services Administration, 2011

University of Michigan: Short Michigan Alcoholism Screening Test—Geriatric Version. Ann Arbor, Regents of the University of Michigan, 1991

Waern M: Alcohol dependence and misuse in elderly suicides. Alcohol Alcohol 38:249–254, 2003

Wagman AM, Allen RP, Upright D: Effects of alcohol consumption upon parameters of ultradian sleep rhythms in alcoholics. Adv Exp Med Biol 85A:601–616, 1977

Werch C: Quantity-frequency and diary measures of alcohol consumption for elderly drinkers. Int J Addict 24:859–865, 1989

Widlitz M, Marin D: Substance abuse in older adults: an overview. Geriatrics 57:29–34, 2002

Wiens AN, Menustik CE, Miller SI, et al: Medical-behavioral treatment for the older alcoholic patient. Am J Drug Alcohol Abuse 9:461–475, 1982

Wilsnack SC, Wilsnack RW: Drinking and problem drinking in U.S. women: patterns and recent trends. Recent Dev Alcohol 12:29–60, 1995

Suggested Readings

Blow FC (consensus panel chair): Substance Abuse Among Older Adults. Treatment Improvement Protocol (TIP) Series 26. Center for Substance Abuse Treatment. Rockville, MD, U.S. Department of Health and Human Services, 1998

Fleming MF, Manwell LB, Barry KL, et al: Brief physician advice for alcohol problems in older adults: a randomized community-based trial. J Fam Pract 48:378–384, 1999

Gfroerer J, Penne M, Pemberton M, et al: Substance abuse treatment need among older adults in 2020: the impact of the aging baby-boom cohort. Drug Alcohol Depend 69:127–135, 2003

Oslin D, Liberto JG, O'Brien J, et al: Naltrexone as an adjunctive treatment for older patients with alcohol dependence. Am J Geriatr Psychiatry 5:324–332, 1997

Satre DD, Mertens JR, Arean PA, et al: Five-year alcohol and drug treatment outcomes of older adults versus middle-aged and younger adults in a managed care program. Addiction 99:1286–1297, 2004

Schonfeld L, Dupree LW: Cognitive-behavioral treatment of older veterans with substance abuse problems. J Geriatr Psychiatry Neurol 13:124–129, 2000

Simoni-Wastila L, Yang HK: Psychoactive drug abuse in older adults. Am J Geriatr Pharmacother 4:380–394, 2006

Substance Abuse and Mental Health Services Administration: Results from the 2010 National Survey on Drug Use and Health: Summary of National Findings (NSDUH Series H-41, HHS Publ No [SMA] 11-4658). Rockville, MD, Substance Abuse and Mental Health Services Administration, 2011

10

Individual and Group Psychotherapy

Thomas R. Lynch, Ph.D.

Dawn E. Epstein, B.S.

Moria J. Smoski, Ph.D.

Psychotherapy has been shown to be an effective treatment for several mental disorders seen in older adults. As a treatment modality, it can be particularly useful for older adult psychiatric patients who cannot or will not tolerate medication or who are dealing with stressful conditions, interpersonal difficulties, limited levels of social support, or recurrent episodes of a disorder. However, it has been estimated that only 10% of older adults in need of psy-

The author M.J.S. was supported by K23-MH087754 from the National Institute of Mental Health.

chiatric services actually receive professional care, and there has been minimal use of mental health services in this age group (Lebowitz et al. 1997; Weissman et al. 1981). African American older adults seek out professional mental health care about one-half as often as their white counterparts do, instead turning to informal support networks as a means of coping (Conner et al. 2010). Older adults report a longer delay in initiation of mental health treatment than do younger cohort groups (Wang et al. 2005).

Many practitioners assume that older adults have negative attitudes toward psychotherapy, but research on attitudes toward treatment in samples of elderly individuals is not conclusive. Contrary to clinical lore, growing descriptive research suggests that older adults may prefer counseling over medication treatment (Conner et al. 2010; Gum et al. 2006). Older adults also have been shown to report a greater number of positive attitudes toward mental health professionals and to be less concerned than younger adults about stigma attached to seeking treatment for depression (Rokke and Scogin 1995). However, older adults prefer that mental health treatment be provided in a primary care context rather than through specialty clinics; favor therapists who understand their existential and spiritual concerns and values; and, as a result of their unique sociohistorical context, often feel more comfortable receiving care from practitioners who share the same race, ethnicity, and religion (Bartels et al. 2004; Chen et al. 2006; Gum et al. 2010; Hinrichsen 2006; Snodgrass 2009). Whenever possible, patient preferences or biases regarding treatment should be considered before referral for psychotherapy.

Given the higher incidence of confounding factors in older adult populations (e.g., declines in sensory functions and speed of processing), age-specific adaptations of standard therapy procedures are advisable. For instance, the pace of therapy should be slower, and fonts for written material should be larger. Providing memory aids such as handouts and session summaries also can be very helpful. Accounting for unique cohort-based differences (e.g., sociohistorical environment, norms and commonly held beliefs, role expectations, illness beliefs, culture) and age-specific stressors (e.g., chronic illness and disability; loss of loved ones and, consequently, sources of support; caregiving responsibilities) is also advisable. In-home mental health services may be a valuable option for those who lack reliable transportation and/or have a medical or physical disability. Alternatively, telephone and Internet-based interventions also may help older adults overcome common treatment barriers (Alexander et al. 2010).

In this chapter, we review the empirical evidence for psychotherapy in older adults, giving consideration to both individual and group-based therapies. The material is organized by type of disorder and, for each disorder, by type of therapy. When possible, we evaluate the evidence with respect to quality of data, generalizability, and long-term effects of treatment.

Depression

Individual Cognitive-Behavioral Therapies

Broadly, cognitive-behavioral therapies aim to help patients engage in meaningful activities and modify depressogenic thinking. Several variants of cognitive-behavioral therapy (CBT) are effective in reducing depressive symptoms in older adults. Individual CBT has a strong track record of treating depression in older adults (Koder et al. 1996; Scogin and McElreath 1994; Serfaty et al. 2009; Thompson and Gallagher 1984; Thompson et al. 1987). Exercise therapy, which uses many of the techniques of behavioral activation, appears to be more effective than psychoeducation in reducing depressive symptoms (Singh et al. 2001) and may even be comparable to medication use (sertraline) in older adults (Babyak et al. 2000; Blumenthal et al. 2007). Group-based exercise interventions also may help to increase older adults' level of social integration and, as a result, reduce depressogenic symptoms and increase psychological well-being (Fox et al. 2007; Salmon 2001). Another variant, problem-solving therapy (PST), is based on a model in which ineffective coping under stress is hypothesized to lead to a breakdown of problem-solving abilities and to subsequent depression (Nezu 1987; Thompson and Gallagher 1984). In an attempt to increase coping and buffer factors, patients are taught a structured multistage format for solving problems that maintain and aggravate depression (Hegel et al. 2002). PST has been found to be effective in treating depression in populations with (Areán et al. 2010) or without (Areán et al. 1993) executive function deficits and can be successfully implemented in a primary care setting (Areán et al. 2010; Hegel et al. 2002; Mynors-Wallis 2001; Unützer et al. 2001; Williams et al. 2000).

Group-Based Cognitive-Behavioral Psychotherapies

Although originally designed to be implemented as an individual therapy, CBT has been successfully modified for a group format. Group-based CBT has been found to be more effective than a wait-list control and slightly more effective than a psychodynamic group therapy (Jarvik et al. 1982; Steuer 1984). It also can be used as an effective augmentation of pharmacotherapy in outpatient (Beutler et al. 1987; but see Wilkinson et al. 2009) and inpatient (Brand and Clingempeel 1992) settings. In dialectical behavior therapy (DBT), another treatment approach that combines cognitive and behavioral strategies, individuals are taught specific skills to increase mindfulness, interpersonal effectiveness, emotion regulation, and distress tolerance. Originally designed to treat chronically suicidal younger adult women, DBT has been modified to treat several difficult-to-treat conditions, including chronic depression in older adults (Lynch et al. 2003). In a study of comorbid depression and personality disorder in older adults, DBT plus medication resulted in a faster reduction in depressive symptoms than did medication alone (Lynch et al. 2007).

Interpersonal Psychotherapy

Interpersonal psychotherapy (IPT) is a problem-focused, manualized treatment that addresses four components that are hypothesized to lead to or maintain depression: 1) grief (e.g., death of a spouse), 2) interpersonal disputes (e.g., conflict with adult children), 3) role transitions (e.g., retirement), and 4) interpersonal deficits (e.g., lack of assertiveness skills). Whatever its etiology, depression is seen to persist in a social context. Techniques used in treatment include role-playing, communication analysis, clarification of the patient's wants and needs, and links between affect and environmental events (Hinrichsen 1997, 2008). Separate treatment manuals for interpersonal therapy in late life and interpersonal maintenance therapy for older patients have been developed that include adaptations specific for use in elderly patients, including flexibility in length of sessions, addressing of long-standing role disputes, and the need to help the patient with practical problems (Frank et al. 1993).

Controlled trials in populations of depressed adults have documented the efficacy of IPT for the treatment of acute depression (Bruce et al. 2004; Frank and Spanier 1995; Hinrichsen 1997), and IPT in the acute treatment of major depressive disorder was found to be as effective as nortriptyline (Sloane et al.

1985). Of additional importance are findings that elderly patients receiving IPT were less likely to drop out of treatment than were those taking nortriptyline, because of the medication's side effects; combined IPT and medication management emerged as the most effective treatment strategy for maintaining treatment gains (Reynolds et al. 1999).

Other Psychotherapeutic Techniques

Various other psychotherapeutic techniques used for the treatment of late-life depression boast less empirical support but warrant mentioning: bibliotherapy, life review and reminiscence psychotherapy, and psychodynamic psychotherapy. Bibliotherapy, or book therapy, emphasizes a skills acquisition approach via selected readings from books and has been shown to be efficacious in the treatment of mild to moderate depression (Floyd et al. 2004; Jamison and Scogin 1995; Naylor et al. 2010; Scogin et al. 1989, 1990). Individuals with depression read books such as *Feeling Good* (Burns 1980) to enhance behavioral skills that combat depression or to modify dysfunctional thoughts. A study by Naylor et al. (2010) compared a physician-delivered behavioral prescription to read *Feeling Good* and a usual care control for depression in a primary care setting. Dysfunctional attitudes and depressive symptoms were similarly reduced in both treatment groups, and perceived life satisfaction and enjoyment increased.

Life review and reminiscence psychotherapy are both based on the patient's reexperiencing of personal memories and significant life experiences. These interventions have been empirically supported as effective therapies in the treatment of late-life depression, with reminiscence therapy showing reductions in depressive symptoms comparable to those with CBT in a meta-analysis performed by Pinquart et al. (2007). Reminiscence therapy is often administered in a group setting with the goal of improving one's self-esteem and sense of social cohesiveness.

Psychodynamic psychotherapy is based on psychoanalytic theory, which views current interpersonal and emotional experience as having been influenced by early childhood experience (Bibring 1952). Revised conceptualizations have emphasized how relationships are internalized and transformed into a sense of self (e.g., Kohut and Wolf 1978; Mahler 1952). During therapy, patients are encouraged to develop insight into past experiences and how these experiences influence their current relationships. Although short-term psychodynamic therapy has been less studied for older adults than other treatments have (e.g., CBT, IPT), there have been several indications that short-term psychodynamic therapy, particularly as conducted by Thompson, Gallagher-Thompson, and colleagues (Gallagher-Thompson and Steffen 1994; Gallagher-Thompson et al. 1990; Thompson et al. 1987), is an effective means to treat depression in older adults.

Anxiety Disorders

Individual Cognitive-Behavioral Therapies

Although pharmacotherapy for late-life anxiety is quite effective, unwanted side effects can limit its utility (Stanley et al. 2009; Wetherell et al. 2011). Research on evidence-based treatments for late-life anxiety is still in its infancy; however, CBT appears to be the best form of psychotherapy to manage the diagnostic and treatment issues that exist in older populations with generalized anxiety disorder (GAD) (Ayers et al. 2007; Stanley and Novy 2000; Stanley et al. 1996, 2004; Wetherell et al. 2003). CBT has been found to be effective for a range of anxiety symptoms (Barrowclough et al. 2001), with effectiveness comparable to that of medication management (Gorenstein et al. 2005). An additional benefit is that CBT can be used to augment medications (Wetherell et al. 2011). Findings from a meta-analysis (Covin et al. 2008) support the conclusion that CBT for GAD is highly effective in reducing GAD's cardinal symptom: pathological worry.

In one example of a randomized trial of GAD treatment, Stanley et al. (2003a) compared the efficacy of CBT with that of a minimal contact condition. The researchers' treatment protocol included education training, relaxation training, cognitive restructuring, and exposure to anxiety-provoking stimuli. CBT participants reported a significant within-group improvement in the severity of GAD symptoms postintervention and at 12-month follow-up. These findings suggest that CBT not only may provide effective immediate therapy but also may promote long-term gains in the management of GAD. Several other randomized trials also have supported the use of CBT for the treatment of GAD (Mohlman et al. 2003; Stanley et al. 1996, 2003b; Wetherell et al. 2003), including in primary care settings (Stanley et al. 2009). Adapting CBT to use in primary care facilities will provide treatment where older adults are most likely to look for it and will facilitate collaboration between CBT therapists and prescription providers, while reducing costs.

Although CBT has strong promise for treating GAD in older adults, further empirical research must be conducted to verify its efficacy in this population and to determine mediators and moderators of treatment response. For example, it appears that CBT is not effective in older adults who have consistently low executive function abilities but is effective in individuals whose executive functioning improves along with their psychological symptoms (Mohlman and Gorman 2004). In addition, and in contrast to younger adult populations, older individuals with more severe anxiety at baseline as well as psychiatric comorbidities showed the greatest benefit from treatment (Wetherell et al. 2005). A greater understanding of the mechanisms and predictors of treatment response will help further refine CBT as an effective treatment for late-life anxiety disorders.

Relaxation Training

The most frequently used and the most well-substantiated treatments for anxiety in older adults are based on behavioral therapies, including relaxation training. Work by DeBerry (1982a, 1982b; DeBerry et al. 1989) showed that progressive muscle relaxation and meditation relaxation techniques reduced anxiety symptoms more effectively than treatment control conditions in older adults. Scogin et al. (1992) assessed the use of progressive muscle relaxation and imaginal relaxation. General symptom improvements were maintained at 1-month follow-up, and gains in treatment responders were maintained at a 1-year follow-up assessment (Rickard et al. 1984). Relaxation training has some advantages for treating mild anxiety in older adults. The strategies can be taught in brief individual or group sessions. Theoretically, the strategies can be delivered during a regular visit to a primary care physician. As with many behavioral strategies, relaxation training has the advantage of masquerading as skills training for patients who might avoid traditional psychotherapy. Also, patients with cognitive deficits, who may have difficulty with more cognitively based strategies, may benefit from purely behavioral strategies.

Substance Use Disorders

Cognitive-Behavioral Therapies

With the exception of alcohol use and prescription drug abuse, most substance use in late life is thought to be an extension of substance use from earlier periods of life into late life (Oslin et al. 2000). Although medical comorbidity becomes an increasing factor in older adults, most substance use in late life is presumed to differ from younger populations' use, because of cohort differences more than developmental differences. Treatment research on substance use in this population, specifically illicit drug use, is lagging but is greatly needed. The "baby boom" cohort is entering old age and is larger than previous cohorts. Moreover, rates of heavy alcohol use and illicit drug use are higher among this cohort than in earlier cohorts (Gfroerer et al. 2003; Lofwall et al. 2008; Wu and Blazer 2011). It has been projected that 5.7 million older adults will need treatment for a substance abuse problem in 2020—a substantial increase from approximately 2.8 million in 2002–2006 (Han et al. 2009; Wu and Blazer 2011).

Research on effective therapy for alcohol-related disorders in older adults is sparse. In the review literature, standard treatment for older adults is to mainstream them into therapeutic groups for adults of any age, such as Alcoholics Anonymous. This treatment choice has not been empirically validated for older adults, and in fact some researchers suggest that older adults will show better treatment gains in peer support groups and age-specific treatment protocols (Dupree et al. 1984; Schonfeld et al. 2000). Wu and Blazer (2011) suggest that substance abuse treatment protocols be age specific, supportive and nonconfrontational, directive, and geared toward the development of interpersonal skills for increased social support.

Although some previous comprehensive cognitive-behavioral interventions have shown promise, they are also plagued with high dropout rates (Schonfeld et al. 2000). Schonfeld et al. (2010) assessed the effectiveness of the Florida Brief Intervention and Treatment for Elders (BRITE) project, a low-cost approach for older adults at risk for illicit and nonillicit substance abuse and misuse. Prescription medication misuse and alcohol abuse were most prevalent in the sample. The treatment protocol involved a brief home-based intervention of one to five sessions that included motivational interviewing, education about relevant substances and consequences of substance use and misuse, reasons to quit drinking, and medication management. Following graduation from the brief intervention, participants completed a 16-session cognitive-behavioral treatment. The BRITE approach resulted in a significant reduction in depression and suicide risk, as well as reduction in alcohol and prescription medication misuse (Schonfeld et al. 2010).

Because primary care physicians are most likely to identify overuse of alcohol in their patients, this is a natural setting for which to develop treatment protocols. Brief counseling by the treating physician has been found to be significantly more effective in reducing alcohol misuse in older adults than has providing a general health booklet (Fleming et al. 1999).

Despite growing awareness that addictive disorders are common among older populations, it remains clear that more research is needed in this area.

Personality Disorders

Cognitive-Behavioral Therapies

Personality disorders are enduring patterns of inner experience (e.g., cognition, affect, impulse control) and behavior (e.g., interpersonal difficulties) that have an onset in adolescence or early adulthood, are stable over time, deviate considerably from normal cultural expectations, and cause distress or impairment in functioning. Meta-analyses have concluded that the prevalence rate of personality disorder in the older adult community is between 10% and 20% (Abrams 1996; Abrams and Horowitz 1999), essentially analogous to the 13% prevalence rate among younger age groups (Torgersen et al. 2001). Overall, the emotionally constricted/risk-averse disorders in Clusters A (paranoid and schizoid personality disorders) and C (obsessive-compulsive, avoidant, and dependent personality disorders) are the most commonly diagnosed in late life (Abrams 1996; Abrams and Horowitz 1999; Kenan et al. 2000; Morse and Lynch 2004), and there are also high rates of the not otherwise specified category compared with other individual personality disorder diagnoses (Abrams 1996; Abrams and Horowitz 1999; Kenan et al. 2000). In addition, personality disorder rates are even higher (approximately 30%) among depressed older adult samples (Abrams 1996; Thompson et al. 1988).

Personality psychopathology generally has been associated with poorer response to treatment—with either antidepressants or psychotherapy—among older adults (Abrams et al. 1994; Lynch et al. 2007; Thompson et al. 1988; Zweig 2008; but see Gum et al. 2007; for a review, also see Gradman et al. 1999). Depressed older adult patients with comorbid personality disorder are four times more likely to experience maintenance or reemergence of depressive symptoms compared with those without personality disorder diagnoses (Morse and Lynch 2004). Despite this, minimal controlled studies of the treatment of personality disorders in late life have been done.

In a randomized clinical trial specifically targeting personality disorders in older adults, Lynch et al. (2007) focused on providing standard DBT in both group and individual sessions following Linehan's (1993) manual. Participants were depressed older adults who had at least one comorbid personality disorder and who failed an 8-week selective serotonin reuptake inhibitor trial. Compared with a medication-only condition, participants who received DBT plus medication management plus clinical management reached remission more quickly than did the medication management plus clinical management group and showed improvements in interpersonal sensitivity and aggression (Lynch et al. 2007). Despite the promising nature of these findings, most of the empirical evidence suggests that the presence of a personality disorder in an older adult seriously compromises treatment. It appears that psychotherapy interventions likely will be enhanced when they target the unique behavioral, cognitive, and interpersonal dynamics associated with older-adult personality disorders.

Dementia

The development of psychosocial interventions for dementia is a complicated area of research. Unlike some of the other disorders discussed in this chapter, dementia is unlikely to remit as a result of psychotherapy. Researchers in this area have struggled to find distinct goals and outcomes on which to focus. Because the dementia as a whole is not expected to abate, researchers have chosen to focus on specific variables in older adults with dementia, such as global quality of life, affective states, disruptive behavioral symptoms, functional impairment, and prevention of self-harm.

Because of the cognitive deterioration experienced by dementia patients, most empirical research on interventions for dementia is based on behavioral strategies and targets caregivers as well as, or in lieu of, the patients themselves.

Studies of psychosocial interventions can be categorized by the treatment outcome goals and by the intervention targets. Typical targets include cognitive functioning, affect, and problematic behaviors, with interventions often attempting to address multiple targets. Reviews of empirically supported interventions by Teri et al. (2005b) and Livingston et al. (2005) provide overviews of current treatment approaches.

Cognitive Stimulation Therapy

Cognitive symptoms such as disorientation and confusion can cause distress and injury in patients and increased stress in caregivers. One proposed psychotherapeutic technique to cope with the cognitive symptoms of dementia is cognitive stimulation therapy. Derived from reality-orientation therapy, which aims to continually reorient patients' attention to the current situation and surroundings by repeating who they are and where they are, cognitive stimulation therapy focuses on improving information-processing abilities. Treatment can take place in formal groups or through training of professional or lay caregivers to administer intervention activities during the course of day-to-day activities. Several randomized controlled studies have found improved performance in patients receiving cognitive stimulation therapy, whether as a stand-alone intervention (Hayslip et al. 2009; Quayhagen et al. 1995; Spector et al. 2001, 2003) or as an augmentation of cholinesterase inhibitor medication (Onder et al. 2005). Cognitive abilities were generally preserved and/or improved in the treatment groups relative to control subjects (Onder et al. 2005; Spector et al. 2003). Relative improvements in mood (Spector et al. 2001) and behavior (Quayhagen et al. 1995) were observed, but not all studies showed improvements in these areas (e.g., Onder et al. 2005; Quayhagen et al. 2000; Spector et al. 2003).

Behavioral Therapies

Individuals with dementia are often at risk for anxiety, depression, or other negative affective states. Several behavioral therapies involving a combination of caregiver training in problem solving and communication and structured behavioral activation for patients have been found to be effective in reducing depressive symptoms (Beck et al. 2004; McCallion et al. 1999; Proctor et al. 1999; Teri et al. 1997, 2003). Behavioral therapy also has a strong history of controlling patients' problem behaviors, such as aggression, withdrawal, or resistance. These therapies generally train those who care for individuals with dementia—whether in the community or in inpatient facilities—to manage patient behavior via principles of operant conditioning. The behavioral interventions found effective in reducing depressive symptoms also have been found to be helpful in reducing problem behaviors (Bourgeois et al. 2002; Proctor et al. 1999; Teri et al. 1997, 2003, 2005a). For example, stimulus preference assessment can be used to identify effective reinforcers for use in individualized behavioral management protocols, which have been found to reduce agitation in residents of long-term-care facilities (Feliciano et al. 2009).

Progressively Lowered Stress Threshold–Based Caregiver Training

Another set of treatments with growing empirical support is based on the progressively lowered stress threshold (PLST) theory (Hall and Buckwalter 1987). From this perspective, the disease processes underlying dementia progressively lower the patient's ability to cope with stressors such as fatigue, change in routine, or physical illness. Treatment consists of educating and training caregivers in managing the patient's environment to minimize such stressors. PLST-based training is effective in reducing problem behaviors (Gerdner et al. 2002; Huang et al. 2003) and caregiver distress over patient behavior problems (Gerdner et al. 2002). Although further research is necessary to match the empirical validation of behavioral therapies for problem behaviors in dementia, the PLST approach shows great promise.

Conclusion

It is evident that psychotherapy offers significant promise for the treatment of psychopathology in elderly persons and at times may be the treatment of choice in terms of both efficacy and patient preference. We encourage practitioners to select treatments that have been tested with randomized clinical trials rather than basing their choices on theoretical preference or ease of application. The use of treatments without this type of empirical support can slow or reduce recovery.

References

Abrams RC: Personality disorders in the elderly. Int J Geriatr Psychiatry 11:759–763, 1996

Abrams RC, Horowitz SV: Personality disorders after age 50: a meta-analytic review of the literature, in Personality Disorders in Older Adults: Emerging Issues in Diagnosis and Treatment. Edited by Rosowsky E, Abrams RC. Mahwah, NJ, Erlbaum, 1999, pp 55–68

Abrams RC, Rosendahl E, Card C, et al: Personality disorder correlates of late and early onset depression. J Am Geriatr Soc 42:727–731, 1994

Alexander CL, Arnkoff DB, Glass CR: Bringing psychotherapy to primary care: innovations and challenges. Clinical Psychology: Science and Practice 17:191–214, 2010

Areán PA, Perri MG, Nezu AM, et al: Comparative effectiveness of social problem-solving therapy and reminiscence therapy as treatments for depression in older adults. J Consult Clin Psychol 61:1003–1010, 1993

Areán PA, Raue P, Mackin RS, et al: Problem solving therapy and supportive therapy in older adults with major depression and executive dysfunction. Am J Psychiatry 167:1391–1398, 2010

Ayers CR, Sorrell JT, Thorp SR, et al: Evidence-based psychological treatments for late-life anxiety. Psychol Aging 22:8–17, 2007

Babyak M, Blumenthal JA, Herman S, et al: Exercise treatment for major depression: maintenance of therapeutic benefit at 10 months. Psychosom Med 62:633–638, 2000

Barrowclough C, King P, Colville J, et al: A randomized trial of the effectiveness of cognitive-behavioral therapy and supportive counseling for anxiety symptoms in older adults. J Consult Clin Psychol 69:756–762, 2001

Bartels SJ, Coakley EH, Zubritsky C, et al: Improving access to geriatric mental health services: a randomized trial comparing treatment engagement with integrated versus enhanced referral care for depression, anxiety, and at-risk alcohol use. Am J Psychiatry 161:1455–1462, 2004

Beck AT, Freeman A, Davis DD: Cognitive Therapy of Personality Disorders, 2nd Edition. New York, Guilford, 2004

Beutler LE, Scogin F, Kirkish P, et al: Group cognitive therapy and alprazolam in the treatment of depression in older adults. J Consult Clin Psychol 55:550–556, 1987

Bibring E: [The problem of depression]. Psyche (Stuttg) 6:82–101, 1952

Blumenthal JA, Babyak MA, Doraiswamy PM, et al: Exercise and pharmacotherapy in the treatment of major depressive disorder. Psychosom Med 69:587–596, 2007

Bourgeois MS, Schulz R, Burgio LD, et al: Skills training for spouses of patients with Alzheimer's disease: outcomes of an intervention study. Journal of Clinical Geropsychology 8:53–73, 2002

Brand E, Clingempeel WG: Group behavioral therapy with depressed geriatric inpatients: an assessment of incremental efficacy. Behav Ther 23:475–482, 1992

Bruce ML, Ten Have TR, Reynolds CF 3rd, et al: Reducing suicidal ideation and depressive symptoms in depressed older primary care patients. JAMA 291:1081–1091, 2004

Burns D: Feeling Good. New York, New American Library, 1980

Chen H, Coakley EH, Cheal K, et al: Satisfaction with mental health services in older primary care patients. Am J Geriatr Psychiatry 14:371–379, 2006

Conner KO, Lee B, Mayers V, et al: Attitudes and beliefs about mental health among African American older adults suffering from depression. J Aging Stud 24:266–277, 2010

Covin R, Ouimet AJ, Seeds PM, et al: A meta-analysis of CBT for pathological worry among clients with GAD. J Anxiety Disord 22:108–116, 2008

DeBerry S: The effects of meditation-relaxation on anxiety and depression in a geriatric population. Psychotherapy: Theory, Research and Practice 19:512–521, 1982a

DeBerry S: An evaluation of progressive muscle relaxation on stress related symptoms in a geriatric population. Int J Aging Hum Dev 14:255–269, 1982b

DeBerry S, Davis S, Reinhard KE: A comparison of meditation-relaxation and cognitive/behavioral techniques for reducing anxiety and depression in a geriatric population. J Geriatr Psychiatry 22:231–247, 1989

Dupree LW, Broskowski H, Schonfeld LI: The Gerontology Alcohol Project: a behavioral treatment program for elderly alcohol abusers. Gerontologist 24:510–516, 1984

Feliciano L, Steers ME, Elite-Marcandonatou A, et al: Applications of preference assessment procedures in depression and agitation management in elders with dementia. Clin Gerontol 32:239–259, 2009

Fleming MFM, Manwell LB, Barry KLP, et al: Brief physician advice for alcohol problems in older adults: a randomized community-based trial. J Fam Pract 48:378–384, 1999

Floyd M, Scogin F, McKendree-Smith NL, et al: Cognitive therapy for depression: a comparison of individual psychotherapy and bibliotherapy for depressed older adults. Behav Modif 28:297–318, 2004

Fox KR, Stathi A, McKenna J, et al: Physical activity and mental well-being in older people participating in the Better Ageing Project. Eur J Appl Physiol 100:591–602, 2007

Frank E, Spanier C: Interpersonal psychotherapy for depression: overview, clinical efficacy, and future directions. Clinical Psychology: Sci ence and Practice 2:349–369, 1995

Frank E, Frank N, Cornes C, et al: Interpersonal psychotherapy in the treatment of late-life depression, in New Applications of Interpersonal Psychotherapy. Edited by Klerman GL, Weissman MM. Washington, DC, American Psychiatric Press, 1993, pp 167–198

Gallagher-Thompson D, Steffen AM: Comparative effects of cognitive-behavioral and brief psychodynamic psychotherapies for depressed family caregivers. J Consult Clin Psychol 62:543–549, 1994

Gallagher-Thompson D, Hanley-Peterson P, Thompson LW: Maintenance of gains versus relapse following brief psychotherapy for depression. J Consult Clin Psychol 58:371–374, 1990

Gerdner LA, Buckwalter KC, Reed D: Impact of a psychoeducational intervention on caregiver response to behavioral problems. Nurs Res 51:363–374, 2002

Gfroerer J, Penne M, Pemberton M, et al: Substance abuse treatment need among older adults in 2020: the impact of the aging baby-boom cohort. Drug Alcohol Depend 69:127–135, 2003

Gorenstein EE, Kleber MS, Mohlman J, et al: Cognitive-behavioral therapy for management of anxiety and medication taper in older adults. Am J Geriatr Psychiatry 13:901–909, 2005

Gradman TJ, Thompson LW, Gallagher-Thompson D: Personality disorders and treatment outcome, in Personality Disorders in Older Adults: Emerging Issues in Diagnosis and Treatment. Edited by Rosowsky E, Abrams RC. Mahwah, NJ, Erlbaum, 1999, pp 69–94

Gum AM, Areán PA, Hunkeler E, et al: Depression treatment preferences in older primary care patients. Gerontologist 46:14–22, 2006

Gum AM, Areán PA, Bostrom A: Low-income depressed older adults with psychiatric comorbidity: secondary analyses of response to psychotherapy and case management. Int J Geriatr Psychiatry 22:124–130, 2007

Gum AM, Ayalon L, Greenberg JM, et al: Preferences for professional assistance for distress in a diverse sample of older adults. Clin Gerontol 33:136–151, 2010

Hall GR, Buckwalter KC: Progressively lowered stress threshold: a conceptual model for care of adults with Alzheimer's disease. Arch Psychiatr Nurs 1:399–406, 1987

Han B, Gfroerer JC, Colliver JD, et al: Substance use disorder among older adults in the United States in 2020. Addiction 104:88–96, 2009

Hayslip B, Paggi K, Poole M, et al: The impact of mental aerobics training on memory impaired older adults. Clin Gerontol 32:389–394, 2009

Hegel MTP, Barrett JE, Cornell JE, et al: Predictors of response to problem solving treatment of depression in primary care. Behav Ther 33:511–527, 2002

Hinrichsen GA: Interpersonal psychotherapy for depressed older adults. J Geriatr Psychiatry 30:239–257, 1997

Hinrichsen GA: Why multicultural issues matter for practitioners working with older adults. Prof Psychol Res Pr 37:29–35, 2006

Hinrichsen GA: Interpersonal psychotherapy as a treatment for depression in late life. Prof Psychol Res Pr 39:306–312, 2008

Huang HL, Shyu YIL, Chen MC, et al: A pilot study on a home-based caregiver training program for improving caregiver self-efficacy and decreasing the behavioral problems of elders with dementia in Taiwan. Int J Geriatr Psychiatry 18:337–345, 2003

Jamison C, Scogin F: The outcome of cognitive bibliotherapy with depressed adults. J Consult Clin Psychol 63:644–650, 1995

Jarvik LF, Mintz J, Steuer JL, et al: Treating geriatric depression: a 26-week interim analysis. J Am Geriatr Soc 30:713–717, 1982

Kenan MM, Kendjelic EM, Molinari VA, et al: Age-related differences in the frequency of personality disorders among inpatient veterans. Int J Geriatr Psychiatry 15:831–837, 2000

Koder DA, Brodaty H, Anstey KJ: Cognitive therapy for depression in the elderly. Int J Geriatr Psychiatry 11:97–107, 1996

Kohut H, Wolf ES: The disorders of the self and their treatment: an outline. Int J Psychoanal 59:413–425, 1978

Lebowitz BD, Pearson JL, Schneider LS, et al: Diagnosis and treatment of depression in late life: consensus statement update. JAMA 278:1186–1190, 1997

Linehan MM: Cognitive-Behavioral Treatment of Borderline Personality Disorder. New York, Guilford, 1993

Livingston G, Johnston K, Katona C, et al: Systematic review of psychological approaches to the management of neuropsychiatric symptoms of dementia. Am J Psychiatry 162:1996–2021, 2005

Lofwall MR, Schuster A, Strain EC: Changing profile of abused substances by older persons entering treatment. J Nerv Ment Dis 196:898–905, 2008

Lynch TR, Morse JQ, Mendelson T, et al: Dialectical behavior therapy for depressed older adults: a randomized pilot study. Am J Geriatr Psychiatry 11:33–45, 2003

Lynch TR, Cheavens JS, Cukrowicz KC, et al: Treatment of older adults with co-morbid personality disorder and depression: a dialectical behavior therapy approach. Int J Geriatr Psychiatry 22:131–143, 2007

Mahler MS: On child psychosis and schizophrenia: autistic and symbiotic infantile psychoses. Psychoanal Study Child 7:286–305, 1952

McCallion P, Toseland RW, Freeman K: An evaluation of a family visit education program. J Am Geriatr Soc 47:203–214, 1999

Mohlman J, Gorman JM: The role of executive functioning in CBT: a pilot study with anxious older adults. Behav Res Ther 43:447–465, 2004

Mohlman J, Gorenstein EE, Kleber M, et al: Standard and enhanced cognitive-behavior therapy for late-life generalized anxiety disorder: two pilot investigations. Am J Geriatr Psychiatry 11:24–32, 2003

Morse JQ, Lynch TR: A preliminary investigation of self-reported personality disorders in late life: prevalence, predictors of depressive severity, and clinical correlates. Aging Ment Health 8:307–315, 2004

Mynors-Wallis LM: Pharmacotherapy is more effective than psychotherapy for elderly people with minor depression or dysthymia. Evidence-Based Healthcare 5:61, 2001

Naylor EV, Antonuccio DO, Litt M, et al: Bibliotherapy as a treatment for depression in primary care. J Clin Psychol Med Settings 17:258–271, 2010

Nezu AM: A problem-solving formulation of depression: a literature review and proposal of a pluralistic model. Clin Psychol Rev 7:121–144, 1987

Onder G, Zanetti O, Giocobini E, et al: Reality orientation therapy combined with cholinesterase inhibitors in Alzheimer's disease: randomised controlled trial. Br J Psychiatry 187:450–455, 2005

Oslin DW, Katz IR, Edell WS, et al: Effects of alcohol consumption on the treatment of depression among elderly patients. Am J Geriatr Psychiatry 8:215–220, 2000

Pinquart M, Duberstein PR, Lyness JM: Effects of psychotherapy and other behavioral interventions on clinically depressed older adults: a meta-analysis. Aging Ment Health 11:645–657, 2007

Proctor R, Burns A, Powell HS, et al: Behavioural management in nursing and residential homes: a randomised controlled trial. Lancet 354:26–29, 1999

Quayhagen MP, Quayhagen M, Corbeil RR, et al: A dyadic remediation program for care recipients with dementia. Nurs Res 44:153–159, 1995

Quayhagen MP, Quayhagen M, Corbeil RR, et al: Coping with dementia: evaluation of four nonpharmacologic interventions. Int Psychogeriatr 12:249–265, 2000

Reynolds CF 3rd, Frank E, Perel JM, et al: Nortriptyline and interpersonal psychotherapy as maintenance therapies for recurrent major depression: a randomized controlled trial in patients older than 59 years. JAMA 281:39–45, 1999

Rickard HC, Scogin F, Keith S: A one-year follow-up of relaxation training for elders with subjective anxiety. Gerontologist 34:121–122, 1984

Rokke PD, Scogin F: Depression treatment preferences in younger and older adults. Journal of Clinical Geropsychology 1:243–257, 1995

Salmon P: Effects of physical exercise on anxiety, depression, and sensitivity to stress: a unifying theory. Clin Psychol Rev 21:33–61, 2001

Schonfeld L, Dupree LW, Dickson-Fuhrmann E, et al: Cognitive-behavioral treatment of older veterans with substance abuse problems. J Geriatr Psychiatry Neurol 13:124–129, 2000

Schonfeld L, King-Kallimanis BL, Duchene DM, et al: Screening and brief intervention for substance misuse among older adults: the Florida BRITE project. Am J Public Health 100:108–114, 2010

Scogin F, McElreath L: Efficacy of psychosocial treatments for geriatric depression: a quantitative review. J Consult Clin Psychol 62:69–73, 1994

Scogin F, Jamison C, Gochneaur K: Comparative efficacy of cognitive and behavioral bibliotherapy for mildly and moderately depressed older adults. J Consult Clin Psychol 57:403–407, 1989

Scogin F, Jamison C, Davis N: Two-year follow-up of bibliotherapy for depression in older adults. J Consult Clin Psychol 58:665–667, 1990

Scogin F, Rickard HC, Keith S, et al: Progressive and imaginal relaxation training for elderly persons with subjective anxiety. Psychol Aging 7:419–424, 1992

Serfaty MA, Hayworth D, Blanchard M, et al: Clinical effectiveness of individual cognitive behavioral therapy for depressed older people in primary care: a randomized controlled trial. Arch Gen Psychiatry 66:1332–1340, 2009

Singh NA, Clements KM, Fiatarone Singh MA: The efficacy of exercise as a long-term antidepressant in elderly subjects: a randomized, controlled trial. J Gerontol A Biol Sci Med Sci 56:M497–M504, 2001

Sloane RB, Staples FR, Schneider LSM: Interpersonal therapy versus nortriptyline for depression in the elderly: case reports and discussion, in Clinical and Pharmacological Studies of Psychiatric Disorders. Edited by Burrows G, Norman TR, Dennerstein L. London, John Libbey, 1985, pp 344–346

Snodgrass J: Toward holistic care: integrating spirituality and cognitive behavioral therapy for older adults. Journal of Religion, Spirituality and Aging 21:219–236, 2009

Spector A, Orrell M, Davies S, et al: Can reality orientation be rehabilitated? Development and piloting of an evidence-based programme of cognition-based therapies for people with dementia. Neuropsychol Rehabil 11:377–379, 2001

Spector A, Thorgrimsen L, Woods B, et al: Efficacy of an evidence-based cognitive stimulation therapy programme for people with dementia: randomised controlled trial. Br J Psychiatry 183:248–254, 2003

Stanley MA, Novy DM: Cognitive-behavior therapy for generalized anxiety in late life: an evaluative overview. J Anxiety Disord 14:191–207, 2000

Stanley MA, Beck JG, Glassco JD: Treatment of generalized anxiety in older adults: a preliminary comparison of cognitive-behavioral and supportive approaches. Behav Ther 27:565–581, 1996

Stanley MA, Beck JG, Novy DM, et al: Cognitive behavioral treatment of late-life generalized anxiety disorder. J Consult Clin Psychol 71:309–319, 2003a

Stanley MA, Hopko DR, Diefenbach GJ, et al: Cognitive-behavioral therapy for older adults with late-life anxiety disorder in primary care: preliminary findings. Am J Geriatr Psychiatry 11:92–96, 2003b

Stanley MA, Diefenbach GJ, Hopko DR: Cognitive behavioral treatment for older adults with generalized anxiety disorder: a therapist manual for primary care settings. Behav Modif 28:73–117, 2004

Stanley MA, Wilson NL, Novy DM, et al: Cognitive behavior therapy for generalized anxiety disorder among older adults in primary care: a randomized clinical trial. JAMA 301:1480–1487, 2009

Steuer JL: Cognitive-behavioral and psychodynamic group psychotherapy in treatment of geriatric depression. J Consult Clin Psychol 52:180–189, 1984

Teri L, Logsdon RG, Uomoto J, et al: Behavioral treatment of depression in dementia patients: a controlled clinical trial. J Gerontol B Psychol Sci Soc Sci 52:P159–P166, 1997

Teri L, Gibbons LE, McCurry SM, et al: Exercise plus behavioral management in patients with Alzheimer disease: a randomized controlled trial. JAMA 290:2015–2022, 2003

Teri L, McCurry SM, Logsdon RG, et al: Training community consultants to help family members improve dementia care: a randomized controlled trial. Gerontologist 45:802–811, 2005a

Teri L, McKenzie G, LaFazia D: Psychosocial treatment of depression in older adults with dementia. Clinical Psychology: Science and Practice 12:303–316, 2005b

Thompson LW, Gallagher D: Efficacy of psychotherapy in the treatment of late-life depression. Advances in Behaviour Research and Therapy 6:127–139, 1984

Thompson LW, Gallagher D, Breckenridge JS: Comparative effectiveness of psychotherapies for depressed elders. J Consult Clin Psychol 55:385–390, 1987

Thompson LW, Gallagher D, Czirr R: Personality disorder and outcome in the treatment of late-life depression. J Geriatr Psychiatry 21:133–146, 1988

Torgersen S, Kringlen E, Cramer V: The prevalence of personality disorders in a community sample. Arch Gen Psychiatry 58:590–596, 2001

Unützer JM, Katon WM, Williams JW Jr, et al: Improving primary care for depression in late life: the design of a multicenter randomized trial. Med Care 39:785–799, 2001

Wang PS, Berglund P, Olfson M, et al: Failure and delay in initial treatment contact after first onset of mental disorders in the National Comorbidity Survey Replication. Arch Gen Psychiatry 62:629–640, 2005

Weissman MM, Myers JK, Thompson WD: Depression and its treatment in a U.S. urban community, 1975–1976. Arch Gen Psychiatry 38:417–421, 1981

Wetherell JL, Gatz M, Craske MG: Treatment of generalized anxiety disorder in older adults. J Consult Clin Psychol 71:31–40, 2003

Wetherell JL, Hopko DR, Diefenbach GJ, et al: Cognitive-behavioral therapy for late-life generalized anxiety disorder: who gets better? Behav Ther 36:147–156, 2005

Wetherell JL, Stoddard JA, White KS, et al: Augmenting antidepressant medication with modular CBT for geriatric generalized anxiety disorder: a pilot study. Int J Geriatr Psychiatry 26:869–875, 2011

Wilkinson P, Alder N, Juszczak E, et al: A pilot randomised controlled trial of a brief cognitive behavioural group intervention to reduce recurrence rates in late life depression. Int J Geriatr Psychiatry 24:68–75, 2009

Williams JW Jr, Barrett J, Oxman T, et al: Treatment of dysthymia and minor depression in primary care: a randomized controlled trial in older adults. JAMA 284:1519–1526, 2000

Wu LT, Blazer DG: Illicit and nonmedical drug use among older adults: a review. J Aging Health 23:481–504, 2011

Zweig RA: Personality disorder in older adults: assessment challenges and strategies. Prof Psychol Res Pr 39:298–305, 2008

Suggested Readings

Barrowclough C, King P, Colville J, et al: A randomized trial of the effectiveness of cognitive-behavioral therapy and supportive counseling for anxiety symptoms in older adults. J Consult Clin Psychol 69:756–762, 2001

Bartels SJ, Coakley EH, Zubritsky C, et al: Improving access to geriatric mental health services: a randomized trial comparing treatment engagement with integrated versus enhanced referral care for depression, anxiety, and at-risk alcohol use. Am J Psychiatry 161:1455–1462, 2004

Bruce ML, Ten Have TR, Reynolds CF 3rd, et al: Reducing suicidal ideation and depressive symptoms in depressed older primary care patients. JAMA 291:1081–1091, 2004

Lebowitz BD, Pearson JL, Schneider LS, et al: Diagnosis and treatment of depression in late life: consensus statement update. JAMA 278:1186–1190, 1997

Livingston G, Johnston K, Katona C, et al: Systematic review of psychological approaches to the management of neuropsychiatric symptoms of dementia. Am J Psychiatry 162:1996–2021, 2005

Lynch TR, Cheavens JS, Cukrowicz KC, et al: Treatment of older adults with co-morbid personality disorder and depression: a dialectical behavior therapy approach. Int J Geriatr Psychiatry 22:131–143, 2007

Mohlman J, Gorman JM: The role of executive functioning in CBT: a pilot study with anxious older adults. Behav Res Ther 43:447–465, 2004

Oslin DW: Evidence-based treatment of geriatric substance abuse. Psychiatr Clin North Am 28:897–911, 2005

Thompson LW, Coon DW, Gallagher-Thompson D, et al: Comparison of desipramine and cognitive/behavioral therapy in the treatment of elderly outpatients with mild-to-moderate depression. Am J Geriatr Psychiatry 9:225–240, 2001

Unützer JM, Katon W, Callahan CM, et al: Collaborative care management of late-life depression in the primary care setting: a randomized controlled trial. JAMA 228:2836–2845, 2002

11

Clinical Psychiatry in the Nursing Home

Joel E. Streim, M.D.

Nursing homes provide long-term care for elderly patients with chronic illness and disability as well as rehabilitation and convalescent care for those recovering from acute illness. As documented in previous reviews (Streim and Katz 2009), clinical studies have consistently provided evidence that the diagnosis, management, and treatment of mental disorders are important components of nursing home care. In this chapter, I review current information on the psychiatric problems that are common in nursing homes and discuss current trends affecting clinical care.

Prevalence of Psychiatric Disorders

Epidemiological studies conducted between 1986 and 1993 uniformly reported high prevalence rates for psychiatric disorders among nursing home residents. On the basis of psychiatric interviews of subjects in randomly selected samples, investigators have found prevalence rates of DSM-III (American Psychiatric Association 1980) or DSM-III-R (American Psychiatric Association 1987) disorders to be as high as 94% (Chandler and Chandler 1988; Rovner et al. 1986; Tariot et al. 1993). A more recent review of epidemiological studies and the 2004 National Nursing Home Survey calculated the median prevalence of dementia as 58% among nursing home residents, a 78% median prevalence of behavioral and psychological symptoms of dementia, a 10% median prevalence of major depression, and a 29% prevalence of depressive symptoms (Seitz et al. 2010). The challenge of providing long-term-care services in nursing homes is therefore complicated by the extensive psychiatric comorbidity found in this setting (Reichman and Conn 2010).

Cognitive Disorders and Behavioral Disturbances

In all studies, the most common psychiatric disorder was dementia, with prevalence rates of 50%–75% (Chandler and Chandler 1988; Katz et al. 1989; Parmelee et al. 1989; Rovner et al. 1986, 1990a; Tariot et al. 1993; Teeter et al. 1976). Alzheimer's disease (DSM-III-R primary degenerative dementia) accounted for about 50%–60% of cases of dementia, and vascular dementia accounted for about 25%–30% (Barnes and Raskind 1980; Rovner et al. 1986, 1990a).

Delirium is common in nursing homes and occurs primarily in patients made more vulnerable by a dementing illness. Available studies indicated that approximately 6%–7% of residents were delirious at the time of evaluation (Barnes and Raskind 1980; Rovner et al. 1986, 1990a). In one study, investigators found that nearly 25% of impaired residents had potentially reversible cognitive disturbance (Sabin et al. 1982); another study found that 6%–12% of residential care patients with dementia actually improved in cognitive performance over the course of 1 year (Katz et al. 1991). A large study of residents with severe cognitive impairment found improvement at 6-month follow-up in 14% of the sample (Buttar et al. 2003). Improvement was associated with the following baseline findings: higher function, antidepressant medication use, and falls. In the nursing home, as in other settings, a common reversible cause of cognitive impairment may be cognitive toxicity from drugs used to treat medical or psychiatric disorders. For residents admitted to the nursing home for post–acute care rehabilitation, unresolved delirium is associated with poor functional recovery (Kiely et al. 2007).

In patients with dementia, combined 1-year prevalence of psychosis, agitation, and depression has been estimated to be between 76% and 82% (Ballard et al. 2001), and 2-year prevalence of neuropsychiatric symptoms was found to be 96.6% (Wetzels et al. 2010). In nursing home populations, psychotic symptoms have been reported in approximately 25%–50% of residents with a primary dementing illness (Berrios and Brook 1985; Chandler and Chandler 1988; Rovner et al. 1986, 1990a; Teeter et al. 1976). Clinically significant depression is seen in approximately 25% of patients with dementia; one-third of such patients have symptoms of secondary major depression (Parmelee et al. 1989; Rovner et al. 1986, 1990a). Dementia complicated by mixed agitation and depression accounts for more than one-third of complicated dementia in nursing home populations and is associated with multiple psychiatric and medical needs, psychotropic drug use, and hospital admissions (Bartels et al. 2003).

A prospective cohort study of nursing home residents with dementia found a point prevalence of agitation or aggression ranging from 20.5% to 29.1%, with a 2-year cumulative prevalence of 53.8%; point prevalence of irritability ranging from 21.4% to 28.2%, with a 2-year cumulative prevalence of 58.1%; and a point prevalence of aberrant motor behavior fluctuating between 18.8% and 26.5%, with a cumulative prevalence of 50.4% (Wetzels et al. 2010). Most psychiatric consultations in long-term-care settings are for the evaluation and treatment of behavioral disturbances such as pacing and wandering, verbal abusiveness, disruptive shouting, physical aggression, destructive acts, and resistance to necessary care (Fenton et al. 2004; Loebel et al. 1991). Behavioral disturbances most frequently occur in patients with dementia, often in those with psychotic symptoms—an association that remains even after controlling for level of cognitive impairment (Rovner et al. 1990b). Agitation and hyperactivity also can be caused by agitated depression (Heeren et al. 2003), as well as delirium, sensory deprivation or overload, occult physical illness, pain, constipation, urinary retention, and adverse drug effects (including akathisia caused by neuroleptics) (Cohen-Mansfield and Billig 1986). Depressive symptoms are associated with disruptive vocalizations in nursing home residents, even after controlling for gender, age, and cognitive status (Dwyer and

Byrne 2000). In a subsequent study comparing verbal and physical nonaggressive agitation, verbal agitation was correlated with female gender, depressed affect, poor performance of activities of daily living, and impaired social functioning (Cohen-Mansfield and Libin 2005).

In addition to agitation, symptoms such as apathy, inactivity, and withdrawal occur among nursing home residents with and without a diagnosis of depression. Apathy has been found to increase over time, with a 2-year cumulative incidence of 42.1% (Wetzels et al. 2010). Although these symptoms are less disturbing to staff and less frequently lead to psychiatric consultation (Fenton et al. 2004), they can be disabling and may be associated with decreases in socialization and self-care.

Depression

Among community-dwelling elderly persons in the United States and Europe, depression increases the risk of nursing home admission (Ahmed et al. 2007; Harris and Cooper 2006; Onder et al. 2007), and this association remains after controlling for age, physical illness, and functional status (Harris 2007). Among elderly persons who reside in nursing homes, depressive disorders represent the second most common psychiatric diagnosis. Most studies in U.S. nursing homes show depression prevalence rates of 15%–50%, depending on what population is studied, what instruments are used, whether major depression or depressive symptoms are being reported, and whether primary depression and depression occurring secondary to dementia are considered together or separately (Baker and Miller 1991; Chandler and Chandler 1988; Hyer and Blazer 1982; Katz et al. 1989; Kaup et al. 2007; Lesher 1986; Levin et al. 2007; Parmelee et al. 1989; Rovner et al. 1986, 1990a, 1991; Tariot et al. 1993; Teeter et al. 1976). DSM-III or DSM-III-R criteria for major depression are met in approximately 6%–10% of all nursing home residents, and in 20%–25% of those who are cognitively intact; the latter figure is an order of magnitude greater than rates among community-dwelling elderly persons (Blazer and Williams 1980; Kramer et al. 1985).

Parmelee et al. (1992a) reported that the 1-year incidence of major depression was 9.4% and that patients with preexisting minor depression were at increased risk; the incidence of minor depression among those who were euthymic at baseline was 7.4%. Depression among nursing home residents tends to be persistent. Ames et al. (1988) found that only 17% of the patients with diagnosable depressive disorders had recovered after an average of 3.6 years of follow-up. Smalbrugge et al. (2006) found persistence of symptoms in two-thirds of residents at 6-month follow-up, although rates were significantly higher in those with more severe symptoms at baseline.

Evidence for morbidity associated with depression comes from studies that showed an increase in pain complaints among residents with depression (Parmelee et al. 1991) and an association between depression and biochemical markers of subnutrition (Katz et al. 1993). Depression in nursing home residents, both with and without dementia, is associated with disability (Kaup et al. 2007). Among individuals admitted to nursing homes for post–acute care rehabilitation, those with depression have poorer functional outcomes (Webber et al. 2005). In addition to its association with morbidity and disability, depression has been found to be associated with an increase in mortality rate, with effect sizes ranging from 1.6 to 3 (Ashby et al. 1991; Katz et al. 1989; Parmelee et al. 1992b; Rovner et al. 1991; Sutcliffe et al. 2007). In addition to the high level of complexity that characterizes major depression among nursing home residents, the evidence of heterogeneity in these patients may reflect the existence of clinically relevant subtypes of depression. The treatment study by Katz et al. (1990) reported that measures of self-care deficits and serum levels of albumin were highly intercorrelated and that both predicted a lack of response to treatment with nortriptyline. Therefore, although this study determined that major depression is a specific, treatable disorder—even in long-term-care patients with medical comorbidity—there is also evidence in this setting for a treatment-relevant subtype of depression characterized by high levels of disability and low levels of serum albumin. Depressed residents with dementia have been found to have a poorer response to treatment with noradrenergic and serotonergic antidepressant drugs (Magai et al. 2000; Oslin et al. 2000; Streim et al. 2000).

Progress in Treatment of Psychiatric Disorders in the Nursing Home

An appreciation of the unique characteristics of nursing home populations—particularly the extremes of old age and the high prevalence rates of cognitive impairment, psychiatric and medical comorbidity, and disability, all in the context of residential long-term-care institutions—has led to increased recognition that results of efficacy studies conducted in general adult outpatient populations may not be readily generalizable to nursing home residents. This recognition points to the need for treatment studies conducted specifically with nursing home patients. Although the number of randomized controlled studies is limited, the body of literature on treatment outcomes in the nursing home is growing.

Nonpharmacological Management of Behavioral Disturbances

Since 1990, numerous studies have been published describing nonpharmacological interventions for behavioral disturbances associated with dementia in the nursing home setting. Few of these were randomized controlled trials. Several nonpharmacological interventions have been shown to be effective, although only behavior management therapies, specific types of caregiver and residential care staff education, and possibly cognitive stimulation appear to have lasting effectiveness (Livingston et al. 2005). One promising approach combined enhanced activities, establishment of and adherence to guidelines for psychotropic medication use, and educational rounds for nursing home staff (Rovner et al. 1996). In a randomized clinical trial, this approach was shown to reduce the prevalence of problem behaviors and the use of antipsychotic drugs and physical restraints. Activities matched to skills and interests of residents with dementia also have been shown to reduce agitation and negative affect (Kolanowski et al. 2005). Individualized consultation for staff nurses about the management of patients with dementia also was shown to diminish the use of physical restraints (Evans et al. 1997). Reductions in agitation were observed in a study of a daytime physical activity intervention combined with a nighttime program to decrease noise and sleep-disruptive nursing care practices (Alessi et al. 1999). Bright light therapy has been shown to increase observed nocturnal sleep time but not to improve agitated behavior in nursing home residents with dementia (Lyketsos et al. 1999). Although some studies have claimed that aromatherapy with lavender oil is effective in reducing agitated behaviors, results have not been consistently replicated when controlling for nonolfactory aspects of treatment in residents with severe dementia (Snow et al. 2004). Other programs decrease behavioral difficulties through individualized modifications in the physical environment (van Weert et al. 2005).

Psychotherapy

The evidence for the efficacy of psychotherapy in other settings suggests that it may be of value for treating mental disorders of aging in nursing home residents whose cognitive abilities allow them to participate. Bharucha et al. (2006) identified and reviewed 18 controlled "talk" psychotherapy studies conducted in nursing home populations and found that most showed at least short-term benefits on measures of mood, hopelessness, perceived control, self-esteem, or other psychological variables. However, the investigators noted that interpretation of findings of many of these studies was limited by small sample sizes, variable study entry criteria, short duration of trials, heterogeneous outcome assessment methods, and lack of detail on intervention methods. Controlled research on psychotherapeutic interventions has included studies of task-oriented versus insight-oriented therapy (Moran and Gatz 1987); reality orientation (Baines et al. 1987); reminiscence groups (Baines et al. 1987; Chao et al. 2006; Goldwasser et al. 1987; McMurdo and Rennie 1993; Orten et al. 1989; Politis et al. 2004; Rattenbury and Stones 1989; Youssef 1990); exercise, activity, and progressive relaxation groups (Bensink et al. 1992; McMurdo and Rennie 1993); supportive group psychotherapy (Goldwasser et al. 1987; Williams-Barnard and Lindell 1992); validation therapy (Tondi et al. 2007; Toseland et al. 1997); cognitive or cognitive-behavioral group therapies (Abraham et al. 1992; Zerhusen et al. 1991); focused visual imagery therapy (Abraham et al. 1997); and a psychosocial activity intervention (Beck et al. 2002). With the exception of the investigations by Abraham and colleagues, patients in most of these studies were not selected on the basis of specific psychiatric symptoms or syndromes but rather on the basis of age, cognitive status, or mobility. Some of these studies reported improvements on measures of communication, behavior, cognitive performance, mood, social withdrawal, physical function, somatic preoccupation, self-esteem, perceived locus of control, quality of life, and life satisfaction.

Pharmacotherapy

Pharmacological treatments are commonly used in nursing homes for dementia and its associated psychological and behavioral symptoms and for depression. Some earlier studies provided evidence for the efficacy of antipsychotic drugs in managing agitation and related symptoms in nursing home residents with dementia, but the effect sizes were often modest, and high placebo response rates were common (Barnes et al. 1982; Schneider et al. 1990; Sunderland and Silver 1988). Subsequently, several multicenter, randomized, double-blind, placebo-controlled clinical trials showed that some of the atypical antipsychotic agents had efficacy for the treatment of psychotic symptoms and agitated behavior in nursing home residents with dementia. These include published studies of risperidone (Brodaty et al. 2003; Katz et al. 1999), olanzapine (Meehan et al. 2002; Street et al. 2000), quetiapine (Zhong et al. 2007), and aripiprazole (Mintzer et al. 2007). Secondary analyses of data from the nursing home trials of risperidone showed that it had antipsychotic effects and also had independent effects on aggression or agitation. Other studies of atypical antipsychotic drugs in nursing home residents with dementia failed to show statistically significant benefits on the a priori designated primary outcome measures related to psychosis or behavioral disturbances (De Deyn et al. 1999, 2005; Mintzer et al. 2006; Streim et al. 2008), although some of these studies found possible benefits on secondary behavioral measures. Widespread interest in studying atypical antipsychotics in the treatment of elderly nursing home residents was partly attributable to the expectation that these agents would be better tolerated than would conventional antipsychotics in this population. For example, early follow-up studies had suggested that risperidone may cause less tardive dyskinesia than do typical antipsychotic agents (Jeste et al. 2000).

These controlled clinical trials have examined only the acute effects of treatment, typically for 6–12 weeks of treatment, and little is known about the effectiveness of treatment for longer periods. However, evidence suggests that the need for and benefit from antipsychotic drug treatment change over the course of months in nursing home patients with dementia. Several double-blind, placebo-controlled studies of antipsychotic drug discontinuation reported that most patients who had been receiving longer-term treatment could be withdrawn from these agents without reemergence of psychosis or agitated behaviors (Bridges-Parlet et al. 1997; Cohen-Mansfield et al. 1999;

Ruths et al. 2004). Therefore, it is important to reevaluate periodically the need for continuing antipsychotic drug treatment.

Since 2003, analyses of safety data from randomized controlled studies of atypical antipsychotic drugs in elderly patients with dementia, including the aforementioned nursing home studies, have found significantly increased risks of cerebrovascular adverse events and mortality in this population. Although elevated risks were not found in every study, pooled analyses showed that the rate of cerebrovascular adverse events (including stroke and transient ischemic attacks) is greater than with placebo. These findings led to regulatory warnings in the United States, Canada, and the United Kingdom regarding the safety of these drugs in elderly patients with dementia.

The U.S. Food and Drug Administration (FDA) also warned that elderly patients with dementia-related psychosis who are given atypical antipsychotics have a risk of death between 1.6 and 1.7 times greater than do those who are given placebo (4.5% vs. 2.6%), with a reminder that atypical antipsychotics are not FDA approved for the treatment of dementia-related psychosis. Consistent with this FDA warning, a meta-analysis by Schneider et al. (2005), which examined results of 15 randomized controlled trials, many of which were conducted in nursing home patients, found that the risk of mortality was 3.5% in elderly patients taking atypical antipsychotics compared with 2.3% in patients taking placebo. Wang et al. (2005) found a significantly higher adjusted risk of death in elderly patients taking conventional antipsychotics compared with those taking atypical antipsychotic medications, regardless of whether the patients had dementia or resided in a nursing home. The investigators suggested that conventional antipsychotic medications not be used to replace atypical agents discontinued in response to FDA warnings.

In light of the concerns about risks of antipsychotic drugs in elderly nursing home residents with dementia, experts in the field have suggested that nonpharmacological approaches be considered first when treating noncognitive behavioral symptoms. However, for those nursing home patients whose behavioral symptoms do not respond to nonpharmacological interventions, the decision to use an atypical antipsychotic should be based on a careful assessment of the individual risk-benefit profile.

Five randomized clinical trials evaluated the efficacy of mood-stabilizing anticonvulsant drugs for the treatment of agitation and aggression in nursing home residents. The first was a study of carbamazepine that showed it to be effective for agitation and aggression but not for psychotic symptoms such as delusions and hallucinations (Tariot et al. 1998). Another trial of carbamazepine found high rates of improvements in patients receiving carbamazepine or placebo, with no significant between-group differences (Olin et al. 2001). Several placebo-controlled studies evaluated divalproex, with few encouraging results, including one trial that was discontinued before completion because of adverse effects in the drug treatment group. Overall, these studies failed to provide evidence for efficacy in reducing agitated behavior (Porsteinsson et al. 2001; Tariot et al. 2001b, 2005). Notably, the tolerability of divalproex was limited by somnolence, weakness, and diminished oral intake in this population of elderly nursing home subjects with dementia.

Acetylcholinesterase inhibitors have been shown to delay the decline in cognitive function in patients with mild to severe Alzheimer's disease, although few studies have been conducted specifically in nursing home samples. One randomized clinical trial of donepezil in nursing home residents showed effects on cognitive performance that were comparable to those observed in less impaired outpatients (Tariot et al. 2001a). A subsequent study reported that donepezil improves cognition and preserves function in Alzheimer's disease patients with severe dementia residing in nursing homes (Winblad et al. 2006). These studies also examined the effects of donepezil on behavioral disturbances, as a secondary outcome measure, and did not find significant benefits. Tariot et al. (2004) reported significant improvement in Neuropsychiatric Inventory scores with the N-methyl-D-aspartate receptor antagonist memantine, but this agent has not been studied prospectively in the nursing home setting. Survival analyses in an observational study have suggested that the addition of memantine to a cholinesterase inhibitor can delay the time to nursing home placement (Lopez et al. 2009).

Several randomized clinical trials have evaluated the effects of antidepressants in nursing home residents. In a placebo-controlled study, a positive response to nortriptyline for treatment of major depression was reported in a long-term-care population with high levels of medical comorbidity (Katz et al. 1990). In another study, patients were randomly assigned to receive regular or low-dose nortriptyline, and significant plasma level–response relations were documented in cognitively intact patients (Streim et al. 2000). However, in patients with dementia, the plasma level–response relation was significantly different, suggesting that the depression occurring in dementia might be a treatment-relevant subtype of depression or a distinct disorder. A controlled antidepressant trial in nursing home residents with late-stage Alzheimer's disease showed no significant benefits of sertraline over placebo (Magai et al. 2000). Available open-label studies of the efficacy of selective serotonin reuptake inhibitors (SSRIs) in nursing home residents with depression have had mixed results, some consistent with the findings of Magai et al. (2000), suggesting that SSRIs may be less effective for depression in patients with dementia than in those who are cognitively intact (Oslin et al. 2000; Rosen et al. 2000; Trappler and Cohen 1996, 1998).

Although the SSRIs, because of their side-effect profile, might be expected to be well tolerated by frail elderly nursing home patients, evidence indicates that these drugs can cause serious adverse events in this population. Thapa et al. (1998) found that the use of SSRIs was associated with a nearly twofold increase in the risk of falls in nursing home residents, comparable with the risk found with tricyclic antidepressant drugs. Investigators in the United Kingdom reported that antidepressant use was associated with better physical functioning but also with greater frequency of falls in residential care patients (Arthur et al. 2002). A randomized, double-blind comparison trial found that venlafaxine was less well tolerated compared with sertraline in frail nursing home patients without conferring more treatment benefits, as might be expected from an agent with mixed serotonergic and noradrenergic effects (Oslin et al. 2003).

Federal Regulations and Psychiatric Care in the Nursing Home

Federal Regulations

The Nursing Home Reform Act was enacted as part of the Omnibus Budget Reconciliation Act of 1987 (Public Law 100-203). This legislation provided for government regulation of the operation of nursing facilities and of the care that they provide (Elon and Pawlson 1992). This legislation directed the Health Care Financing Administration—reorganized and renamed in 2001 as the Centers for Medicare and Medicaid Services (CMS)—to issue regulations (Health Care Financing Administration 1991) that would operationalize the laws and to develop guidelines (Centers for Medicare and Medicaid Services

2007) that would assist federal and state surveyors in interpreting the regulations. Mental health screening, assessment, care planning, and treatment are addressed under sections of the regulations that pertain to resident assessment, resident rights and facility practices, and quality of care (Health Care Financing Administration 1991, 1992a, 1992b).

Regulations requiring comprehensive assessment for all residents (Health Care Financing Administration 1991) have led to development of a uniform Resident Assessment Instrument, which includes the Minimum Data Set (MDS) (Morris et al. 1990), an updated version of which was implemented in 2010 (Centers for Medicare and Medicaid Services 2010). This instrument must be administered on a regular basis by members of an interdisciplinary health care team (Health Care Financing Administration 1992c). Areas of assessment relevant to mental illness and behavior include mood, cognition, communication, functional status, medications, and other treatments. Responses on the MDS may indicate changes in a patient's clinical status that warrant further evaluation and point to a possible need for changes in the treatment plan.

Regulations related to resident rights and facility practices restrict the use of physical restraints and antipsychotic drugs when they are "administered for purposes of discipline or convenience and not required to treat the resident's medical symptoms" (Health Care Financing Administration 1991, p. 48,875). Regulations related to quality of care further require that residents not receive "unnecessary drugs" and specify that antipsychotic medications may not be given "unless these are necessary to treat a specific condition as diagnosed and documented in the clinical record" (p. 48,910). The guidelines based on these regulations further limit the use of antipsychotic medications, antianxiety agents, sedative-hypnotics, and related medications (Centers for Medicare and Medicaid Services 2011). For each of these classes, the guidelines specify a list of acceptable indications, upper limits for daily dosages, requirements for monitoring treatment and adverse effects, and time frames for attempting dosage reductions and discontinuation. These guidelines are periodically updated to reflect new clinical knowledge and the availability of new drugs approved by the FDA (Centers for Medicare and Medicaid Services 2011).

To minimize concerns about federal interference with medical practice, the current guidelines include qualifying statements that recognize cases in which strict adherence to prescribing limits or gradual dosage reduction or discontinuation is "clinically contraindicated." Thus, the physician's options for treating nursing home residents need not be unduly restricted by the regulations if the clinical rationale—explaining that the benefits of treatment (in terms of symptom relief, improved health status, or improved functioning) outweigh the risks—is clearly documented in the medical record. Although the facility, not the physician, is accountable for compliance with the regulations, the physician's clinical reasoning and judgment play a critical role in the process of ensuring quality care.

To enable surveyors to compare individual facilities within the same state, the CMS introduced quality indicators derived from MDS data (Nursing Home Quality Indicators Development Group 1999). There are 24 quality indicators in 11 different domains, including behavior and emotional problems, cognitive patterns, and psychotropic drug use.

Whenever a review in any of these areas results in a citation of deficiency, a plan of correction must be developed and submitted for approval. This system is a first step in monitoring quality of care, although the face validity of some of the quality indicators has been questioned, and the results of quality surveys may be difficult to interpret. Nevertheless, the results from every nursing home survey are available for public inspection, and consumers of nursing home services (and their families) can access the quality indicator reports online.

Subacute Care in Nursing Homes

Over the past 30 years, many patients have been discharged to nursing homes that serve as step-down facilities, providing subacute medical treatment, convalescent care, and rehabilitation services. It has been estimated that subacute-care patients constitute about one-third of nursing home admissions in the United States (Jones et al. 2009; Leon et al. 1997).

In general, short-stay residents differ from long-term-care patients in that the former are younger; more likely to be admitted directly from an acute-care hospital; less likely to have irreversible cognitive impairment, incontinence, or ambulatory dysfunction; and more likely to have a primary diagnosis of hip fracture, stroke, or cancer. The objectives of mental health care for short-stay patients are to search for delirium and reversible causes of cognitive impairment, and to treat disorders such as depression and anxiety that can be impediments to rehabilitation and recovery; these goals are similar to those of traditional consultation-liaison psychiatry in the general hospital. For subacute-care patients in nursing homes, an investment in psychiatric care can lead to improved participation in rehabilitation efforts, with more efficient recovery and return to independent functioning and more rapid discharge to the community.

References

Abraham IL, Neundorfer MM, Currie LJ: Effects of group interventions on cognition and depression in nursing home residents. Nurs Res 41:196–202, 1992

Abraham IL, Onega LL, Reel SJ, et al: Effects of cognitive group interventions on depressed frail nursing home residents, in Depression in Long Term and Residential Care: Advances in Research and Treatment. Edited by Rubinstein RL, Lawton MP. New York, Springer, 1997, pp 154–168

Ahmed A, Lefante CM, Alam N: Depression and nursing home admission among hospitalized older adults with coronary artery disease: a propensity score analysis. Am J Geriatr Cardiol 16:76–83, 2007

Alessi CA, Yoon EJ, Schelle JF, et al: A randomized trial of a combined physical activity and environmental intervention in nursing home residents: do sleep and agitation improve? J Am Geriatr Soc 47:784–791, 1999

American Psychiatric Association: Diagnostic and Statistical Manual of Mental Disorders, 3rd Edition. Washington, DC, American Psychiatric Association, 1980

American Psychiatric Association: Diagnostic and Statistical Manual of Mental Disorders, 3rd Edition, Revised. Washington, DC, American Psychiatric Association, 1987

Ames D, Ashby D, Mann AH, et al: Psychiatric illness in elderly residents of Part III homes in one London borough: prognosis and review. Age Ageing 17:249–256, 1988

Arthur A, Matthews R, Jagger C, et al: Factors associated with antidepressant treatment in residential care: changes between 1990 and 1997. Int J Geriatr Psychiatry 17:54–60, 2002

Ashby D, Ames D, West CR, et al: Psychiatric morbidity as predictor of mortality for residents of local authority homes for the elderly. Int J Geriatr Psychiatry 6:567–575, 1991

Baines S, Saxby P, Ehlert K: Reality orientation and reminiscence therapy. Br J Psychiatry 151:222–231, 1987

Baker FM, Miller CL: Screening a skilled nursing home population for depression. J Geriatr Psychiatry Neurol 4:218–221, 1991

Ballard CG, Margallo-Lana M, Fossey J, et al: A 1-year follow-up study of behavioral and psychological symptoms in dementia among people in care environments. J Clin Psychiatry 62:631–636, 2001

Barnes R, Raskind MA: DSM-III criteria and the clinical diagnosis of dementia: a nursing home study. J Gerontol 36:20–27, 1980

Barnes R, Veith R, Okimoto J, et al: Efficacy of antipsychotic medications in behaviorally disturbed dementia patients. Am J Psychiatry 139:1170–1174, 1982

Bartels SJ, Horn SD, Smout RJ, et al: Agitation and depression in frail nursing home elderly patients with dementia: treatment characteristics and service use. Am J Geriatr Psychiatry 11:231–238, 2003

Beck CK, Vogelpohl TS, Rasin JH, et al: Effects of behavioral interventions on disruptive behavior and affect in demented nursing home residents. Nurs Res 51:219–228, 2002

Bensink GW, Godbey KL, Marshall MJ, et al: Institutionalized elderly: relaxation, locus of control, self-esteem. J Gerontol Nurs 18:30–36, 1992

Berrios GE, Brook P: Delusions and psychopathology of the elderly with dementia. Acta Psychiatr Scand 75:296–301, 1985

Bharucha AJ, Dew MA, Miller MD, et al: Psychotherapy in long-term care: a review. J Am Med Dir Assoc 7:568–580, 2006

Blazer DG, Williams CD: Epidemiology of dysphoria and depression in an elderly population. Am J Psychiatry 137:439–444, 1980

Bridges-Parlet S, Knopman D, Steffes S: Withdrawal of neuroleptic medications from institutionalized dementia patients: results of a double-blind, baseline-treatment-controlled pilot study. J Geriatr Psychiatry Neurol 10:119–126, 1997

Brodaty H, Ames D, Snowdon J, et al: A randomized placebo-controlled trial of risperidone for the treatment of aggression, agitation, and psychosis of dementia. J Clin Psychiatry 64:134–143, 2003

Buttar AB, Mhyre J, Fries BE, et al: Six-month cognitive improvement in nursing home residents with severe cognitive impairment. J Geriatr Psychiatry Neurol 16:100–108, 2003

Centers for Medicare and Medicaid Services: State Operations Manual, Appendix PP: Guidance to Surveyors for Long Term Care Facilities. Baltimore, MD, Centers for Medicare and Medicaid Services, 2007. Available at: http://www.cms.hhs.gov/manuals/Downloads/som107ap_pp_guidelines_ltcf.pdf. Accessed August 6, 2008.

Centers for Medicare and Medicaid Services: Nursing home quality initiative: MDS 3.0 technical information. Baltimore, MD, Centers for Medicare and Medicaid, 2010. Available at: http://www.cms.gov/Medicare/Quality-Initiatives-Patient-Assessment-Instruments/NursingHomeQualityInits/NHQIMDS30TechnicalInformation.html. Accessed June 20, 2013.

Centers for Medicare and Medicaid Services: State Operations Manual, Appendix PP—Guidance to Surveyors for Long Term Care Facilities; Rev 70. January 7, 2011. Available at: https://www.cms.gov/manuals/Downloads/som107ap_pp_guidelines_ltcf.pdf. Accessed June 22, 2013

Chandler JD, Chandler JE: The prevalence of neuropsychiatric disorders in a nursing home population. J Geriatr Psychiatry Neurol 1:71–76, 1988

Chao SY, Liu HY, Wu CY, et al: The effects of group reminiscence therapy on depression, self esteem, and life satisfaction of elderly nursing home residents. J Nurs Res 14:36–45, 2006

Cohen-Mansfield J, Billig N: Agitated behaviors in the elderly: a conceptual review. J Am Geriatr Soc 34:711–721, 1986

Cohen-Mansfield J, Libin A: Verbal and physical non-aggressive agitated behaviors in elderly persons with dementia: robustness of syndromes. J Psychiatr Res 39:325–332, 2005

Cohen-Mansfield J, Lipson S, Werner P, et al: Withdrawal of haloperidol, thioridazine, and lorazepam in the nursing home: a controlled, double-blind study. Arch Intern Med 159:1733–1740, 1999

De Deyn PP, Rabheru K, Rasmussen A, et al: A randomized trial of risperidone, placebo, and haloperidol for behavioral symptoms of dementia. Neurology 53:946–955, 1999

De Deyn PP, Katz IR, Brodaty H, et al: Management of agitation, aggression, and psychosis associated with dementia: a pooled analysis including three randomized, placebo-controlled double-blind trials in nursing home residents treated with risperidone. Clin Neurol Neurosurg 107:497–508, 2005

Dwyer M, Byrne GJ: Disruptive vocalization and depression in older nursing home residents. Int Psychogeriatr 12:463–471, 2000

Elon R, Pawlson LG: The impact of OBRA on medical practice within nursing facilities. J Am Geriatr Soc 40:958–963, 1992

Evans LK, Strumpf NE, Allen-Taylor SL, et al: A clinical trial to reduce restraints in nursing homes. J Am Geriatr Soc 45:675–681, 1997

Fenton J, Raskin A, Gruber-Baldini AL, et al: Some predictors of psychiatric consultation in nursing home residents. Am J Geriatr Psychiatry 12:297–304, 2004

Goldwasser AN, Auerbach SM, Harkins SW: Cognitive, affective, and behavioral effects of reminiscence group therapy of demented elderly. Int J Aging Hum Dev 25:209–222, 1987

Harris Y: Depression as a risk factor for nursing home admission among older individuals. J Am Med Dir Assoc 8:14–20, 2007

Harris Y, Cooper JK: Depressive symptoms in older people predict nursing home admission. J Am Geriatr Soc 54:593–597, 2006

Health Care Financing Administration: Medicare and Medicaid: Requirements for Long Term Care Facilities, Final Regulations. Fed Regist 56:48865–48921, 1991

Health Care Financing Administration: Medicare and Medicaid Programs: Preadmission Screening and Annual Resident Review. Fed Regist 57:56450–56504, 1992a

Health Care Financing Administration: Medicare and Medicaid: Resident Assessment in Long Term Care Facilities. Fed Regist 57:61614–61733, 1992b

Health Care Financing Administration: State Operations Manual: Provider Certification (Transmittal No 250). Washington, DC, Health Care Financing Administration, 1992c

Heeren O, Borin L, Raskin A, et al: Association of depression with agitation in elderly nursing home residents. J Geriatr Psychiatry Neurol 16:4–7, 2003

Hyer L, Blazer DG: Depressive symptoms: impact and problems in long term care facilities. International Journal of Behavioral Gerontology 1:33–44, 1982

Jeste DV, Okamoto A, Napolitano J, et al: Low incidence of persistent tardive dyskinesia in elderly patients with dementia treated with risperidone. Am J Psychiatry 157:1150–1155, 2000

Jones AL, Dwyer LL, Bercovitz AR, Strahan GW: The National Nursing Home Survey: 2004 overview. National Center for Health Statistics. Vital Health Stat 13(167), 2009. Available at: http://www.cdc.gov/nchs/data/series/sr_13/sr13_167.pdf. Accessed June 22, 2013.

Katz IR, Lesher E, Kleban M, et al: Clinical features of depression in the nursing home. Int Psychogeriatr 1:5–15, 1989

Katz IR, Simpson GM, Curlik SM, et al: Pharmacological treatment of major depression for elderly patients in residential care settings. J Clin Psychiatry 51(suppl):41–48, 1990

Katz IR, Parmelee P, Brubaker K: Toxic and metabolic encephalopathies in long-term care patients. Int Psychogeriatr 3:337–347, 1991

Katz IR, Beaston-Wimmer P, Parmelee PA, et al: Failure to thrive in the elderly: exploration of the concept and delineation of psychiatric components. J Geriatr Psychiatry Neurol 6:161–169, 1993

Katz IR, Jeste DV, Mintzer JE, et al: Comparison of risperidone and placebo for psychosis and behavioral disturbances associated with dementia: a randomized, double-blind trial. J Clin Psychiatry 60:107–115, 1999

Kaup BA, Loreck D, Gruber-Baldini AL, et al: Depression and its relationship to function and medical status, by dementia status, in nursing home admissions. Am J Geriatr Psychiatry 15:438–442, 2007

Kiely DK, Jones RN, Bergmann MA, et al: Association between delirium resolution and functional recovery among newly admitted postacute facility patients. J Gerontol A Biol Sci Med Sci 62:107–108, 2007

Kolanowski AM, Litaker M, Buettner L: Efficacy of theory-based activities for behavioral symptoms of dementia. Nurs Res 54:219–228, 2005

Kramer M, German PS, Anthony JC, et al: Patterns of mental disorders among the elderly residents of eastern Baltimore. J Am Geriatr Soc 33:236–245, 1985

Leon J, Cheng M, Dunbar J: Trends in Special Care: The 1995 National Nursing Home Census of Sub-Acute Units. U.S. Dept of Health and Human Services, Office of Disability, Aging and Long-Term Care Policy and Project Hope Center for Health Affairs, September 1997. Available at: http://aspe.hhs.gov/daltcp/reports/sctrend.htm#figure1. Accessed June 22, 2013.

Lesher E: Validation of the Geriatric Depression Scale among nursing home residents. Clinics in Gerontology 4:21–28, 1986

Levin CA, Wei W, Akincigil A, et al: Prevalence and treatment of diagnosed depression among elderly nursing home residents in Ohio. J Am Med Dir Assoc 8:585–594, 2007

Livingston G, Johnston K, Katona C, et al: Systematic review of psychological approaches to the management of neuropsychiatric symptoms of dementia. Am J Psychiatry 162:1996–2021, 2005

Loebel JP, Borson S, Hyde T, et al: Relationships between requests for psychiatric consultations and psychiatric diagnoses in long-term care facilities. Am J Psychiatry 148:898–903, 1991

Lopez OL, Becker JT, Wahed AS, et al: Long-term effects of the concomitant use of memantine with cholinesterase inhibition in Alzheimer disease. J Neurol Neurosurg Psychiatry 80:600–607, 2009

Lyketsos CG, Lindell Veiel L, Baker A, et al: A randomized, controlled trial of bright light therapy for agitated behaviors in dementia patients residing in long-term care. Int J Geriatr Psychiatry 14:520–525, 1999

Magai C, Kennedy G, Cohen CI, et al: A controlled clinical trial of sertraline in the treatment of depression in nursing home patients with late-stage Alzheimer's disease. Am J Geriatr Psychiatry 8:66–74, 2000

McMurdo MET, Rennie L: A controlled trial of exercise by residents of old people's homes. Age Ageing 22:11–15, 1993

Meehan KM, Wang H, David SR, et al: Comparison of rapidly acting intramuscular olanzapine, lorazepam, and placebo: a double-blind, randomized study in acutely agitated patients with dementia. Neuropsychopharmacology 26:494–504, 2002

Mintzer J, Greenspan A, Caers I, et al: Risperidone in the treatment of psychosis of Alzheimer disease: results from a prospective clinical trial. Am J Geriatr Psychiatry 14:280–291, 2006

Mintzer JE, Tune LE, Breder CD, et al: Aripiprazole for the treatment of psychoses in institutionalized patients with Alzheimer dementia: a multicenter, randomized, double-blind, placebo-controlled assessment of three fixed doses. Am J Geriatr Psychiatry 15:918–931, 2007

Moran JA, Gatz M: Group therapies for nursing home adults: an evaluation of two treatment approaches. Gerontologist 27:588–591, 1987

Morris JN, Hawes C, Fries BE, et al: Designing the national Resident Assessment Instrument for nursing homes. Gerontologist 30:293–307, 1990

Nursing Home Quality Indicators Development Group: Facility Guide for the Nursing Home Quality Indicators. National Data System. September 28, 1999. Available at: www.cms.hhs.gov/MinimumDataSets20/Downloads/CHSRA%20QI%20Fact%20Sheet.pdf. Accessed August 6, 2008.

Olin JT, Fox LS, Pawluczyk S, et al: A pilot randomized trial of carbamazepine for behavioral symptoms in treatment-resistant outpatients with Alzheimer disease. Am J Geriatr Psychiatry 9:400–405, 2001

Omnibus Budget Reconciliation Act of 1987, Pub. L. No. 100-203. Subtitle C: Nursing home reform

Onder G, Liperoti R, Soldato M, et al: Depression and risk of nursing home admission among older adults in home care in Europe: results from the Aged in Home Care (AdHOC) study. J Clin Psychiatry 68:1392–1398, 2007

Orten JD, Allen M, Cook J: Reminiscence groups with confused nursing center residents: an experimental study. Soc Work Health Care 14:73–86, 1989

Oslin DW, Streim JE, Katz IR, et al: Heuristic comparison of sertraline with nortriptyline for the treatment of depression in frail elderly patients. Am J Geriatr Psychiatry 8:141–149, 2000

Oslin DW, Ten Have TR, Streim JE, et al: Probing the safety of medications in the frail elderly: evidence from a randomized clinical trial of sertraline and venlafaxine in depressed nursing home residents. J Clin Psychiatry 64:875–882, 2003

Parmelee PA, Katz IR, Lawton MP: Depression among institutionalized aged: assessment and prevalence estimation. J Gerontol 44:M22–M29, 1989

Parmelee PA, Katz IR, Lawton MP: The relation of pain to depression among institutionalized aged. J Gerontol 46:P15–P21, 1991

Parmelee PA, Katz IR, Lawton MP: Depression and mortality among institutionalized aged. J Gerontol 47:P3–P10, 1992a

Parmelee PA, Katz IR, Lawton MP: Incidence of depression in long-term care settings. J Gerontol 47:M189–M196, 1992b

Politis AM, Vozzella S, Mayer LS, et al: A randomized, controlled, clinical trial of activity therapy for apathy in patients with dementia residing in long-term care. Int J Geriatr Psychiatry 19:1087–1094, 2004

Porsteinsson AP, Tariot PN, Erb R, et al: Placebo-controlled study of divalproex sodium for agitation in dementia. Am J Geriatr Psychiatry 9:58–66, 2001

Rattenbury C, Stones MJ: A controlled evaluation of reminiscence and current topics discussion groups in a nursing home context. Gerontologist 29:768–771, 1989

Reichman WE, Conn DK: Nursing home psychiatry: is it time for a reappraisal? Am J Geriatr Psychiatry 18:1049–1053, 2010

Rosen J, Mulsant BH, Pollock BG: Sertraline in the treatment of minor depression in nursing home residents: a pilot study. Int J Geriatr Psychiatry 15:177–180, 2000

Rovner BW, Kafonek S, Filipp L, et al: Prevalence of mental illness in a community nursing home. Am J Psychiatry 143:1446–1449, 1986

Rovner BW, German PS, Broadhead J, et al: The prevalence and management of dementia and other psychiatric disorders in nursing homes. Int Psychogeriatr 2:13–24, 1990a

Rovner BW, Lucas-Blaustein J, Folstein MF, et al: Stability over one year in patients admitted to a nursing home dementia unit. Int J Geriatr Psychiatry 5:77–82, 1990b

Rovner BW, German PS, Brant LJ, et al: Depression and mortality in nursing homes. JAMA 265:993–996, 1991

Rovner BW, Steele CD, Shmuely Y, et al: A randomized trial of dementia care in nursing homes. J Am Geriatr Soc 44:7–13, 1996

Ruths S, Straand J, Nygaard HA, et al: Effect of antipsychotic withdrawal on behavior and sleep/wake activity in nursing home residents with dementia: a randomized, placebo-controlled, double-blinded study. The Bergen District Nursing Home Study. J Am Geriatr Soc 52:1737–1743, 2004

Sabin TD, Vitug AJ, Mark VH: Are nursing home diagnosis and treatment inadequate? JAMA 248:321–322, 1982

Schneider LS, Pollock VE, Lyness SA: A meta-analysis of controlled trials of neuroleptic treatment in dementia. J Am Geriatr Soc 38:553–563, 1990

Schneider LS, Dagerman KS, Insel P: Risk of death with atypical antipsychotic drug treatment for dementia: meta-analysis of randomized placebo-controlled trials. JAMA 294:1934–1943, 2005

Seitz D, Purandare N, Conn D: Prevalence of psychiatric disorders among older adults in long-term care homes: a systematic review. Int Psychogeriatr 22:1025–1039, 2010

Smalbrugge M, Jongenelis L, Pot AM, et al: Incidence and outcome of depressive symptoms in nursing home patients in the Netherlands. Am J Geriatr Psychiatry 14:1069–1076, 2006

Snow LA, Hovanec L, Brandt J: A controlled trial of aromatherapy for agitation in nursing home patients with dementia. J Altern Complement Med 10:431–437, 2004

Street JS, Clark WS, Gannon KS, et al: Olanzapine treatment of psychotic and behavioral symptoms in patients with Alzheimer disease in nursing care facilities: a double-blind, randomized, placebo-controlled trial. Arch Gen Psychiatry 57:968–976, 2000

Streim JE, Katz IR: Psychiatric aspects of long-term care, in Comprehensive Textbook of Psychiatry, 9th Edition, Vol II. Edited by Sadock BJ, Sadock VA, Ruiz P. Philadelphia, PA, Lippincott Williams & Wilkins, 2009, pp 4195–4200

Streim JE, Oslin DW, Katz IR, et al: Drug treatment of depression in frail elderly nursing home residents. Am J Geriatr Psychiatry 8:150–159, 2000

Streim JE, Porsteinsson AP, Breder CD, et al: A randomized, double-blind, placebo-controlled study of aripiprazole for the treatment of psychosis in nursing home patients with Alzheimer's disease. Am J Geriatr Psychiatry 16:537–550, 2008

Sunderland T, Silver MA: Neuroleptics in the treatment of dementia. Int J Geriatr Psychiatry 3:79–88, 1988

Sutcliffe C, Burns A, Challis D, et al: Depressed mood, cognitive impairment, and survival in older people admitted to care homes in England. Am J Geriatr Psychiatry 15:708–715, 2007

Tariot PN, Podgorski CA, Blazina L, et al: Mental disorders in the nursing home: another perspective. Am J Psychiatry 150:1063–1069, 1993

Tariot PN, Erb R, Podgorski CA, et al: Efficacy and tolerability of carbamazepine for agitation and aggression in dementia. Am J Psychiatry 155:54–61, 1998

Tariot PN, Cummings JL, Katz IR, et al: A randomized, double-blind, placebo-controlled study of the efficacy and safety of donepezil in patients with Alzheimer's disease in the nursing home setting. J Am Geriatr Soc 49:1590–1599, 2001a

Tariot PN, Schneider LS, Mintzer J, et al: Safety and tolerability of divalproex sodium in the treatment of signs and symptoms of mania in elderly patients with dementia: results of a double-blind, placebo-controlled trial. Curr Ther Res Clin Exp 62:51–67, 2001b

Tariot PN, Farlow MR, Grossberg GT, et al: Memantine treatment in patients with moderate to severe Alzheimer disease already receiving donepezil: a randomized controlled trial. JAMA 291:317–324, 2004

Tariot PN, Raman R, Jakimovich L, et al: Divalproex sodium in nursing home residents with possible or probable Alzheimer disease complicated by agitation: a randomized, controlled trial. Am J Geriatr Psychiatry 13:942–949, 2005

Teeter RB, Garetz FK, Miller WR, et al: Psychiatric disturbances of aged patients in skilled nursing homes. Am J Psychiatry 133:1430–1434, 1976

Thapa PB, Gideon P, Cost TW, et al: Antidepressants and the risk of falls among nursing home residents. N Engl J Med 339:875–882, 1998

Tondi L, Ribani L, Bottazzi M, et al: Validation therapy (VT) in nursing home: a case-control study. Arch Gerontol Geriatr 44 (suppl 1):407–411, 2007

Toseland RW, Diehl M, Freeman K, et al: The impact of validation group therapy on nursing home residents with dementia. J Appl Gerontol 61:31–50, 1997

Trappler B, Cohen CI: Using fluoxetine in "very old" depressed nursing home residents. Am J Geriatr Psychiatry 4:258–262, 1996

Trappler B, Cohen CI: Use of SSRIs in "very old" depressed nursing home residents. Am J Geriatr Psychiatry 6:83–89, 1998

van Weert JC, van Dulmen AM, Spreeuwenberg PM, et al: Behavioral and mood effects of Snoezelen integrated into 24-hour dementia care. J Am Geriatr Soc 53:24–33, 2005

Wang PS, Schneeweiss S, Avorn J, et al: Risk of death in elderly users of conventional vs. atypical antipsychotic medications. N Engl J Med 353:2335–2341, 2005

Webber AP, Martin JL, Harker JO, et al: Depression in older patients admitted for postacute nursing home rehabilitation. J Am Geriatr Soc 53:1017–1022, 2005

Wetzels RB, Zuidema SU, de Jonghe JFM, et al: Course of neuropsychiatric symptoms in residents with dementia in nursing homes over 2-year period. Am J Geriatr Psychiatry 18:1054–1065, 2010

Williams-Barnard CL, Lindell AR: Therapeutic use of "prizing" and its effect on self-concept of elderly clients in nursing homes and group homes. Issues Ment Health Nurs 13:1–17, 1992

Winblad B, Kilander L, Eriksson S, et al: Donepezil in patients with severe Alzheimer's disease: double-blind, parallel-group, placebo-controlled study. Lancet 367:1057–1065, 2006

Youssef FA: The impact of group reminiscence counseling on a depressed elderly population. Nurse Pract 15:32–38, 1990

Zerhusen JD, Boyle K, Wilson W: Out of the darkness: group cognitive therapy for depressed elderly. J Psychosoc Nurs Ment Health Serv 29:16–21, 1991

Zhong KX, Tariot PN, Mintzer J, et al: Quetiapine to treat agitation in dementia: a randomized, double-blind, placebo-controlled study. Curr Alzheimer Res 4:81–93, 2007

Suggested Readings

American Geriatrics Society, American Association for Geriatric Psychiatry: The American Geriatrics Society and American Association for Geriatric Psychiatry recommendations for policies in support of quality mental health care in U.S. nursing homes. J Am Geriatr Soc 51:1299–1304, 2003

Bharucha AJ, Dew MA, Miller MD, et al: Psychotherapy in long-term care: a review. J Am Med Dir Assoc 7:568–580, 2006

Centers for Medicare and Medicaid Services: State Operations Manual, Appendix PP: Guidance to Surveyors for Long Term Care Facilities. Baltimore, MD, Centers for Medicare and Medicaid, Rev 70, January 7, 2011. Available at: www.cms.gov/Regulations-and-Guidance/Guidance/Manuals/downloads/som107ap_pp_guidelines_ltcf.pdf. Accessed October 1, 2012.

Sink KM, Holden KF, Yaffe K: Pharmacological treatment of neuropsychiatric symptoms of dementia: a review of the evidence. JAMA 293:596–608, 2005

Snowden M, Sato K, Roy-Byrne P: Assessment and treatment of nursing home residents with depression or behavioral symptoms associated with dementia: a review of the literature. J Am Geriatr Soc 51:1305–1317, 2003

Streim JE, Katz IR: Federal regulations and the care of patients with dementia in the nursing home. Med Clin North Am 78:895–909, 1994

Index

*Page numbers printed in **boldface** type refer to tables or figures.*